Advances in Neurosurgical Procedures - Unveiling New Horizons

Edited by Amit Agrawal

Published in London, United Kingdom

Advances in Neurosurgical Procedures - Unveiling New Horizons
http://dx.doi.org/10.5772/intechopen.1003452
Edited by Amit Agrawal

Contributors
Ahmed Shawky Abdelgawaad, Alejandro Enriquez-Marulanda, Amit Agarwal, Amit Agrawal, Anil Kumar Sharma, Ankita Jain, Ariel Sacknovitz, Azmi Nasser, Bhoresh Dhamija, Cameron Rawanduzy, Ching-Hsiang Hsieh, Chirag Gandhi, Efstathios Papavassiliou, Elad Mashiach, Fernando De Nigris Vasconcellos, Fernando Terry, Forough Yazdanian, Geet Shukla, Ha Dai Duong, Hayley Donaldson, Jitender Chaturvedi, Justin Santarelli, Kung Chia Li, Linh Duy Nguyen, Max S. Fleisher, Michael K. Rosner, Mihit Kalawatia, Osman Fikret Sönmez, Punit Pandya, Sabrina Zeller, Sauson Soldozy, Shang-Chih Lin, Steven Tominey, Ting-Hua Liao, Yu-Kun Xu, Yücel Doğruel, Ziev B. Moses

First published in London, United Kingdom, 2025 by IntechOpen
IntechOpen is the global imprint of INTECHOPEN LIMITED, registered in England and Wales, registration number: 11086078, 167-169 Great Portland Street, London, W1W 5PF, United Kingdom

For EU product safety concerns: IN TECH d.o.o., Prolaz Marije Krucifikse Kozulić 3, 51000 Rijeka, Croatia, info@intechopen.com or visit our website at intechopen.com.

British Library Cataloguing-in-Publication Data
A catalogue record for this book is available from the British Library

Advances in Neurosurgical Procedures - Unveiling New Horizons
Edited by Amit Agrawal
p. cm.
Print ISBN 978-1-83634-161-1
Online ISBN 978-1-83634-160-4
eBook (PDF) ISBN 978-1-83634-162-8

Meet the editor

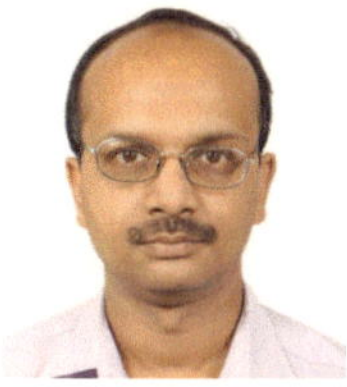

Dr. Agrawal completed his neurosurgery training at the National Institute of Mental Health and Neurosciences in Bangalore, India, in 2003. Dr. Agrawal is a self-motivated, enthusiastic, and results-oriented professional with over 21 years of rich experience in research and development, as well as teaching and mentoring in the field of neurosurgery. He is proficient in managing and leading teams to run successful process operations and has experience developing procedures and service standards of excellence. He has attended and participated in numerous international and national symposia and conferences, delivering lectures on a wide range of topics. He has published over 1,000 articles in the medical field, covering a wide range of topics in national and international journals. His expertise lies in identifying training needs, designing effective training modules, and executing them efficiently, even with limited resources. He has excellent communication, presentation, and interpersonal skills with proven abilities in teaching and training for various academic and professional courses. Currently, he is working at the All India Institute of Medical Sciences, Bhopal, Madhya Pradesh, India.

Contents

Preface **IX**

Section 1
Advances in Surgical Techniques and Approaches **1**

Chapter 1 **3**
Introductory Chapter: Advancement in Neurosurgery
by Amit Agrawal

Chapter 2 **7**
Glioma Resection in Functional Areas Using Diffusion Tensor Imaging-Based Tractography and Neuro-Navigation
by Ha Dai Duong and Linh Duy Nguyen

Chapter 3 **23**
The Supracerebellar Approach for Pineal and Brainstem Lesions: Advantages and Limitations
by Yücel Doğruel and Osman Fikret Sönmez

Chapter 4 **41**
The Supraorbital "Keyhole" Approach (SOKHA) for Skull Base Lesions
by Anil Kumar Sharma, Jitender Chaturvedi, Mihit Kalawatia and Amit Agarwal

Section 2
Innovations in Spine Surgery **51**

Chapter 5 **53**
Locking Lumbar Interbody Cementation: Biomechanics, Manual Reduction, Surgical Techniques, and Long-Term Results
by Kung Chia Li, Ching-Hsiang Hsieh, Ting-Hua Liao, Shang-Chih Lin and Yu-Kun Xu

Chapter 6 **83**
Endoscopic Lumbar Rhizotomy for Facetogenic Pain
by Azmi Nasser

Chapter 7 95
Anterior Approach to the Cervical Spine: Past, Present, and Future
by Max S. Fleisher and Michael K. Rosner

Chapter 8 111
Lumbar Disc Surgery: Advances in the Last Few Decades
by Ahmed Shawky Abdelgawaad

Chapter 9 129
Lumbar Fusion for Spondylosis: Indications and Techniques for Interbody Fusion, Comparing TLIF, PLIF, Extreme Lateral, ALIF and Oblique/Approach
by Bhoresh Dhamija and Steven Tominey

Section 3
Emerging Technologies in Neurosurgery 145

Chapter 10 147
Advanced Imaging and Augmented Reality in Neurosurgery: Bridging Innovation and Precision
by Elad Mashiach, Sauson Soldozy, Ariel Sacknovitz, Ankita Jain, Hayley Donaldson, Sabrina Zeller, Geet Shukla, Cameron Rawanduzy, Fernando De Nigris Vasconcellos, Chirag Gandhi and Justin Santarelli

Chapter 11 181
Foundations of Robotic Spine Surgery: Emerging Technologies and Future Directions
by Fernando Terry, Alejandro Enriquez-Marulanda, Punit Pandya, Forough Yazdanian, Efstathios Papavassiliou and Ziev B. Moses

Preface

Advances in Neurosurgical Procedures – Unveiling New Horizons explores the latest developments in neurosurgery, focusing on key innovations that are transforming surgical practices. The volume is organized into three sections: surgical techniques, spine surgery innovations, and emerging technologies.

The first section, *Advances in Surgical Techniques and Approaches*, covers new methods for treating brain and skull base conditions. It discusses the integration of advanced imaging and neuro-navigation to improve precision and the shift toward minimally invasive approaches for complex brain lesions.

The second section, *Innovations in Spine Surgery*, highlights advancements in spinal procedures, including new lumbar and cervical spine surgery techniques. It focuses on minimally invasive methods and spinal fusion technologies to improve outcomes and reduce recovery times.

The third section, *Emerging Technologies in Neurosurgery*, examines how augmented reality, robotics, and advanced imaging enhance surgical precision and enable more personalized treatments in brain and spine surgeries.

This volume provides a comprehensive look at current trends in neurosurgery, offering insights into the evolving landscape of surgical practices and technologies.

Amit Agrawal
Department of Neurosurgery,
All India Institute of Medical Sciences,
Saket Nagar, Bhopal, Madhya Pradesh, India

Section 1

Advances in Surgical Techniques and Approaches

Chapter 1

Introductory Chapter: Advancement in Neurosurgery

Amit Agrawal

1.Introduction

Neurosurgery is a complex and critical medical discipline that requires precision and dedication for the diagnosis and management of diseases and disorders affecting the brain, spinal cord, and peripheral nervous system [1]. The practice of neurosurgery is undergoing extensive and diverse changes, supported by continuous exposure to clinical material, advancements in technical skills, and the acquisition of pre-, intra-, and postoperative clinical data, which guide decision making in clinical practice [2, 3].

2. Evolution of neurosurgery

The evolution of neurosurgery can be viewed as a timeline that includes the Pre-Cushing Era, Cushing Era, Yasargil Era, Endoscopic Era, and Robotic Era [4], and in the future, it is anticipated that the AI-based approaches shall help in making patient-oriented outcome-based decisions [5]. Ongoing advances include insights into clinical approaches through data collection methods, a deeper understanding of genetics and pathophysiology, novel imaging modalities such as 3D imaging, innovative techniques for monitoring physiological parameters, surgical methods including neuronavigation and robot-assisted surgeries, and outcome assessments across various disease processes [6, 7].

3. Scope

The scope of neurosurgical advances includes developing techniques to precisely localize brain lesions or areas of interest as needed in functional neurosurgery to deliver precise radiation while preserving the normally functioning neural tissue (**Table 1**) [4]. To drive advances in these areas, various sub-groups can be identified—for example, frameless stereotaxy, interventional magnetic resonance imaging for real-time intraoperative imaging, robotics in spinal surgery, neuroendoscopy with specialized instruments, and methods for performing subthalamic stimulation to create lesions for the management of movement disorders [9].

4. Postoperative care

It can be anticipated that a comprehensive postoperative care that will include the rehabilitation process shall help in improving the overall outcomes and

• Augmented reality (AR) system
• Behavioral neuroscience
• Cellular and molecular neuroscience
• Cognitive and computational neuroscience
• Endovascular embolization technology
• Fluorescence imaging technology
• Functional neurosurgery, that is, deep brain stimulation (DBS)
• Gene therapy
• Gut-brain connection
• Minimally invasive three-dimensional (3D) endoscope
• Multimodality monitoring
• Neural engineering
• Neuroimaging
• Neuronavigation system
• Robotic systems
• Teleneurosurgery
• Woundless stereotactic ablative radiotherapy (SABR)

Table 1.
Scope of advancements [8].

bringing person back to normal life and integrate into society. This will need well-equipped critical care units, rapid recognition of complication and timely intervention to manage these complications with facilities to pediatric neurosurgical cases as well [10].

5. Challenges

While we continue to discuss advancements, we must also anticipate the challenges, particularly how to provide high-quality neurosurgical care in regions with limited resources. The major challenges anticipated include accessibility, affordability, the need to develop infrastructure, prevention of medical malpractice, and the provision of continuous and comprehensive training and education opportunities [11]. In addition, there may be service delivery related challenges which may include shortage of trained professionals, lack of infrastructure, limited availability of medications and associated comorbidities those may further increase the complexity of health care needs of an individual and overall outcomes [11].

6. Synthetic data generation

An evolving concept in neurosurgical care is the use of synthetic data solutions, designed to enhance care by providing detailed image simulations needed for preoperative planning. These solutions also aim to support the availability of mixed reality environments required for precision and patient-specific surgical training [3].

7. Artificial intelligence

Recently, collaboration among health care and technical experts' artificial intelligence (AI) has been incorporated to support neurosurgical decision making and thus to extend the scope of high-quality care to a wider group of individuals [1]. Although AI use is gaining momentum; however, there is a need to ensure that this is used ethically and the patients should be safe [2].

8. Conclusions

In summary, the current book tries to bring experts and share their expertise on ongoing advances in various fields of neurosurgery, including cervical and lumbar spine fusion methods, surgical management of gliomas and other cranial tumors, imaging methods, neuronavigation guided surgical approaches, use of augmented reality in neurosurgery, endoscopic approaches to perform lumbar rhizotomy, robotic spine surgery and keyhole approaches to skull base lesions.

Author details

Amit Agrawal
Department of Neurosurgery, All India Institute of Medical Sciences, Bhopal, Madhya Pradesh, India

*Address all correspondence to: dramitagrawal@gmail.com; dramitagrawal@hotmail.com

References

[1] Kuo CH, Tu TH, Chen KT. Editorial: Advanced technological applications in neurosurgery. Frontiers in Surgery. 2023;**10**:1277997

[2] Kazemzadeh K, Akhlaghdoust M, Zali A. Advances in artificial intelligence, robotics, augmented and virtual reality in neurosurgery. Frontiers in Surgery. 2023;**10**:1241923

[3] Bouras A. The emerging applications of synthetic data in neurosurgery research and practice: A systematic review. medRxiv [Preprint]. 2024. DOI: 10.1101/2024.03.04.24303724

[4] Souza FS, Silva RPS, Junior LSB, Azevedo Filho HRC. The evolution of neurosurgery throughout the ages: From trepanations in prehistory to the robotic era. Arquivos Brasileiros de Neurocirurgia: Brazilian Neurosurgery. 2022;**41**(02):e153-e1e8

[5] Lo P-C, Kung W-M. Innovation, advances and updates in neurosurgery. Signa Vitae. 2022;**18**(2):1-7

[6] Pandey P, Steinberg GK. Neurosurgical advances in the treatment of moyamoya disease. Stroke. 2011;**42**(11):3304-3310

[7] Wakabayashi T, Fujii M, Kajita Y, Natsume A, Maezawa S, Yoshida J. Advanced new neurosurgical procedure using integrated system of intraoperative MRI and neuronavigation with multimodal neuroradiological images. Nagoya Journal of Medical Science. 2009;**71**(3-4):101-107

[8] Mohamed AA, Sargent E, Williams C, Karve Z, Nair K, Lucke-Wold B. Advancements in neurosurgical intraoperative histology. Tomography [Internet]. 2024;**10**(5):693-704

[9] Powell M. Recent advances-neurosurgery. British Medical Journal. 1999;**318**(7175):35-38

[10] Bonfield CM, Basem J, Cochrane DD, Singhal A, Steinbok P. Examining the need for routine intensive care admission after surgical repair of nonsyndromic craniosynostosis: A preliminary analysis. Journal of Neurosurgery. Pediatrics. 2018;**22**(6):616-619

[11] Chandankhede AR, Thombre SD. Advancements and challenges in neurosurgical practice in India: Where do we stand? Cureus. 2023;**15**(4):e37738

Chapter 2

Glioma Resection in Functional Areas Using Diffusion Tensor Imaging-Based Tractography and Neuro-Navigation

Ha Dai Duong and Linh Duy Nguyen

Abstract

Gliomas located in critical brain regions, such as the motor and language areas, present significant challenges in neurosurgery due to the elevated risk of causing neurological deficits during intervention. Diffusion tensor imaging (DTI)-based tractography has emerged as a valuable tool for both preoperative planning and intraoperative navigation, facilitating the identification of essential white matter tracts to help preserve functional integrity. This chapter provides a comprehensive overview of the application of DTI tractography combined with neuro-navigation in glioma resections within critical functional areas. The foundational principles of DTI are explored, with a focus on its role in reconstructing fiber tracts and key neural pathways. Current clinical research is reviewed, highlighting its contribution to achieving higher rates of gross total resection (GTR) while minimizing postoperative complications. Additionally, the limitations of DTI tractography, such as image distortion caused by peritumoral edema or tumor infiltration, are examined along with technical strategies designed to address these challenges.

Keywords: diffusion tensor imaging (DTI), tractography, neuro-navigation, eloquent, glioma resection, functional area

1. Introduction

Diffusion tensor imaging (DTI) is an advanced imaging technique derived from diffusion-weighted magnetic resonance imaging (MRI), designed to measure both the direction and extent of water diffusion within tissues. This method is particularly valuable for visualizing the architecture of nerve fiber pathways in the brain, a process known as fiber tract imaging. Fiber tract imaging generates detailed two- and three-dimensional representations of the brain's neural networks [1].

In the context of brain tumors, DTI plays a crucial role in identifying whether nerve fiber tracts have been infiltrated or displaced by the tumor, providing essential data for treatment planning. Furthermore, diffusion-weighted MRI offers significant insights into various intracranial pathological conditions that standard MRI may struggle to assess effectively, including tumor characterization, inflammatory processes, and white matter abnormalities [2, 3].

2. Methods

This chapter synthesizes current knowledge on the clinical use of diffusion tensor imaging (DTI) and diffusion tensor tractography (DTT) in glioma surgery, particularly in functional brain regions. A comprehensive literature review was conducted using major databases to identify studies on the integration of these techniques in both preoperative and intraoperative settings. Key topics explored include imaging advancements, tractography's role in identifying white matter tracts, and strategies for functional preservation during glioma surgery. Challenges such as brain shift and the differentiation between tumor and healthy tissue were also addressed, emphasizing the importance of combining technical insights with clinical data to optimize resection outcomes while minimizing neurological impairments.

3. DTI acquisition protocol

To perform diffusion tensor imaging (DTI), the patient is first positioned and selected for appropriate diagnostic pulse sequences, usually including T1, T2, and FLAIR sequences. The cutting directions include axial (transverse), coronal (horizontal), and sagittal (vertical). The patient then undergoes conventional diffusion-weighted imaging, and the apparent diffusion coefficient (ADC) map is calculated to assess the lesion. Additionally, depending on the detected lesions, necessary pulse sequences may be conducted, such as T2* sequences to detect whether bleeding has occurred. The next step is to select the fiber tract imaging (tensor) pulse sequences and choose the direction based on the orientation of the axons to be examined.

At our institution, MRI imaging was conducted using a 3 Tesla MRI scanner equipped with a head coil. The standard imaging protocol included axial or sagittal T1-weighted sequences (T1W, TR/TE: 2325/25 ms), axial fluid-attenuated inversion recovery (FLAIR, TR/TE: 8500/117 ms), coronal T2 gradient echo (T2 GE), and axial diffusion-weighted imaging (DWI, TR/TE: 5202/78 ms, matrix size 116 × 116, slice thickness 5 mm). To enhance contrast, gadolinium-based contrast medium (0.1 mmol/kg) was injected intravenously using an 18–20 G needle, followed by post-contrast T1W imaging in three planes: axial, coronal, and sagittal.

The DTI acquisition protocol employed a single-shot echo-planar imaging (EPI) sequence in the axial plane. Key parameters included a TR/TE of 7000/84 ms, 4 mm slice thickness, 0.4 mm inter-slice gap, 128 × 128 matrix, and a field of view (FOV) of 260 × 260 mm. Diffusion data were collected in 27 directions with b-values of 0 and 1000 s/mm^2. The entire acquisition process lasted approximately 3 minutes. Imaging data were transferred to Workstation 4.7 (GE Medical System) for post-processing, where fractional anisotropy (FA) maps and color-coded orientation maps were generated using a matrix of eigenvalues and eigenvectors. Fiber tracts were color-mapped with red, green, and blue, representing left-right, anterior-posterior, and superior-inferior directions, respectively [4–6].

4. Diffusion tensor tractography (DTT)

Techniques for mapping neural connections in the brain have evolved significantly over time. Early approaches were lesion-based, focusing on identifying pathways through retrograde or anterograde degeneration following brain injury. Later advancements introduced the use of molecular tracers, such as horseradish peroxidase, alongside other markers including fluorescent dyes, lectins, neurotrophins, neurotoxins, dextrans, carbocyanine dyes, latex microspheres, and certain viral vectors. While effective in visualizing neural pathways, these methods are highly invasive and often necessitate histological analysis, which involves sacrificing experimental animals to examine the distribution of the tracers in the brain tissue [7].

Magnetic resonance imaging (MRI) incorporating tensor-based metrics, such as fractional anisotropy (FA) maps and color-coded maps, is collectively referred to as diffusion tensor imaging (DTI). An advanced application derived from DTI is tractography, a technique enabling the non-invasive visualization of specific white matter pathways and brain connections for clinical purposes. While diffusion tensor tractography (DTT) is technically a subset of DTI, it is often treated as a distinct method due to its specific focus on fiber tract reconstruction and pathway analysis [8].

DTI and DTT have expanded the possibilities for exploring neural structures and assessing alterations caused by brain disorders. DTT, a non-invasive imaging technique, enables the mapping of nerve fiber tracts by integrating the directional data of individual voxels into pathways that link distant regions of the brain. This method allows for the analysis of fiber tract trajectory, shape, structural integrity, anatomical positioning, and connectivity patterns. Furthermore, DTT can simultaneously generate three-dimensional representations of white matter regions and detect connectivity disruptions. By visualizing fiber pathways across the brain, DTT offers insights beyond the capabilities of standard imaging modalities or conventional histological methods. It specifically refers to the 3D reconstruction of white matter tracts based on diffusion-weighted MRI data, most often derived from DTI sequences [9–11].

5. The role of DTI in glioma surgery

The primary goal of glioma resection surgery is to obtain histological diagnosis and achieve maximal tumor volume reduction. Due to the unclear boundaries in gliomas, gross total resection is preferred over partial resection or biopsy for diagnosis. With accurate histological diagnosis, the prognosis for the patient as well as the optimal treatment regimen can be established. Treatment regimens may include adjuvant radiotherapy and/or chemotherapy. Maximal tumor volume reduction aims to reduce the number of cells that could potentially progress to higher-grade tumors and enhance the effectiveness of adjuvant therapies by altering cell dynamics and reducing the number of chemotherapy-resistant cells. In fact, the extent of resection of high-grade and low-grade gliomas has been shown to correlate with survival. Regarding quality of life, up to 53% of glioma patients show improved neurological function after tumor resection. Resection of gliomas may also reduce dependence on steroid treatment for edema and anticonvulsants [10].

DTI is just one important component of the preoperative planning process. There are several sources of preoperative localization data, which consider the risks near functional regions necessary for preserving neurological function. These data sources include clinical manifestations, functional anatomy in standard imaging, preoperative functional mapping techniques (including DTI), intraoperative white matter functional testing, and intraoperative cortical mapping. Each of these information sources is often imperfect when used alone but can be very important when combined with other sources [2].

Preoperative planning techniques include DTI, functional MRI, positron emission tomography (PET), conventional MRI, spectral MRI, and computed tomography (CT). The goal of these techniques is to preoperatively identify spatial relationships between the boundaries of the lesion and functional brain areas. The primary focus of these techniques is the DTI and functional MRI duo. DTI assesses white matter, while functional MRI assesses functional cortical areas. The value of DTI and functional MRI data in a specific case often depends on the location of the lesion [12].

However, most commonly, DTI and functional MRI provide useful and complementary information. Researchers have found that combining DTI, anatomical imaging, and functional MRI outperforms anatomical imaging combined with only functional MRI for preoperative risk assessments of functional systems. The optimal use of these techniques for preoperative planning requires an understanding of functional anatomy and dysfunction.

5.1 DTI in preoperative planning for eloquent gliomas

Gliomas are the most common type of brain tumors that infiltrate diffusely into the surrounding white matter. Conventional MRI is typically used to locate and describe the characteristics of tumors [13]. However, routine MRI does not provide accurate information about infiltration into the surrounding white matter tracts. Diffusion tensor imaging (DTI) is a non-invasive MRI technique that measures the integrity of white matter, and fiber tractography is used to visualize the preferred diffusion directions of white matter tracts. DTI allows for the identification of white matter regions adjacent to eloquent gliomas, enabling maximal tumor resection while preserving functional areas. The relationship of the tumor with white matter tracts (displacement, edema, infiltration, and destruction) is one of the most important early applications of DTI. Fiber tracts may be infiltrated in areas that appear normal, and regions of the brain with abnormal imaging may show intact fibers anatomically. In planning surgery for motor cortex gliomas, surgery is supported by knowledge of the proximity and relative position of the tumor to adjacent white matter areas [14].

Preoperative planning and evaluation of surrounding white matter regions are critical steps to allow for the complete resection of eloquent gliomas while avoiding recurrence and the loss of important brain functions [3, 15, 16]. Conventional MRI shows lesions without providing any accurate information about the involvement and integrity of the white matter surrounding the tumor. Diffusion tensor imaging (DTI) is currently the only available non-invasive tool that displays the disruption of white matter areas due to fractional anisotropy (FA) changes and fiber tractography in patients with gliomas [17, 18]. Therefore, it is crucial to accurately delineate the white matter tracts, especially the corticospinal tract, for preoperative planning and decision-making regarding surgical intervention.

DTI originates from diffusion weighted imaging (DWI), which is based on the random diffusion of water within each pixel. However, DTI supplements directional information and provides three maps: apparent diffusion coefficient (ADC), FA map, and direction-encoded color (DEC) map. ADC is a three-dimensional pixel-wise measure of diffusion intensity. FA measures the preferred direction of diffusion and is represented by a numeric value ranging from 0 to 1. High FA values indicate a high degree of directional preference (anisotropic), such as in highly organized white matter regions, while low FA values indicate less preferred directionality, such as in gray matter and cerebrospinal fluid, which have an FA of 0 (isotropic). The color-encoded maps are created from FA calculations, and conventionally, blue highlights regions moving in the up-down direction, green highlights the anterior-posterior direction, and red highlights the left-right direction. Fiber tract color tracking can be performed using various computational algorithms based on preferred diffusion directions in three-dimensional pixels, allowing for a 3D display of neural regions. The correlation between FA and tumor cell density remains controversial, as this effect poses challenges for neurosurgeons and may lead to overestimating the destruction of nerve fibers. Many studies have evaluated the value of FA in predicting the destruction of fiber tracts in white matter regions due to tumor infiltration on DTT. Four types of relationships between the tumor and the area are classified: displacement, edema, infiltration, and destruction (**Figure 1**) [19].

Quantitative assessment of white matter tracts using DTI is more useful than morphological assessment. The purpose of DTI/DTT is to evaluate the regions affected by the tumor and use this information to guide neurosurgeons in maximizing tumor resection, thereby minimizing postoperative neurological deficits and the likelihood of tumor recurrence [20, 21].

5.2 Neurosurgery planning: DTI for non-invasive 3D visualization

DTI allows for non-invasive 3D visualization prior to surgery, guiding the planning for brain lesions in functional motor areas, both on the surface and in deeper subcortical regions (**Figure 2**). Maximally resecting gliomas reduces the risk of tumor recurrence, while chemoradiotherapy may lead to the loss of critical brain functions and poor quality of life [22]. Assessing the extent of tumor infiltration preoperatively is crucial for neurological outcomes and has been shown to be a key independent prognostic factor. The precise location of the white matter tracts related to the tumor aids neurosurgeons in preoperative planning by determining the surgical approach and identifying the extent of tumor resection while preserving motor functions. Functional MRI reveals critical motor and speech cortical areas using specific patterns but does not accurately reflect the involvement of white matter regions, only assessing cortical functional areas [23, 24]. DTI provides in-vivo microstructural tissue information by measuring water diffusion for a given three-dimensional pixel

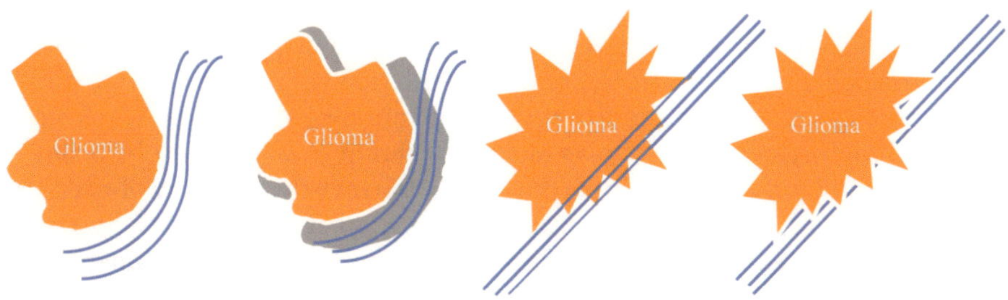

Figure 1.
Pattern of DTI fiber tracts damage: displacement, edema, infiltration, and destruction.

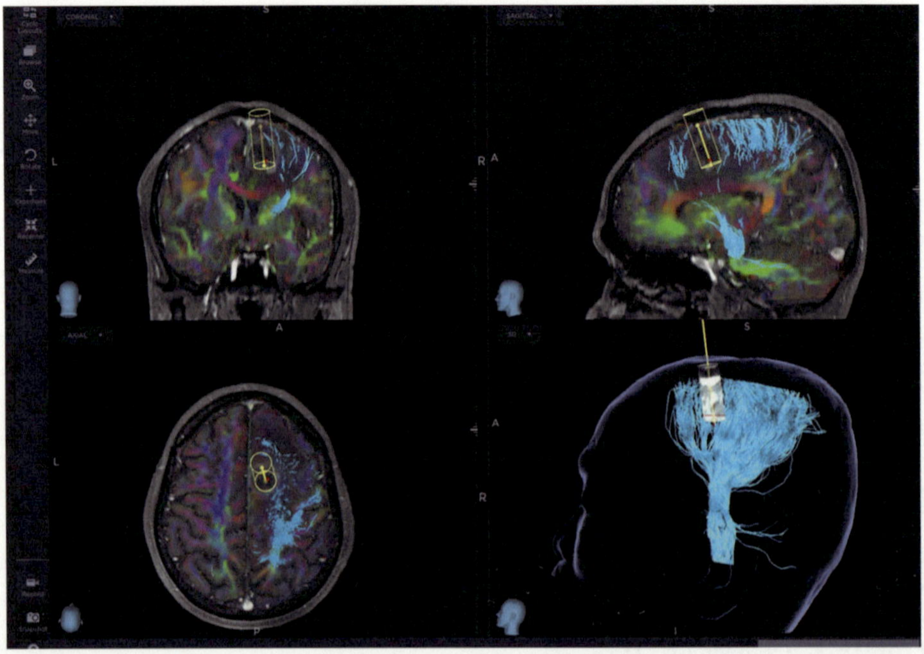

Figure 2.
Preoperative planning for eloquent glioma resection with DTI-based tractography reconstruction.

according to fractional anisotropy (FA) and mean diffusion (MD) values. The first images of nerve fiber tracts were produced in 1991 by Aaron Filler and colleagues, and the clinical utility of DTI/DTT was established in 2002 for brain tumor patients [25]. Damage to the motor corticospinal tract and language tracts during surgery correlates with postoperative language and motor deficits. Yu and colleagues demonstrated the relationship between white matter regions and tumors on DTI postoperatively to assess surgical outcomes in brain tumor patients. The authors found that the extent of tumor resection and improvement in postoperative function in the group with preoperative DTT planning was significantly higher than in the control group [20]. Min and colleagues reported that reduced FA values and the distance between the corticospinal tract and the brain tumor were optimal factors for predicting corticospinal tract damage caused by brain tumors [21]. DTI can be applied in the operating room, and in some cases, the corticospinal tract that is not identified preoperatively can be monitored during surgery due to changes in local tumor effects on adjacent areas. DTI-based surgical planning in selected patients may provide an alternative to awake surgery [26].

Reconstruction and analysis of preoperative DTI imaging data have some limitations, mainly related to the differences in the reduction of fractional anisotropy values due to actual neoplastic infiltration or edema surrounding the tumor [10]. Recent advances in high-resolution diffusion imaging techniques on 3.0 Tesla MRI and improved imaging reconstruction methods may enhance the accuracy of preoperative imaging. Research by Amitesh Dubey and colleagues demonstrates that evaluating white matter tracts is an essential part of integrated preoperative assessment because analyzing the relationship between the tumor and functional tracts on DTI allows for better surgical planning, guiding the surgical approach and maximizing the extent of resection while preserving neurological function [27].

5.3 Application combined with neuro-navigation

The navigation system applies the principle of frameless radiation therapy; the patient's MRI images are reconstructed using the system's software, and the patient is placed within the infrared spectrum of the camera, allowing for an easy comparison of the lesion's position on the imaging with reality, thanks to the reference systems that the machine has pre-calibrated with high accuracy, with an error of no more than 2 mm [28].

The neuro-navigation system during surgery accurately identifies the position of the brain tumor relative to the skull, allowing the surgeon to decide on the smallest incision on the skin and the most direct approach to the tumor. Clearly identifying the boundaries of the tumor with healthy brain tissue minimizes brain damage, especially for tumors with structures similar to healthy brain tissue, such as low-grade gliomas [29].

Combining diffusion tensor imaging (DTI) preoperatively and neuro-navigation aids in identifying white matter tracts during surgery for glioma in the motor region. For each patient, the anatomical images of the tumor and associated cortical tracts are assessed within an integrated dataset of both DTI maps and 3-D functional MRI (fMRI) using registration software. The tumor's margins are outlined using 3D navigated MRI scans, while the cortical tracts are segmented and constructed using the FA map. Initially, the white matter regions are segmented in the FA map using a predefined threshold to create a 3D model of the cortical tracts on automated software.

The neuro-navigation system is registered after the patient is secured on the positioning frame. The position of the probe in the surgical space is displayed on the workstation screen, corresponding to the position in the MRI imaging space. Both the FA maps from DTI and the 3-D navigational MRI datasets are transferred to the workstation via CD or USB. The integrated imaging is then modeled with software for surgical guidance. When the software merges two components—the T1 contrast-enhanced MRI and DTI images—the structural images of the white matter regions in the operational image are integrated with the anatomical images in the reference imaging sequence so that the slices of both datasets can be accurately merged into one view. During the creation of the merged image set, automatic registration merging is frequently performed. This sophisticated computational process allows for accurate image synthesis, but sometimes, PointMerge registration may need to be performed first, followed by the use of AutoMerge technique. The merging process demonstrates high accuracy (with a mean registration error of less than 2 mm) [30]. The merging mode is used to visualize the integrated image set. Both image sequences are displayed simultaneously in a combination of intensities to facilitate setup within neuro-navigation procedures. Image integration is beneficial for displaying tumor contours and surgical pathways, as well as for combining and visualizing white matter tracts during surgery. Furthermore, to optimize image display, the 3-D white matter tract portion and reconstruction process are semi-automatically performed on the corresponding scalp, cortex, tumor, and white matter structures (**Figure 3**).

Neuro-navigation during surgery has become a routine procedure [31]. Before draping the surgical field, the tumor contour is marked and drawn onto the patient's scalp, allowing for minimal skin incision and more detailed planning for the bone flap procedure. After opening the skull, the tumor outline and adjacent pyramidal tracts are indirectly re-identified through the dura mater, and the dura is opened to align with the identified tumor. Once the dura is opened, the central sulcus is identified using

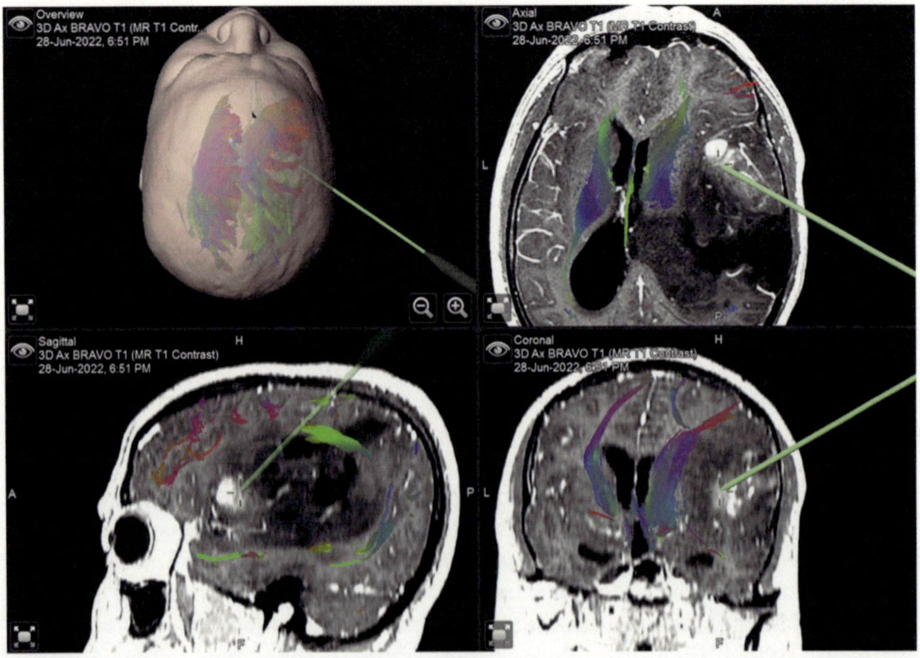

Figure 3.
Neuro-navigation with DTI-based tractography for tumor resection and fiber tract preservation. The navigation probe (green) indicates tumor margins and critical fiber tracts in real-time across axial, sagittal, coronal, and 3D views, ensuring accurate resection and functional preservation.

the navigation probe on the preoperative MRI and DTI images. The projection of the pyramidal tract onto the cortical surface is navigated with the probe to verify the location of the central sulcus area. The craniotomy is then determined based on the precise location of the tumor as well as the anatomical structure of the pyramidal tract in the integrated image space. The tumor is subsequently completely resected; meanwhile, the pyramidal tract associated with the lesion is preserved as much as possible without risking additional motor deficits. Throughout the tumor resection, cerebrospinal fluid drainage, lateral ventricle opening, brain retraction, and the use of anti-edema medications may displace the brain, making neuro-navigation less accurate [32].

Long-term follow-up results of surgeries for gliomas in the motor region have demonstrated that extensive tumor resection can be performed with the support of functional neuro-navigation based on DTI, particularly in patients with high-grade gliomas, consistent with reducing the likelihood of postoperative motor deficits due to pyramidal tract injury. Considering the quality of life for patients, the 6-month KPS score evaluation shows significantly higher KPS scores in patients undergoing glioma resection (both low-grade and high-grade gliomas) using DTI-based functional neuro-navigation compared to those using standard neuro-navigation [32]. Treatment for patients with gliomas focuses on selecting treatment modalities that prolong survival while minimizing neurological damage and maintaining an appropriate quality of life. In the current decade, although still controversial, the majority of studies support the survival advantages conferred by maximal resection of both low-grade and high-grade gliomas [33–36]. For gliomas in or adjacent to the motor cortex and subcortical pyramidal tracts, the surgical principle is to achieve maximal safe resection.

In previous studies, DTI has been used in brain tumor patients primarily to classify tissue characteristics and understand the impact of tumor growth on the microstructural integrity of surrounding brain tissue. Additionally, DTI has been utilized to guide tumor surgery, providing necessary pathways for surgeons and influencing surgical methods [1, 10, 27, 34, 37, 38]. Extensive research on DTI in glioma surgery has been conducted recently, mainly focusing on evaluating brain tumor resection, often combined with other modalities, for instance, in conjunction with functional MRI. So far, no single technique has become the standard for adequately assessing brain tumor resection [39]. Various methods have been developed and utilized alongside DTI, primarily to ensure effectiveness, as DTI has been shown to have several limitations and potential errors [40]. Some studies even claim that DTI provides little additional information for brain mapping, which is crucial in neurosurgery.

Wu et al. reported a randomized controlled trial involving 49 glioma patients associated with pyramidal tracts who were randomly assigned to a study group (DTI-guided neuro-navigation) and a control group (traditional neuro-navigation) [19]. Patients in the study group underwent 3D navigation MRI studies with DTI and T1 sequences. The major white matter regions were constructed from DTI datasets and merged with the anatomical structure on T1-weighted images. The relationship between the tumors and adjacent pyramidal tracts was segmented and reconstructed for three-dimensional visualization. Tumors were completely resected in 12 patients (50.0%) in the control group and 20 patients (80.0%) in the study group ($P < 0.05$). Severe contralateral weakness postoperatively or hemiplegia due to pyramidal tract injury occurred in 75.0% of cases in the control group, while only 20.0% of patients in the study group experienced this ($P < 0.01$). The average Karnofsky performance scale (KPS) scores were 69.58 ± 23.49 and 84.80 ± 23.49 in the control and study groups, respectively ($P < 0.05$). The rate of excellent outcomes (KPS score = 90–100) was 37.5% in the control group and 72.0% in the trial group ($P < 0.05$) [32].

Alexopoulos et al. investigated neurosurgeons' decision-making processes in preoperative planning, analyzing DTI and preoperative MRI images, and making decisions regarding brain tumor resection. However, after analyzing DTI imaging data from some patients, they found that this technique did not influence surgical strategy. Nevertheless, it helped support surgical decision-making, transitioning from total resection to partial resection, a decision initially based solely on routine MRI, leading to better surgical outcomes [41]. Similarly, Buchmann observed that the visualization of white matter tracts on DTI did not impact surgical planning or the surgical process. However, DTI/DTT visualization allowed neurosurgeons to adjust their surgical approach in one of the analyzed cases [1]. In contrast to Alexopoulos and Buchmann, Xiao et al. found that there was a change in surgical methods in over a quarter of patients based on DTI results in their study of cortical-spinal tract imaging. According to DTI data, the choice of surgical methods was more diverse and specific compared to before DTI results, prioritizing better approaches [42].

Currently, neuro-navigation in surgery provides surgeons with surgical orientation, aiding in the accurate approach to tumors and identifying surrounding functional structures. However, the real-time positional changes of the brain during surgery remain the most significant factor affecting the accuracy of neuro-navigation, leading to residual tumors and severe neurological deficits. In addition to preventative measures, intraoperative mapping of subcortical pathways, three approaches can be utilized to address this issue: intraoperative MRI, software registration, and pre-deformation mapping [28, 37, 38, 42, 43].

Surgical outcomes for gliomas in the motor region are evaluated based on the gross total resection rate and patients' postoperative neurological function. Currently, several articles have reported improvements based on the increasing rate of gross total resection decisions and improved postoperative neurological deficits when DTI is integrated as a preoperative planning tool. Many studies have concluded that with the help of DTI, modifications to initial preoperative plans can be made primarily to change outcomes in terms of maximizing tumor removal. Furthermore, optimal surgical decisions for tumor resection have been made for patients, primarily in cooperation with determining the degree of infiltration of gliomas into white matter tracts and finding the best surgical method or altering the initial surgical plan during surgery. The use of DTI to improve postoperative outcomes primarily leads to improvements in neurological deficit conditions. Several studies agree that this can predict postoperative deficits and preserve function [33, 44–47].

Due to the inability to refer to precise anatomical literature for each case, neuro-navigation combined with diffusion tensor imaging (DTI) in surgery has proven to be a valuable tool for maximizing tumor resection. Aiming to balance the unavoidable changes in the brain that occur during the resection of intracranial tumors, subcortical stimulation directly indicates the functional locations of related neural structures, such as the pyramidal tract. However, guidance from direct subcortical stimulation also carries many errors related to stimulation parameters and tissue, patient responses, and assessment techniques, leading to false-positive and false-negative results. Today, to address these situations, each researcher proposes their own rules based on experience, often combining both techniques. The preferred rule for surgeons is to stop tumor resection when subcortical stimulation produces a positive motor response or if the stimulation site is within 2 mm of the pyramidal tract as displayed on DTI imaging. From this perspective, a related issue with DTI-guided neuro-navigation in surgery is accurately determining tumor volume and the anatomy of the pyramidal tract [42, 48, 49].

6. Conclusion

The integration of diffusion tensor imaging (DTI)-based tractography with neuro-navigation represents a significant advancement in the surgical management of gliomas within eloquent brain areas. By reconstructing fiber tracts and providing a comprehensive visualization of neural networks, DTI facilitates maximal tumor resection while minimizing the risk of iatrogenic deficits. Clinical evidence underscores the benefits of this approach, demonstrating improved rates of gross total resection and reduced postoperative morbidity compared to traditional methods. Despite inherent challenges such as signal distortions from peritumoral edema or infiltration, ongoing technical refinements continue to enhance the accuracy and reliability of DTI tractography. Furthermore, the synergy between DTI and neuro-navigation systems allows for real-time adjustments during surgery, ensuring optimal outcomes for patients. As research and technology progress, the application of DTI in neurosurgery is poised to become increasingly integral, offering enhanced precision in tumor removal and better preservation of vital brain functions. Ultimately, the adoption of DTI-based tractography marks a pivotal step toward safer and more effective neurosurgical interventions, significantly improving the quality of life for individuals afflicted with gliomas.

Author details

Ha Dai Duong[1] and Linh Duy Nguyen[2]*

1 Hanoi Medical University, Hanoi, Vietnam

2 Can Tho University of Medicine and Pharmacy, Can Tho, Vietnam

*Address all correspondence to: ndlinh@ctump.edu.vn

References

[1] Buchmann N, Gempt J, Stoffel M, Foerschler A, Meyer B, Ringel F. Utility of diffusion tensor-imaged (DTI) motor fiber tracking for the resection of intracranial tumors near the corticospinal tract. Acta Neurochirurgica. 2011;**153**:68-74; discussion 74. DOI: 10.1007/s00701-010-0817-0

[2] Hecke WV, Emsell L, Sunaert S, editors. Diffusion Tensor Imaging: A Practical Handbook. New York, NY: Springer New York; 2016. DOI: 10.1007/978-1-4939-3118-7

[3] Soni N, Mehrotra A, Behari S, Kumar S, Gupta N. Diffusion-tensor imaging and tractography application in pre-operative planning of intra-axial brain lesions. Cureus. 2017;**9**:e1739. DOI: 10.7759/cureus.1739

[4] Ius T, Somma T, Baiano C, Guarracino I, Pauletto G, Nilo A, et al. Risk assessment by pre-surgical tractography in left hemisphere low-grade gliomas. Frontiers in Neurology. 2021;**12**:1-13

[5] Jellison BJ, Field AS, Medow J, Lazar M, Salamat MS, Alexander AL. Diffusion tensor imaging of cerebral white matter: A pictorial review of physics, fiber tract anatomy, and tumor imaging patterns. AJNR. American Journal of Neuroradiology. 2004;**25**:356-369

[6] Duy Hung N, Duy Linh N, Ha Vi N, Van Anh NT, Dinh Hieu N, Dai Ha D, et al. Predictive value of preoperative diffusion tensor imaging for evaluating postoperative outcomes of supratentorial glioma in the motor function area. Therapeutics and Clinical Risk Management. 2023;**19**:269-278. DOI: 10.2147/TCRM.S402622

[7] Dauguet J, Peled S, Berezovskii V, Delzescaux T, Warfield SK, Born R, et al. Comparison of fiber tracts derived from in-vivo DTI tractography with 3D histological neural tract tracer reconstruction on a macaque brain. NeuroImage. 2007;**37**:530-538. DOI: 10.1016/j.neuroimage.2007.04.067

[8] O'Donnell LJ, Westin C-F. An introduction to diffusion tensor image analysis. Neurosurgery Clinics of North America. 2011;**22**:185–viii. DOI: 10.1016/j.nec.2010.12.004

[9] García MSA, Anaya JSH. Diffusion tensor tractography in cerebral white matter. In: Kaoud HAE, editor. Canine Medicine—Recent Topics and Advanced Research. London, UK: InTech; 2016. DOI: 10.5772/66249

[10] Bello L, Gambini A, Castellano A, Carrabba G, Acerbi F, Fava E, et al. Motor and language DTI fiber tracking combined with intraoperative subcortical mapping for surgical removal of gliomas. NeuroImage. 2008;**39**:369-382. DOI: 10.1016/j.neuroimage.2007.08.031

[11] Bagadia A, Purandare H, Misra BK, Gupta S. Application of magnetic resonance tractography in the perioperative planning of patients with eloquent region intra-axial brain lesions. Journal of Clinical Neuroscience. 2011;**18**:633-639. DOI: 10.1016/j.jocn.2010.08.026

[12] Pope WB, editor. Glioma Imaging: Physiologic, Metabolic, and Molecular Approaches. Cham: Springer International Publishing; 2020. DOI: 10.1007/978-3-030-27359-0

[13] Prabhakar H, Devarajan SLJ. Imaging in Clinical Neurosciences for

Non-radiologists: An Atlas. 1st ed. Boca Raton, FL: CRC Press; 2021

[14] Ono Y, Chernov MF, Muragaki Y, Maruyama T, Abe K, Iseki H. Imaging of intracranial gliomas. In: Chernov MF, Muragaki Y, Kesari S, McCutcheon IE, editors. Progress in Neurological Surgery. Vol. 30. S. Karger AG Publisher; 2018. pp. 12-62. DOI: 10.1159/000464376

[15] Sollmann N, Zhang H, Kloth C, Zimmer C, Wiestler B, Rosskopf J, et al. Modern preoperative imaging and functional mapping in patients with intracranial glioma. RöFo - Fortschritte Auf Dem Gebiet Der Röntgenstrahlen Und Der Bildgebenden Verfahren. 2023;**195**:989-1000. DOI: 10.1055/a-2083-8717

[16] Ibrahim AS, Gomaa M, Sakr H, Elzaher YA. Role of diffusion tensor imaging in characterization and preoperative planning of brain neoplasms. The Egyptian Journal of Radiology and Nuclear Medicine. 2013;**44**:297-307. DOI: 10.1016/j.ejrnm.2013.02.011

[17] Alexander AL, Lee JE, Lazar M, Field AS. Diffusion tensor imaging of the brain. Neurotherapeutics. 2007;**4**:316-329. DOI: 10.1016/j.nurt.2007.05.011

[18] Li S, Xiao W, Tong Z, Li L, Zhang Y. The use of diffusion tensor imaging in the differentiation and surgical planning of suprasellar hypothalamic-opticochiasmatic glioma and craniopharyngioma in children. World Neurosurgery. 2024:474-482. DOI: 10.1016/j.wneu.2024.09.074

[19] Hattingen E, Pilatus U, editors. Brain Tumor Imaging. Berlin, Heidelberg: Springer Berlin Heidelberg; 2016. DOI: 10.1007/978-3-642-45040-2

[20] Yu CS, Li KC, Xuan Y, Ji XM, Qin W. Diffusion tensor tractography in patients with cerebral tumors: A helpful technique for neurosurgical planning and postoperative assessment. European Journal of Radiology. 2005;**56**:197-204. DOI: 10.1016/j.ejrad.2005.04.010

[21] Min Z-G, Niu C, Zhang Q-L, Zhang M, Qian Y-C. Optimal factors of diffusion tensor imaging predicting corticospinal tract injury in patients with brain tumors. Korean Journal of Radiology. 2017;**18**:844-851. DOI: 10.3348/kjr.2017.18.5.844

[22] Chernov MF, Muragaki Y, Kesari S, McCutcheon IE, editors. Intracranial Gliomas Part II—Adjuvant Therapy. Vol. 31. S. Karger AG Publisher; 2018. DOI: 10.1159/isbn.978-3-318-06059-1

[23] Magill ST, Han SJ, Li J, Berger MS. Resection of primary motor cortex tumors: Feasibility and surgical outcomes. Journal of Neurosurgery. 2018;**129**:961-972. DOI: 10.3171/2017.5.JNS163045

[24] Szmuda T, Kierońska S, Ali S, Słoniewski P, Pacholski M, Dzierżanowski J, et al. Tractography-guided surgery of brain tumours: What is the best method to outline the corticospinal tract? Folia Morphologica. 2021;**80**:40-46. DOI: 10.5603/FM.a2020.0016

[25] Filler A. The History, Development and Impact of Computed Imaging in Neurological Diagnosis and Neurosurgery: CT, MRI, and DTI. Nature Precedings Publisher; 2009. DOI: 10.1038/npre.2009.3267.3

[26] Briggs RG, Nix CE, Conner AK, Palejwala AH, Smitherman AD, Teo C, et al. An awake contralateral, transcallosal approach for deep-seated gliomas of the basal ganglia. World Neurosurgery. 2019;**130**:e880-e887. DOI: 10.1016/j.wneu.2019.07.031

[27] Dubey A, Kataria R, Sinha V. Role of diffusion tensor imaging in brain tumor surgery. Asian Journal of Neurosurgery. 2018;**13**:302-306. DOI: 10.4103/ajns.AJNS_226_16

[28] González-Darder JM, González-López P, Talamantes F, Quilis V, Cortés V, García-March G, et al. Multimodal navigation in the functional microsurgical resection of intrinsic brain tumors located in eloquent motor areas: Role of tractography. Neurosurgical Focus. 2010;**28**:E5. DOI: 10.3171/2009.11.FOCUS09234

[29] Tamura M, Kurihara H, Saito T, Nitta M, Maruyama T, Tsuzuki S, et al. Combining pre-operative diffusion tensor images and intraoperative magnetic resonance images in the navigation is useful for detecting white matter tracts during glioma surgery. Frontiers in Neurology. 2022;**12**

[30] Azagury DE, Dua MM, Barrese JC, Henderson JM, Buchs NC, Ris F, et al. Image-guided surgery. Current Problems in Surgery. 2015;**52**:476-520. DOI: 10.1067/j.cpsurg.2015.10.001

[31] Ganslandt O, Behari S, Gralla J, Fahlbusch R, Nimsky C. Neuronavigation: Concept, techniques and applications. Neurology India. 2002;**50**:244

[32] Wu J-S, Zhou L-F, Tang W-J, Mao Y, Hu J, Song Y-Y, et al. Clinical evaluation and follow-up outcome of diffusion tensor imaging-based functional neuronavigation: A prospective, controlled study in patients with gliomas involving pyramidal tracts. Neurosurgery. 2007;**61**:935-948; discussion 948-949. DOI: 10.1227/01.neu.0000303189.80049.ab

[33] Schramm J. Advances and Technical Standards in Neurosurgery: Low-Grade Gliomas. Vienna: Springer; 2010

[34] Mato D, Velasquez C, Gómez E, Marco De Lucas E, Martino J. Predicting the extent of resection in low-grade glioma by using intratumoral tractography to detect eloquent fascicles within the tumor. Neurosurgery. 2021;**88**:E190-E202. DOI: 10.1093/neuros/nyaa463

[35] Sollmann N, Zhang H, Fratini A, Wildschuetz N, Ille S, Schröder A, et al. Risk assessment by presurgical tractography using navigated TMS maps in patients with highly motor- or language-eloquent brain tumors. Cancers (Basel). 2020;**12**:E1264. DOI: 10.3390/cancers12051264

[36] Zhylka A, Sollmann N, Kofler F, Radwan A, De Luca A, Gempt J, et al. Tracking the corticospinal tract in patients with high-grade glioma: Clinical evaluation of multi-level fiber tracking and comparison to conventional deterministic approaches. Frontiers in Oncology. 2021;**11**:761169. DOI: 10.3389/fonc.2021.761169

[37] Zhang W, Ille S, Schwendner M, Wiestler B, Meyer B, Krieg SM. Tracking motor and language eloquent white matter pathways with intraoperative fiber tracking versus preoperative tractography adjusted by intraoperative MRI–based elastic fusion. Journal of Neurosurgery. 2022;**137**:1114-1123. DOI: 10.3171/2021.12.JNS212106

[38] Baker CM, Burks JD, Briggs RG, Smitherman AD, Glenn CA, Conner AK, et al. The crossed frontal aslant tract: A possible pathway involved in the recovery of supplementary motor area syndrome. Brain and Behavior: A Cognitive Neuroscience Perspective. 2018;**8**:e00926. DOI: 10.1002/brb3.926

[39] Li Y, Hou Y, Li Q, Tang J, Lu J. Optimized tractography mapping and quantitative evaluation of pyramidal

tracts for surgical resection of insular gliomas: A correlative study with diffusion tensor imaging–derived metrics and patient motor strength. Journal of Digital Imaging. 2022;**35**.356-364. DOI: 10.1007/s10278-021-00578-4

[40] Faust K. Distinct displacements of the optic radiation based on tumor location revealed using preoperative diffusion tensor imaging. Journal of Neurosurgery. 2016). Available from: https://thejns.org/view/journals/j-neurosurg/124/5/article-p1343.xml;**124**(5) [Accessed: July 30, 2023]

[41] Alexopoulos G, Cikla U, El Tecle N, Kulkarni N, Pierson M, Mercier P, et al. The value of white matter tractography by diffusion tensor imaging in altering a neurosurgeon's operative plan. World Neurosurgery. 2019;**132**:e305-e313. DOI: 10.1016/j.wneu.2019.08.168

[42] Xiao X, Kong L, Pan C, Zhang P, Chen X, Sun T, et al. The role of diffusion tensor imaging and tractography in the surgical management of brainstem gliomas. Neurosurgical Focus. 2021;**50**:E10. DOI: 10.3171/2020.10.FOCUS20166

[43] Youmans JR, Winn HR. Youmans & Winn Neurological Surgery. 7th ed. Philadelphia, PA: Elsevier; 2017

[44] Mair MJ, Geurts M, Van Den Bent MJ, Berghoff AS. A basic review on systemic treatment options in WHO grade II-III gliomas. Cancer Treatment Reviews. 2021;**92**:102124. DOI: 10.1016/j.ctrv.2020.102124

[45] Samuel N, Vetkas A, Pancholi A, Sarica C, Loh A, Germann J, et al. A network-based approach to glioma surgery: Insights from functional neurosurgery. Cancers. 2021;**13**:6127. DOI: 10.3390/cancers13236127

[46] Radwan AM, Sunaert S, Schilling K, Descoteaux M, Landman BA, Vandenbulcke M, et al. An atlas of white matter anatomy, its variability, and reproducibility based on constrained spherical deconvolution of diffusion MRI. NeuroImage. 2022;**254**:119029. DOI: 10.1016/j.neuroimage.2022.119029

[47] Zhu F-P, Wu J-S, Song Y-Y, Yao C-J, Zhuang D-X, Xu G, et al. Clinical application of motor pathway mapping using diffusion tensor imaging tractography and intraoperative direct subcortical stimulation in cerebral glioma surgery: A prospective cohort study. Neurosurgery. 2012;**71**:1170-1184. DOI: 10.1227/NEU.0b013e318271bc61

[48] Holodny AI. Diffusion tensor tractography of the motor white matter tracts in man: Current controversies and future directions. Annals of the New York Academy of Sciences. 2005;**1064**:88-97. DOI: 10.1196/annals.1340.016

[49] Ortiz KJ, Hawayek MI, Middlebrooks EH, Sabsevitz DS, Garcia DP, Quinones-Hinojosa A, et al. Intraoperative direct stimulation identification and preservation of critical white matter tracts during brain surgery. World Neurosurgery. 2021;**146**:64-74. DOI: 10.1016/j.wneu.2020.10.100

Chapter 3

The Supracerebellar Approach for Pineal and Brainstem Lesions: Advantages and Limitations

Yücel Doğruel and Osman Fikret Sönmez

Abstract

The supracerebellar approach is a crucial surgical technique for accessing pineal and posterior brainstem lesions. Originally introduced by Krause and modified by Stein and Yaşargil, this approach provides a direct operative corridor to the pineal region, posterior third ventricle, and tectum, facilitating the resection of various pathologies, including pineal tumors, astrocytomas, and vascular lesions. The paramedian and lateral variants of the approach offer increased surgical freedom and favorable angles of access, minimizing cerebellar retraction and reducing the risk of postoperative complications. Endoscopic-assisted techniques have improved the approach by enhancing visualization, allowing for minimally invasive procedures, and faster recovery times. However, challenges remain, particularly with the proximity of critical structures like the superior medullary velum and the deep venous system, which can limit the rostral extent of tumor resection. Additionally, intraoperative risks such as venous air embolism are concerns, especially in the sitting or semi-sitting positions. Despite these limitations, the supracerebellar approach remains highly effective and versatile. This chapter examines the anatomical considerations, surgical techniques, and clinical applications of the supracerebellar approach, highlighting its advantages and limitations. Through a comprehensive review of historical perspectives and current advancements, we aim to underscore the significance of this technique in the surgical management of posterior fossa lesions.

Keywords: operative corridor, paramedian, posterior brainstem, tectum, tentorium

1. Introduction

The supracerebellar approaches for accessing pineal and brainstem lesions have unique advantages and some challenges. These approaches provide a corridor that allows for direct access to the pineal region and posterior third ventricle, which are often challenging surgical targets due to their deep-seated locations and proximity to critical neurovascular structures. One of the primary advantages of the supracerebellar approach is its ability to facilitate access to lesions located in the pineal region without the need for extensive retraction of the cerebellum, which can lead to postoperative complications such as cerebellar swelling and neurological deficits. For instance, the paramedian variant of the supracerebellar inftra tentorial (SCIT) approach has been shown to provide a more favorable angle for accessing the pineal gland and surrounding structures, thereby minimizing the risk of damage to adjacent neural tissues [1, 2]. This approach allows surgeons to navigate around the cerebellar vermis and superior cerebellar peduncles, which are often obstacles in traditional surgical routes [1, 3].

However, despite its advantages, the supracerebellar approach has its limitations. The complexity of the surrounding anatomy, particularly the deep venous system and brainstem, introduces significant challenges during surgery. The presence of critical vascular structures, such as the vein of Galen and the deep venous complex, requires careful planning and precise implementation to minimize the risk of intraoperative complications [4, 5].

Recent advancements in surgical techniques, including the integration of endoscopic methods, have further enhanced the efficacy of the supracerebellar approach. Endoscopic-assisted techniques offer improved visualization of the surgical field, enabling surgeons to perform less invasive resections with a high degree of precision [6, 7]. Combining microscopic and endoscopic approaches has demonstrated favorable outcomes, particularly in complex tumors that displace critical vascular structures [4, 8]. Additionally, the use of 3D exoscopes has been reported to improve both ergonomics and visualization during surgery, making the SCIT approach more accessible to a broader range of neurosurgeons [9, 10].

2. Historical perspective

The classic midline supracerebellar approach was first introduced by Fedor Krause [11]. This approach was later modified by Stein to access the pineal region [12]. As a variation of the midline approach, the paramedian approach was developed by Yaşargil to access the pineal region, tectum, thalamus, and the posterior mediobasal temporal region, with the addition of a tentorial incision [13–15]. Yasargil first used the paramedian route to approach the superior cerebellar artery aneurysms [16]. In 1990, the lateral corridor of the supracerebellar approach was described by Van den Bergh [17]. Later, it was reported that lesions in the superior and inferior colliculus, superior and middle cerebellar peduncles, and quadrangular lobules of the cerebellum could be safely operated on using this approach [18].

3. Indications for the supracerebellar approaches

The supracerebellar approach, particularly the infratentorial variant, is a well-established surgical technique primarily indicated for accessing lesions located in the pineal region and other midline structures of the posterior fossa. This approach provides direct access to tumors such as pinealomas, meningiomas, and other neoplasms situated in the vicinity of the cerebellum and brainstem, facilitating effective surgical intervention while minimizing cerebellar retraction and associated complications [19, 20]. Moreover, surgical resection of pineal region tumors using this approach has been shown to improve survival rates and reduce recurrence [21, 22]. The paramedian variant of the supracerebellar approach offers additional advantages, including a more favorable angle of access and reduced manipulation of surrounding neural structures, contributing to improved postoperative outcomes [23, 24].

This approach also effectively exposes pineal region lesions such as germ cell tumors, pineoblastomas, astrocytomas, and rarer lesions like meningiomas, epidermoid tumors, and pilocytic astrocytomas. It serves as an alternative, and often preferred, technique for resecting posterior third ventricular and thalamic tumors [1, 25, 26]. Additionally, vascular lesions, including tentorial arteriovenous fistulae and malformations, can be addressed using this approach, along with intraparenchymal posterolateral mesencephalic lesions, such as cavernous malformations and pilocytic astrocytomas, as well as distal superior cerebellar artery aneurysms [25]. The trans-tentorial extension of the paramedian supracerebellar approach enables the removal of the supratentorial component of petrous apex meningiomas without requiring a second-stage subtemporal surgery. It can also resect posterior hippocampal cavernous malformations, arteriovenous malformations, astrocytomas, and metastases [25].

In addition to tumor resection, the supracerebellar approach is indicated for conditions such as vascular lesions and certain types of cysts, including thalamic hemorrhage with extension into the brainstem, showcasing its versatility in addressing a variety of pathologies in the posterior fossa [27]. The development of endoscopic-assisted versions of this approach has further enhanced its utility, allowing for minimally invasive techniques that reduce the need for extensive craniotomies and the associated risks of morbidity [28].

The anatomical considerations for the supracerebellar approach are crucial for its successful application. Surgeons must be vigilant about the surrounding vascular

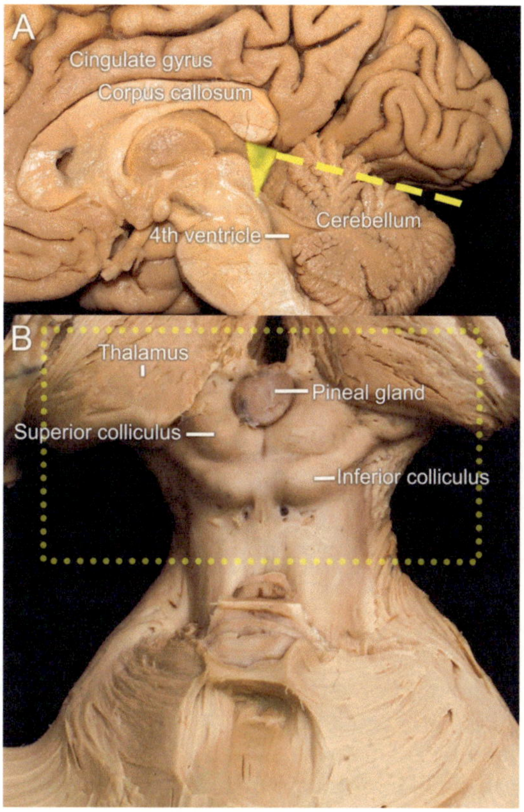

Figure 1.
The surgical trajectory of the supracerebellar approaches. A. The dashed lines indicate the trajectory of the approach, while the yellow triangle marks the accessible areas in the lateral view of a medial brain specimen. B. The accessible areas are highlighted by a yellow quadrangle in the posterior view of the pineal region in a dissected cadaveric specimen.

structures, such as the superior petrosal vein and the bridging veins on the cerebellar surface, as injury can result in significant complications, including hemorrhage and infarction [29, 30]. The approach typically involves creating a bone opening just beneath the transverse sinus, which requires careful preoperative planning to avoid vascular injury [31]. Overall, the supracerebellar infratentorial approach remains an effective and versatile technique for a range of midline lesions, particularly in the pineal region. Its applications extend beyond tumor resection to include vascular and hemorrhagic conditions, with advancements in endoscopic techniques further enhancing its safety profile. The surgical trajectory of the supracerebellar approaches is illustrated in **Figure 1**.

4. Preoperative assessment

The radiologic assessment should include an evaluation of the patient's tentorial angle. Additionally, since the procedure requires moderate neck flexion, the patient's neck length, range of motion, age, and weight should be assessed, as the degree of neck flexion varies [32]. A radiologic cervical evaluation should also be performed to check for degenerative diseases.

Each patient undergoes a routine physical examination and laboratory testing before surgery [32]. One of the most significant complications of the supracerebellar approach is venous air embolism, particularly in the sitting or semi-sitting position, as these positions increase the risk. Therefore, preoperative transthoracic echocardiography should be performed. In the presence of a patent foramen ovale or right-to-left shunt, other positions should be considered, as the sitting or semi-sitting positions may be contraindicated for these patients. However, it is essential to note that transthoracic echocardiography may miss some patients [32]. Consequently, if surgery is planned to be performed in the sitting position, intraoperative transesophageal echocardiography should also be prepared when available. It is worth noting that previous esophageal interventions may contraindicate the use of transesophageal echocardiographic monitoring [32].

The risk of venous air embolism, although low, persists in other positions during supracerebellar approaches. An important example was reported by Cucchiara, where no intraoperative deaths were recorded in a series of 3827 cases performed in the sitting position [33]. However, one postoperative death was possibly related to venous air embolism. In their own neurosurgical practice, the only intraoperative death associated with venous air embolism occurred in the prone position.

5. Surgical steps

5.1 Surgical positioning

The supracerebellar approaches can be performed with the patient sitting, semi-sitting, lateral, prone oblique, or prone position [29, 34, 35]. The semi-sitting position offers improved gravitational drainage of cerebrospinal fluid and blood from the surgical field, resulting in a cleaner and more unobstructed view of the lesion [32]. Additional advantages of the semi-sitting position include enabling the surgeon to perform micromanipulation with both hands rather than dedicating one hand to aspiration, enhancing anatomical orientation, reducing intracranial pressure, and requiring less retraction. For patients in the semi-sitting position, head elevation of up to 30° is considered safe in neurosurgical practice. However, elevations beyond this are directly correlated with an

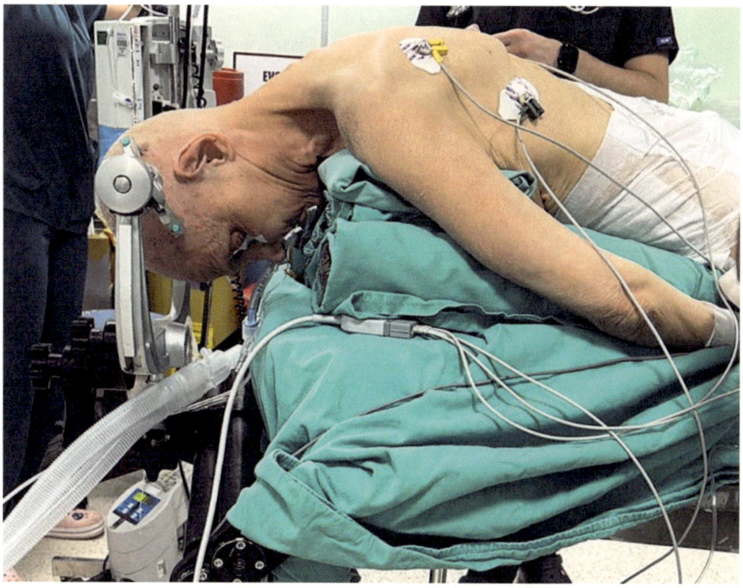

Figure 2.
Modified concorde position. This position can be utilized when the semi-sitting position is not feasible. It facilitates endoscope-assisted surgery, allowing direct placement of the endoscope screen for optimal visualization.

increased risk of venous air embolism [32]. Therefore, following endotracheal intubation, transesophageal echocardiography monitoring is essential to detect potential air embolism, particularly when the patient is positioned in a sitting or semi-sitting posture.

Recently, a new surgical position known as the dynamic lateral semi-sitting position has been described for supracerebellar approaches [36]. This position aims to reduce the risk of venous air embolism associated with traditional sitting and semi-sitting positions. Initially, while the patient's head was held securely, the patient was turned to a lateral decubitus position. The head was then rotated 15° toward the lower shoulder and elevated 40°, with the Mayfield 3-pin head holder fixed. This position is maintained throughout the extradural part of the surgery. After the dura mater incision and hemostasis, the body section of the operating table is tilted up by 40°, resulting in a head angle of 80°. The resection is performed after further elevating the patient's body, allowing the head to maintain an angle similar to the semi-sitting position.

Based on our experience, an alternative option is the modified Concorde position, which can be particularly useful when sitting is contraindicated or the surgical microscope is not suitable for the sitting position (**Figure 2**). One advantage of this position is that it facilitates endoscope-assisted surgery, allowing for the direct placement of the endoscope screen for optimal visualization.

5.2 Incision and craniotomy

Classically, a midline, paramedian, or lateral linear incision is made from the level of the inion to the level of the C1 vertebra (**Figure 3**). The subcutaneous tissues are dissected using monopolar cautery, and the cervical muscles are retracted laterally. Once adequate exposure is achieved, hemostasis is performed. A median, paramedian, or lateral suboccipital craniotomy is then carried out by placing three burr holes, depending on the chosen surgical route (**Figure 4A**). The bone edges can be treated with bone wax to avoid the aspiration of air by any diplopic tissue.

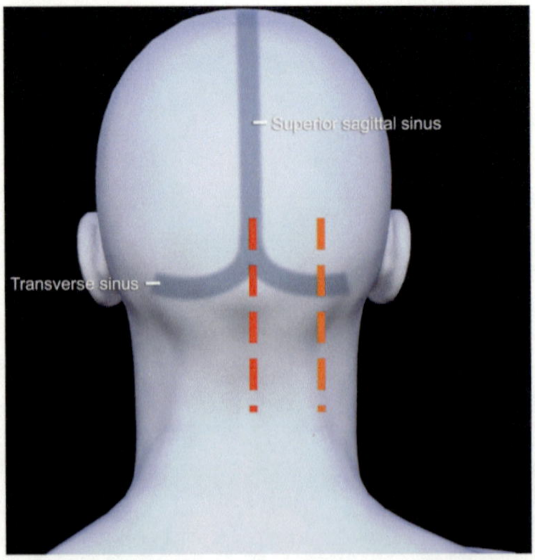

Figure 3.
Surgical incisions for supracerebellar approaches in the suboccipital region. The red dashed lines represent the median incision, while the orange lines indicate the paramedian incision.

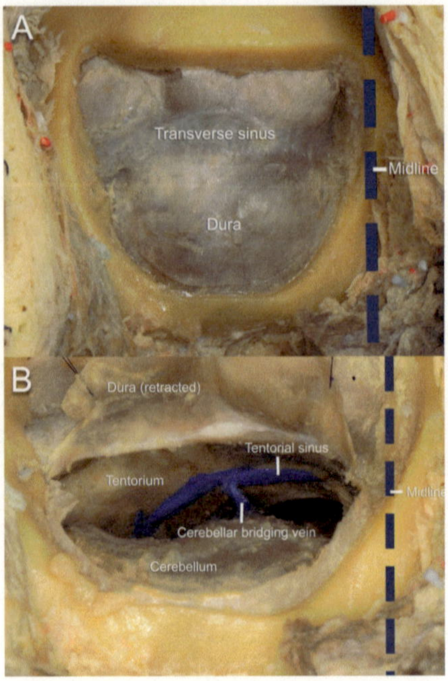

Figure 4.
The paramedian suboccipital craniotomy and dural opening for the supracerebellar approach in a cadaveric specimen. A. The paramedian craniotomy is illustrated. B. The dura is opened and retracted superiorly, while the cerebellum is retracted inferiorly, allowing visualization of the supracerebellar surface.

The dura is typically incised in a Y-shape or semicircular fashion. In the Y-shaped dural incision, the right and left parts of the dura are suspended laterally, while the upper part is suspended upwards In this incision, cerebrospinal fluid (CSF) can be directly released from the cisterna magna after the dural opening. If a semicircular incision is planned, making two dural incisions may increase surgical safety. The first incision is placed over the lower aspect of the craniotomy to release CSF from the cisterna magna, allowing relaxation of the posterior fossa. The second incision is made approximately 15 mm below the transverse sinus, with the ends curving upward, closer to the sinus [37]. In this incision, the dura is suspended upward to expose the supracerebellar corridor (**Figure 4B**). Before the dural incision, Doppler ultrasound is useful for identifying the occipital sinus, and the incision can be adjusted if a dominant occipital sinus is present [38]. The Doppler ultrasound also helps determine the exact location of the transverse sinus, and the identified sinus routes are marked with a surgical pen to avoid sinus injury during dural opening.

In the sitting position and its variants, gravity causes the cerebellum to descend, thereby opening the supracerebellar space without the need for retraction. In contrast, cerebellum retraction may be necessary when the patient is in the prone position; this retraction should be performed gently.

5.3 Microsurgical approach

Under the surgical microscope, arachnoid bands and arachnoid villi between the tentorium and the superior cerebellar surface are carefully dissected. Bridging veins between the superior surface of the cerebellum and the tentorium become visible as these bands are separated (**Figure 5**). Preserving these veins as much as possible is recommended, as predicting whether major venous infarction may occur following their interruption is challenging due to the significant venous variation in this region [20, 29]. Additionally, these veins may bleed due to tension created during the opening of the supracerebellar space and related complications. To reduce this risk, veins can be mobilized using the arachnoid dissection technique or the recently described tentorial cut technique [29]. In midline approaches, it is essential to note that these veins are consistently encountered along the surgical route, and their sacrifice may be inevitable.

In the next step, the arachnoid of the quadrigeminal cistern is dissected. These arachnoid attachments may be thickened, requiring sharp dissection under high magnification [20]. The cisternal space should be opened at the level of the cerebellar culmen to avoid injuring the venous or arterial structures. The arachnoid membrane is opened using scissors, but coagulation should be performed before cutting this layer. The arachnoid opening is then extended laterally to both the left and right sides to expose the

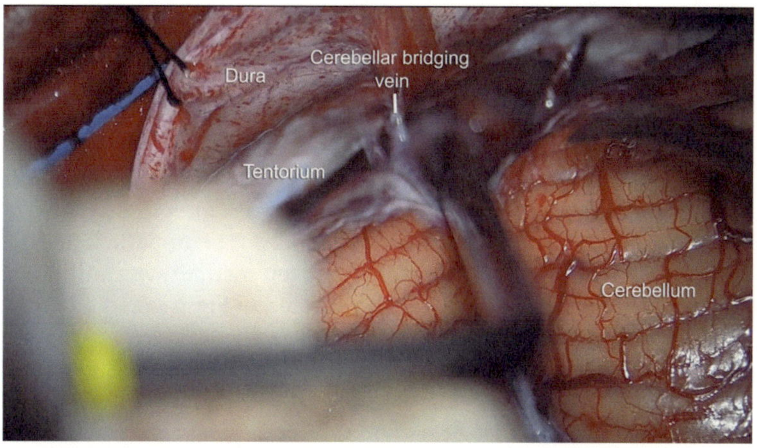

Figure 5.
The anatomy of the supracerebellar surface. The supracerebellar surface, tentorium, and cerebellar bridging veins are shown in a patient during surgery.

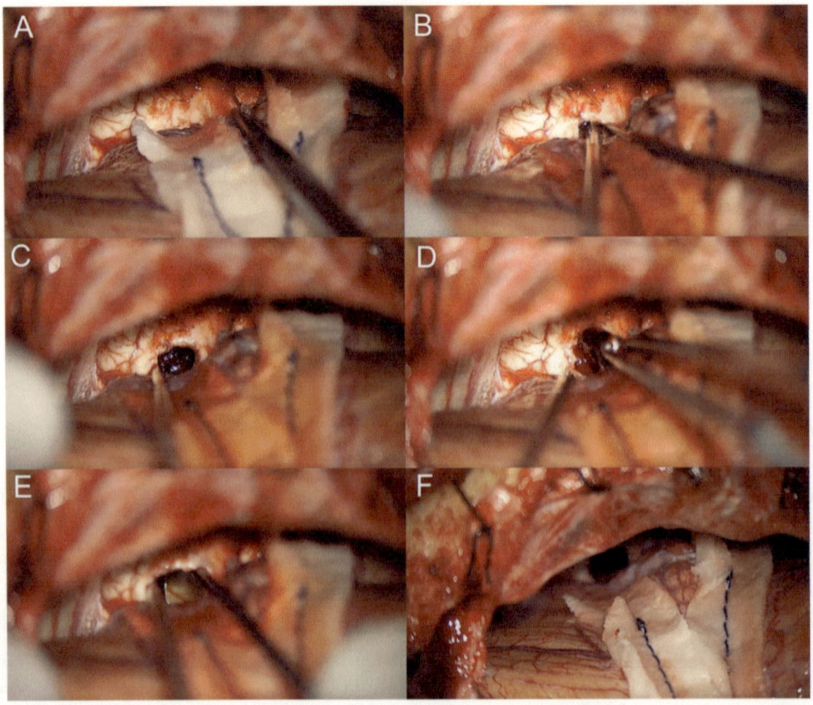

Figure 6.
Surgical steps of the supracerebellar infratentorial approach for brainstem lesions. A. The brainstem is visualized through the supracerebellar corridor. B. A small incision is made on the brainstem to access the lesion. C. The lesion is displayed within the surgical cavity. D. The lesion is carefully dissected and removed. E. The surgical cavity is shown after achieving hemostasis. F. The surgical corridor is illustrated following the resection.

right and left basilar veins, as well as the inferior part of the vein of Galen [39]. The vein of Galen and the internal cerebral veins are positioned superior to the tumor, while the veins of Rosenthal drain laterally into the vein of Galen. These vessels are generally located outside the tumor field, reducing the risk of injury. Initially, before opening the arachnoid and freeing the cerebellum from its adhesions to the brainstem, the surgical trajectory is directed toward the vein of Galen. Once the cerebellum is mobilized and retracted, the trajectory can be adjusted to align through the central axis of the tumor. The posterior aspect of the tumor becomes visible and is often vascularized by branches of the choroidal arteries. A small portion of the posterior tumor surface is cauterized and incised to facilitate internal debulking. Depending on the tumor's consistency, debulking may be performed using suction, cautery, tumor forceps, ring curettes, or a Cavitron with a long-curved tip. A sample of the tumor is sent for frozen section diagnosis to inform intraoperative decision-making. However, neuropathologists often find it challenging to characterize these tumors from frozen sections, warranting caution in clinical decisions [20]. Surgical steps are demonstrated in **Figure 6**.

5.4 Complications

Given the unpredictable venous drainage and the surgical assumption that bridging veins can be sacrificed without consequence, venous-related complications may arise. The clinical spectrum of these complications can vary widely. Many patients report self-limiting dizziness, headaches, and nausea, which may represent milder venous complications due to venous stasis following vein sacrifice [40]. The downward displacement of the cerebellum can cause compression of the cerebellar tonsils at the level of the foramen magnum, potentially resulting in ischemic injury to the cerebellum and brainstem. The use of retractors may increase this risk by adding to the compression. Additionally, surgical site infections, CSF fistula, and meningitis may also occur [39].

6. Illustrative cases

6.1 Illustrative case 1

A 46-year-old woman with a 20-year history of a pontine mass presented with progressive hearing loss and facial paralysis. MRI revealed an epidermoid tumor located

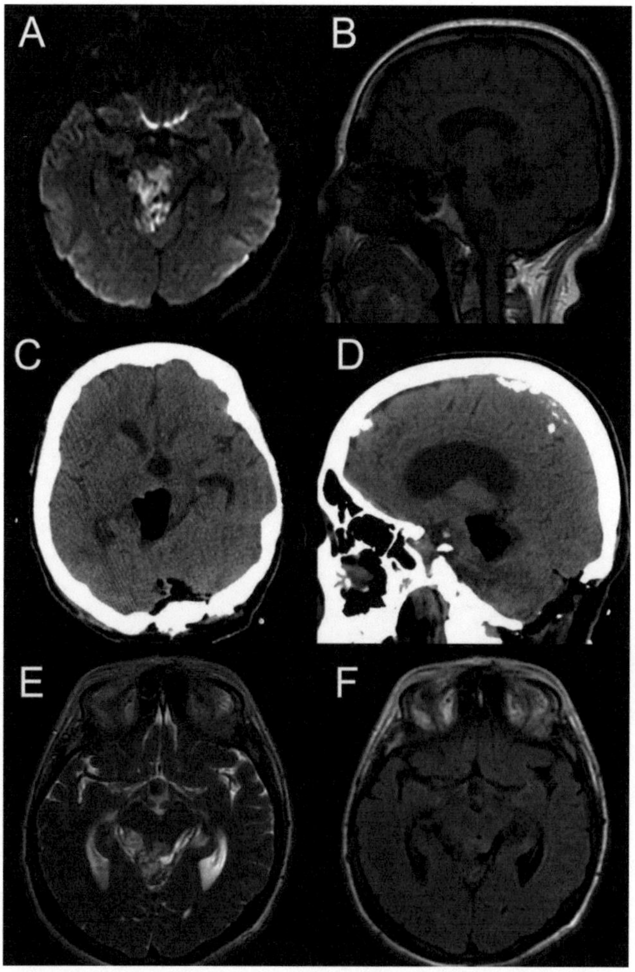

Figure 7.
Preoperative and postoperative imaging of the illustrative case 1 with an epidermoid tumor located posterior and lateral to the tectum. A. Axial diffusion MRI demonstrating the restricted lesion. B. Sagittal T1 MRI showing the lesion. C. Postoperative axial CT scan indicating resection of the lesion. D. Postoperative sagittal CT scan confirming resection of the lesion. E. Late postoperative axial T2 MRI showing no residual tumor or recurrence. F. Late postoperative axial FLAIR MRI confirming no residual tumor or recurrence.

posterior and lateral to the tectum. The patient underwent surgery via a right paramedian supracerebellar approach, resulting in the complete excision of the lesion (**Figure 7**).

6.2 Illustrative case 2

A 19-year-old male patient, initially evaluated 4 years ago for headaches, was found to have a pineal mass and associated hydrocephalus at an external center. A ventriculoperitoneal shunt was placed to address the hydrocephalus, and the patient was followed up. He presented to our clinic with new-onset seizures, and an MRI revealed the progression of the pineal mass. The patient was admitted for surgery and underwent a supracerebellar infratentorial approach for tumor resection. The mass was completely excised. Histopathological examination reported the tumor as pleomorphic xanthoastrocytoma (**Figure 8**).

6.3 Illustrative case 3

A 74-year-old male was admitted with altered consciousness following a 15-day history of slow speech. Neurological examination and imaging studies revealed a mass lesion at the midline level of the mesencephalon, measuring 49 × 37 × 46 mm. The lesion exhibited peripheral nodular enhancement and hyperintense cystic components on T2-weighted MRI sequences. Given the clinical presentation and imaging findings, the patient underwent a surgical intervention via a supracerebellar infratentorial approach (**Figure 9**).

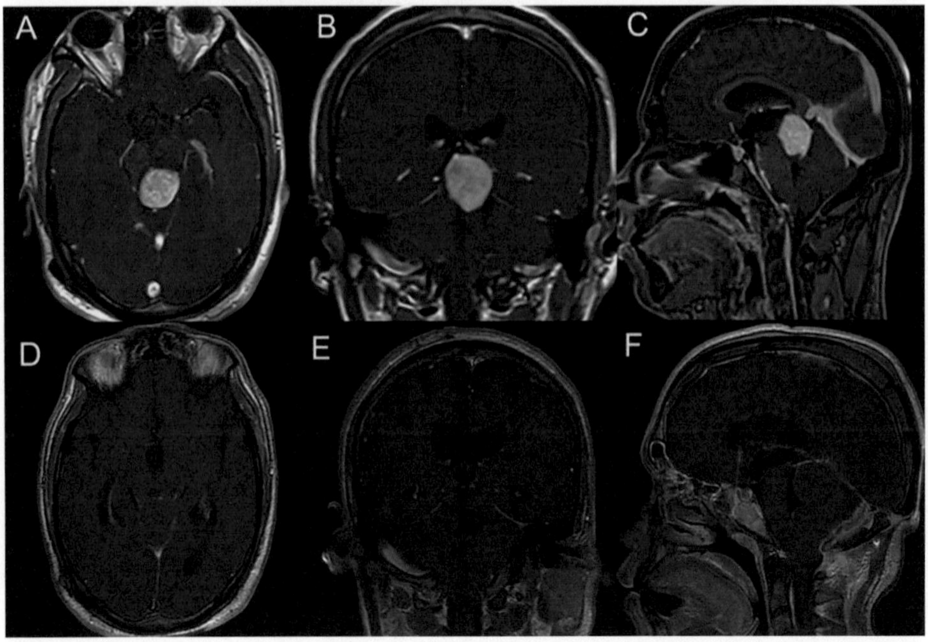

Figure 8.
This figure illustrates the preoperative and postoperative imaging of the illustrative case 2 with a pineal region pleomorphic xanthoastrocytoma. Panels A, B, and C display the preoperative axial, coronal, and sagittal images, respectively. Panels D, E, and F show the corresponding postoperative axial, coronal, and sagittal images of the patient.

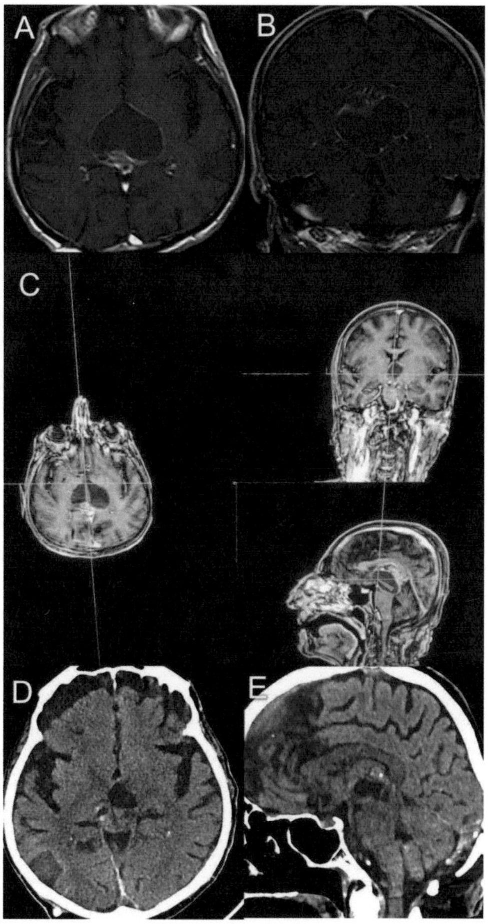

Figure 9.
Preoperative and postoperative imaging of the illustrative case 3, along with intraoperative neuronavigation images. Panel A shows the preoperative axial MRI, while Panel B displays the preoperative coronal MRI. Panel C illustrates the intraoperative neuronavigation image. Postoperative imaging is depicted in Panel D, which presents the axial CT, and Panel E, which shows the sagittal CT.

7. Advantages and limitations of the supracerebellar approaches

The supracerebellar approach presents a range of significant advantages and limitations for the surgical management of posterior fossa lesions, particularly those involving the pineal region, midbrain, and posterior third ventricle. Among its notable advantages, this approach allows for a shorter working distance to the target lesion, thereby enhancing surgical efficiency. It facilitates the preservation of critical neurovascular structures and minimizes the risk of cortical injury while also providing superior visualization of the surgical field. Additionally, the approach enables early control of major venous drainage, which is crucial in managing complex vascular lesions. The inherent anatomical corridor between the cerebellum and the tentorium serves as a direct yet minimally invasive pathway to deep-seated brain structures, thus improving the safety profile of the procedure. Advancements in neuronavigation and intraoperative imaging technologies further enhance the applicability of this technique, allowing for the extension of the approach to encompass a broader spectrum of pathologies.

However, despite these advantages, the supracerebellar approach remains underutilized in contemporary neurosurgical practice. The conical shape of the supracerebellar space limits lateral control of tumor extension, presenting challenges in managing tumor resection. While it is possible to open the tentorium from below, achieving hemostatic control in venous lakes can be difficult, with the risk of catastrophic bleeding. The sacrifice of bridging veins poses additional risks, as predicting the consequences of their interruption is inherently challenging. Such sacrifices can lead to ischemic lesions exacerbated by pressure exerted by cerebellar retractors [39]. Although respecting the precentral venous system is generally considered less critical, it is noteworthy that this system can vary in its formation, as reported by Pendl. In 59% of cases, it may consist of a single vein, while in 27%, it can be paired, and in others, it may be a more complex system [41]. Sparing this venous system is easier when formed by a distinct single vein, allowing the surgeon to navigate between sides more effectively. In contrast, when dealing with a multiple vein system, preserving the vessels becomes more challenging; in such instances, coagulating these veins may be a safer strategy to avoid rupture and air embolism and to maintain hemostasis during tumor dissection. Therefore, careful preoperative assessment and constant monitoring during surgery are crucial for minimizing these risks while maximizing the advantages of the supracerebellar approach.

8. Conclusions

The supracerebellar approach continues to play a critical role in the surgical management of both the pineal region and brainstem lesions, offering distinct advantages in terms of direct access to deep-seated tumors, reduced cerebellar retraction, and the preservation of critical neurovascular structures. Its inherent advantages, including direct access to deep-seated brain tumors, reduced working distance, and the ability to preserve vital neurovascular elements, make it an attractive option in neurosurgical practice. Particularly, the infratentorial variant represents a significant advancement in neurosurgical techniques for accessing the pineal region and brainstem lesions. The ongoing evolution of surgical techniques, including the incorporation of endoscopic methods and advanced imaging technologies, continues to enhance the safety and effectiveness of the supracerebellar approaches for pineal and brainstem lesions.

However, despite its advantages, the supracerebellar approach is not without limitations. The complexity of the surrounding anatomy and the potential for complications necessitate a thorough understanding of the approach's challenges. In particular, the deep venous system and proximity to the brainstem present significant obstacles during surgery, including difficulties with lateral tumor control, unpredictable venous drainage, and the potential for ischemic complications due to bridging vein sacrifice.

Careful preoperative assessment, combined with advanced imaging techniques and meticulous intraoperative management, is essential to navigate these complexities effectively. Ultimately, the successful application of the supracerebellar approach hinges on the surgeon's ability to balance the benefits and risks, ensuring optimal patient outcomes while advancing the capabilities of neurosurgery in managing challenging lesions of the posterior fossa.

Conflict of interest

The authors declare no conflict of interest.

Author details

Yücel Doğruel and Osman Fikret Sönmez*
Tepecik Training and Research Hospital, Health Sciences University, İzmir, Türkiye

*Address all correspondence to: sonmezof@yahoo.com

References

[1] Aboul-Enein H, El-Aziz Sabry AA, Hafez Farhoud A. Supracerebellar infratentorial approach with paramedian expansion for posterior third ventricular and pineal region lesions. Clinical Neurology and Neurosurgery. 2015;**139**:100-109. DOI: 10.1016/j.clineuro.2015.08.009 [published Online First: 20150925]

[2] Kulwin C, Matsushima K, Malekpour M, Cohen-Gadol A. Lateral supracerebellar infratentorial approach for microsurgical resection of large midline pineal region tumors: Techniques to expand the operative corridor. Journal of Neurosurgery. 2016;**124**(1):269-276. DOI: 10.3171/2015.2.jns142088

[3] Choque-Velasquez J, Resendiz-Nieves J, Jahromi BR, et al. Midline and paramedian supracerebellar infratentorial approach to the pineal region: A comparative clinical study in 112 patients. World Neurosurgery. 2020;**137**:e194-e207. DOI: 10.1016/j.wneu.2020.01.137

[4] Ding Y, Sun L, Hu Y-k, et al. Combined microscopic and endoscopic surgery for pineal region meningiomas using the occipital-parietal transtentorial approach. Frontiers in Oncology. 2022;**12**:828361. DOI: 10.3389/fonc.2022.828361

[5] Matsuo S, Baydın S, Güngör A, et al. Midline and off-midline infratentorial supracerebellar approaches to the pineal gland. Journal of Neurosurgery. 2016;**126**(6):1984-1994. DOI: 10.3171/2016.7.jns16277

[6] Fluss R, Kobets AJ, Altschul D, Nakhla J, Lasala P. Laparoscope-assisted guidance to the pineal region. Cureus. 2020;**12**(7):e9085. DOI: 10.7759/cureus.9085

[7] Felbaum DR, Syed HR, Ryan JE, Jean WC, Anaizi A. Endoscope-assisted combined supracerebellar infratentorial and endoscopic transventricular approach to the pineal region: A technical note. Cureus. 2016;**8**(3):e520. DOI: 10.7759/cureus.520

[8] Xie T. Endoscopic supracerebellar infratentorial transpineal approach for posterior-medial thalamic lesions: Surgical technique and clinical experience. Operative Neurosurgery. 2024;**27**(2):187-193. DOI: 10.1227/ons.0000000000001114

[9] Roa JA, Schüpper AJ, Yaeger K, Hadjipanayis C. Use of the 3D exoscope for the supracerebellar infratentorial approach in the concorde position: An effective and ergonomic alternative. Illustrative cases. Journal of Neurosurgery Case Lessons. 2022;**3**(19):CASE21626. DOI: 10.3171/case21626

[10] Hua W. Neurosurgical application of pineal region tumor resection with 3D 4K exoscopy via infratentorial approach: A retrospective cohort study. International Journal of Surgery. 2023;**109**(12):4062-4072. DOI: 10.1097/js9.0000000000000707

[11] Krause F. Chirurgie des gehirns und rückenmarks nach eigenen erfahrungen. Berlin: Urban & Schwarzenberg; 1911

[12] Stein BM. The infratentorial supracerebellar approach to pineal lesions. Journal of Neurosurgery. 1971;**35**(2):197-202. DOI: 10.3171/jns.1971.35.2.0197

[13] Voigt K, Yasargil MG. Cerebral cavernous haemangiomas or cavernomas. Incidence, pathology, localization, diagnosis, clinical features and treatment. Review of the literature and report of an unusual case. Neurochirurgia (Stuttgart). 1976;**19**(2):59-68. DOI: 10.1055/s-0028-1090391

[14] Yasargil MG. Microneurosurgery, Volume III B: AVM of the Brain, Clinical Considerations, General and Special Operative Techniques, Surgical Results, Nonoperated Cases, Cavernous and Venous Angiomas, Neuroanesthesia. Stuttgart: Thieme; 1988

[15] Yasargil MG. Microneurosurgery, Volume IV B: Microneurosurgery of CNS Tumors. Stuttgart: Thieme; 1996

[16] Yasargil MG. Microneurosurgery, Volume I: Microsurgical Anatomy of the Basal Cisterns and Vessels of the Brain, Diagnostic Studies, General Operative Techniques and Pathological Considerations of the Intracranial Aneurysms. Stuttgart: Thieme; 1984

[17] Van den Bergh R. Lateral-paramedian infratentorial approach in lateral decubitus for pineal tumours. Clinical Neurology and Neurosurgery. 1990;**92**(4):311-316. DOI: 10.1016/0303-8467(90)90056-b

[18] Ogata N, Yonekawa Y. Paramedian supracerebellar approach to the upper brain stem and peduncular lesions. Neurosurgery. 1997;**40**(1):101-104; discussion 04-5. DOI: 10.1097/00006123-199701000-00023

[19] Pan Y, Wang C, Xiao-ping D, Lu Y. The Krause approach: MRI measurements in the Chinese population. Journal of Clinical Neuroscience. 2011;**18**(6):794-797. DOI: 10.1016/j.jocn.2010.10.017

[20] Tahta A, Akalan N. Supracerebellar infratentorial approach, indications, and technical pitfalls. Advances and Technical Standards in Neurosurgery. 2023;**46**:53-64. DOI: 10.1007/978-3-031-28202-7_3

[21] Bechri H, Oudrhiri MY, Louraoui SM, et al. Papillary tumor of the pineal region: Is stereotactic radiosurgery efficient for this rare entity? Surgical Neurology International. 2021;**12**:386. DOI: 10.25259/sni_613_2020

[22] Zhu Y, Xiong Z, Zhang T, Chen J. Clinical efficacy of endoscopic infratentorial supracerebellar approach for pineal region tumors: A retrospective case-control study. Contrast Media & Molecular Imaging. 2022;**2022**:5702309. DOI: 10.1155/2022/5702309

[23] Fernández-Miranda JC. Paramedian supracerebellar approach in semi-sitting position for endoscopic resection of pineal cyst: 2-dimensional operative video. Operative Neurosurgery. 2018;**16**(3):E79-E79. DOI: 10.1093/ons/opy216

[24] Merrill S, Bendok BR. Commentary: Pineal region hemangioblastoma resection through paramedian supracerebellar approach: 2-dimensional operative video. Operative Neurosurgery. 2021;**21**(1):E36-E37. DOI: 10.1093/ons/opab127

[25] Cohen-Gadol AA. The paramedian supracerebellar approach: A less disruptive and more flexible operative corridor to the pineal and posterior upper brainstem regions. World Neurosurgery. 2020;**143**:647-657. DOI: 10.1016/j.wneu.2020.07.232

[26] Serra C, Türe H, Yaltırık CK, Harput MV, Türe U. Microneurosurgical removal of thalamic lesions: Surgical results and considerations from a large, single-surgeon consecutive series. Journal

of Neurosurgery. 2021;**135**(2):458-468. DOI: 10.3171/2020.6.Jns20524 [published Online First: 20201002]

[27] Sun E. An endoscopic-assisted contralateral paramedian supracerebellar infratentorial approach in the treatment of thalamic hemorrhage with hematoma extension into the brainstem: A case report. Frontiers in Surgery. 2023;**10**:1277990. DOI: 10.3389/fsurg.2023.1277990

[28] Shahinian HK, Ra Y. Fully endoscopic resection of pineal region tumors. Journal of Neurological Surgery Part B: Skull Base. 2013;**74**(03):114-117. DOI: 10.1055/s-0033-1338165

[29] Berker BB, Dogruel Y, Gungor A, et al. Preserving the cerebellar hemispheric tentorial bridging veins through a novel tentorial cut technique for supracerebellar approaches. Journal of Neurosurgery. 2024;**140**(1):260-270. DOI: 10.3171/2023.5.JNS23657 [published Online First: 20230714]

[30] Watanabe T, Igarashi T, Fukushima T, Yoshino A, Katayama Y. Anatomical variation of superior petrosal vein and its management during surgery for cerebellopontine angle meningiomas. Acta Neurochirurgica. 2013;**155**(10):1871-1878. DOI: 10.1007/s00701-013-1840-8

[31] Jean WC. The paramedian supracerebellar infratentorial approach: 2-dimensional operative video. Operative Neurosurgery. 2023;**26**(1):100. DOI: 10.1227/ons.0000000000000913

[32] Ture H, Harput MV, Bekiroglu N, Keskin O, Koner O, Ture U. Effect of the degree of head elevation on the incidence and severity of venous air embolism in cranial neurosurgical procedures with patients in the semisitting position. Journal of Neurosurgery. 2018;**128**(5):1560-1569. DOI: 10.3171/2017.1.JNS162489 [published Online First: 20170714]

[33] Cucchiara RF. Safety of the sitting position. Anesthesiology. 1984;**61**(6):790. DOI: 10.1097/00000542-198412000-00041

[34] de Oliveira JG, Parraga RG, Chaddad-Neto F, Ribas GC, de Oliveira EP. Supracerebellar transtentorial approach-resection of the tentorium instead of an opening-to provide broad exposure of the mediobasal temporal lobe: Anatomical aspects and surgical applications: Clinical article. Journal of Neurosurgery. 2012;**116**(4):764-772. DOI: 10.3171/2011.12.JNS111256 [published Online First: 20120113]

[35] Kocaoglu M, Acar F. The supracerebellar transtentorial approach in the prone position. Turkish Neurosurgery. 2021;**31**(2):290-295. DOI: 10.5137/1019-5149.JTN.31433-20.5

[36] Durmuş YE, Kaval B, Demirgil BT, et al. Dynamic lateral semisitting position for supracerebellar approaches: Technical note and case series. Operative Neurosurgery. 2023;**25**(2):103-111

[37] Ture U, Harput MV, Kaya AH, et al. The paramedian supracerebellar-transtentorial approach to the entire length of the mediobasal temporal region: An anatomical and clinical study. Laboratory investigation. Journal of Neurosurgery. 2012;**116**(4):773-791. DOI: 10.3171/2011.12.JNS11791 [published Online First: 20120120]

[38] Erol G, Çavuşoğlu N, Sevgi UT, et al. Occipital sinus-sparing linear paramedian dural incision: A technical note and case series for median suboccipital approach. World Neurosurgery. 2024;**184**:e121-ee28.

DOI: 10.1016/j.wneu.2024.01.070 [published Online First: 20240119]

[39] Mottolese C, Szathmari A, Ricci-Franchi AC, Gallo P, Beuriat PA, Capone G. Supracerebellar infratentorial approach for pineal region tumors: Our surgical and technical considerations. Neurochirurgie. 2015;**61**(2-3):176-183. DOI: 10.1016/j.neuchi.2014.02.004 [published Online First: 20140524]

[40] Jakola AS, Bartek J Jr, Mathiesen T. Venous complications in supracerebellar infratentorial approach. Acta Neurochirurgica. 2013;**155**(3):477-478. DOI: 10.1007/s00701-012-1614-8 [published Online First: 20130112]

[41] Pendl G. Infratentorial approach to mesencephalic tumors. In: Clinical Microneurosurgery. Stuttgart: Georg Thieme; 1976. pp. 143-150

Chapter 4

The Supraorbital "Keyhole" Approach (SOKHA) for Skull Base Lesions

Anil Kumar Sharma, Jitender Chaturvedi, Mihit Kalawatia and Amit Agarwal

Abstract

Lesions located around the sellar region and central skull base are suitable for the application of the supraorbital keyhole approach. A wide and diverse group of pathologies can be addressed, including tumors (meningiomas, craniopharyngiomas, pituitary adenomas, etc.) and vascular abnormalities (e.g., aneurysms, arteriovenous malformations, and cavernous haemangiomas). The goal of "keyhole" surgery is not merely to perform a small incision and craniotomy, but to permit adequate access to skull base lesions while maintaining a minimally invasive approach. The supraorbital "keyhole" approach is not only less invasive but also equally efficacious, though proper patient selection is key to achieving the best possible outcomes. In summary, the transciliary supraorbital craniotomy (SOKHA) offers a balance of cosmetic outcomes, minimal invasiveness, and surgical efficacy, offering access to deep skull lesions. The approach should be selected based on tumor anatomy, including aspects such as size and laterality, as well as the surgeon's expertise. SOKHA has consistently shown promising results in terms of tumor resection, along with cosmetic outcomes, when performed correctly after proper training.

Keywords: supraorbital "keyhole" approach, SOKHA, skull base lesions, skull base tumors, craniotomy

1. Introduction

With advanced diagnostic and surgical tools, such as magnetic resonance imaging (MRI), advanced microscopy, and high-definition endoscopy, it has become much easier and safer to approach deep skull base lesions through small incisions and keyhole craniotomies. Transciliary supraorbital craniotomy for such lesions has also become increasingly popular worldwide [1–4]. The supraorbital "keyhole" approach is not only less invasive but also equally efficacious, though proper patient selection is the key to achieving the best possible outcomes.

2. Indications

Lesions located around the sellar region and central skull base are suitable for the application of the supraorbital keyhole approach. A wide and diverse group of pathologies can be addressed, including tumors (meningiomas, craniopharyngiomas, pituitary adenomas, etc.) and vascular abnormalities (e.g., aneurysms, arteriovenous malformations, and cavernous haemangiomas).

2.1 Surgical steps and description

2.1.1 Patient positioning

The patient is placed supine on the operating table; the head is fixed in a three-pin Mayfield holder and the neck is kept in extension with the head above the heart level to facilitate venous drainage during surgery. The head is then rotated to the contralateral side, with the degree of rotation depending on the precise location of the lesion.

- 15° for ipsilateral Sylvian fissure lesions,
- 20° for lateral suprasellar lesions,
- 30° for anterior suprasellar lesions, and
- 60° for lesions in the olfactory groove or cribriform plate region.

This positioning allows the frontal lobe to fall away from the anterior fossa floor, therefore, minimizing the amount of frontal lobe retraction (**Figure 1**).

2.1.2 Incision

The eyebrows are preserved. Usually, a skin incision is placed lateral to the supraorbital foramen running within the eyebrow and extending towards the frontozygomatic suture. It is crucial to check the medial extension of the incision beyond the supraorbital nerve to prevent frontal numbness (**Figure 1**). A 3–4 cm skin incision is made within the

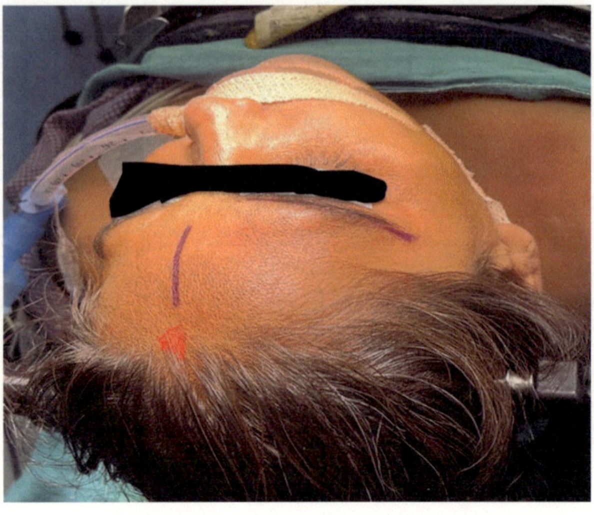

Figure 1.
Intraoperative position and planning incision.

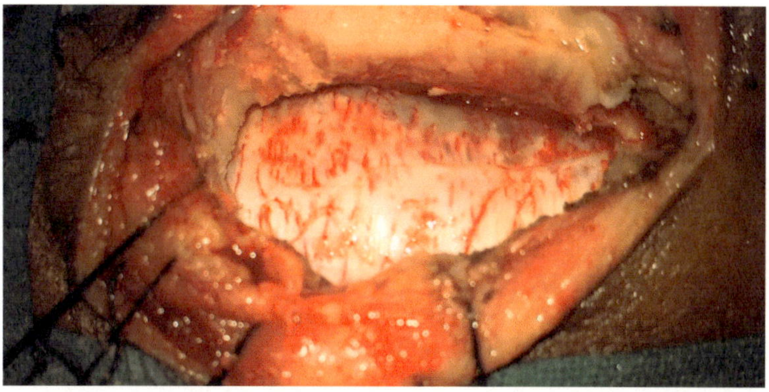

Figure 2.
After eyebrow skin incision, the subcutaneous tissue dissection, and craniotomy is completed.

eyebrow, and the subcutaneous tissue and frontal fascia are subsequently cut. The skin flaps are retracted temporarily using stitches to attain optimal exposure of the occipitofrontal, orbicular, and temporal muscles. After exposure, the frontalis muscle is cut parallel to the orbital rim. This is followed by careful dissection of the orbicularis oculi muscle along with the frontotemporal attachment of the temporalis muscle (**Figure 2**).

2.1.3 Craniotomy and surgical procedure

A small portion of the temporalis muscle and fascia at the superior temporal line is bluntly dissected. A single burr hole is made behind the frontal bone zygomatic

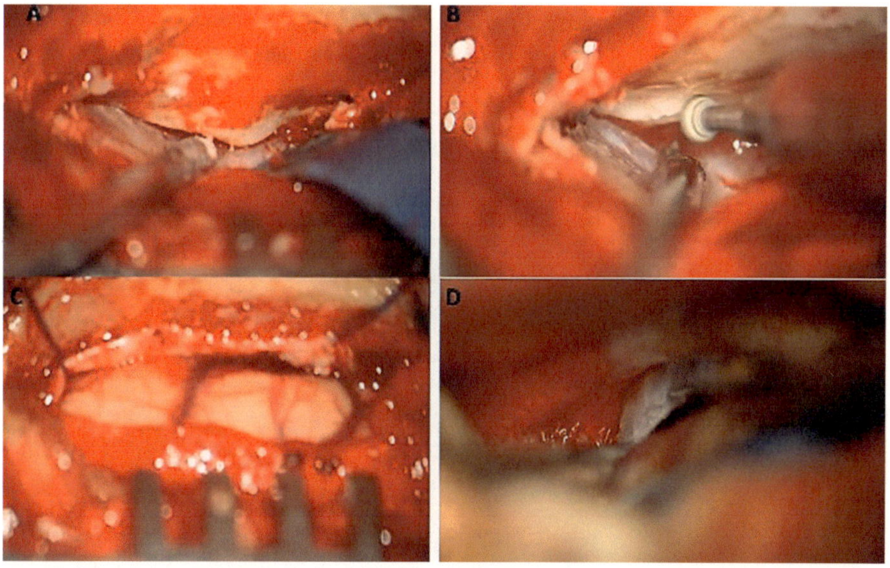

Figure 3.
(A, B) After removal of the bone flap, the inner edge of the bone should be removed. Drilling of the inner edge of the supraorbital rim after removal of the bone flap allows excellent intracranial visualization, easy introduction, and maneuvering of micro-instruments to the site small osseous extensions of the orbital roof should also be removed extradurally. (C) The dura is opened with the base at the orbital rim and reflected inferiorly with a stitch. (D) The CSF cisterns are opened to allow CSF egress to facilitate brain relaxation.

process (keyhole position) to create a bone flap of approximately 2.0 cm × 2.5 cm. It is important to ensure a craniotomy at least 1.5–2 cm in width, which is paramount in the manipulation of micro-instruments. It is also crucial to recognize a breach of the frontal sinus, as this can be a source of CSF leak post-operatively if not adequately addressed. Therefore, bone wax should be used to seal off any small breach of the frontal sinus, and betadine-soaked gel foam to seal off larger defects. Any osseous extension of the orbital roof can also be leveled with a high-speed drill. This not only improves visualization but also allows greater access to instruments during the surgical procedure (**Figure 3A** and **B**). The dura is opened in a "C"-shaped fashion with the base at the orbital rim and reflected inferiorly with a stitch (**Figure 3C**). The microscope is brought into the field, the frontal lobe is gently lifted with a cottonoid, and the CSF cisterns are opened to allow CSF egress to facilitate brain relaxation (**Figure 3D**). Following brain relaxation, the primary procedure may be performed safely with no or minimal use of fixed retractors on the brain. The intradural lesion is resected with a standard micro-surgical technique (**Figure 4**).

2.1.4 Postoperative care

Post-operatively, proper closure of the dura is essential to prevent CSF leaks and infections. A watertight Dural closure is critical and the Dural leaflets are reapproximated with a 4-0 Prolene in a running fashion. The craniotomy bone flap is replaced with a burr hole cover and two titanium square plates to restore the contour of the supraorbital ridge for an optimal cosmetic result. The pericranium and muscle flap are then closed primarily, followed by the final closure of the skin using a subcuticular stitch. This technique provides enhanced cosmetic results without compromising surgical efficacy.

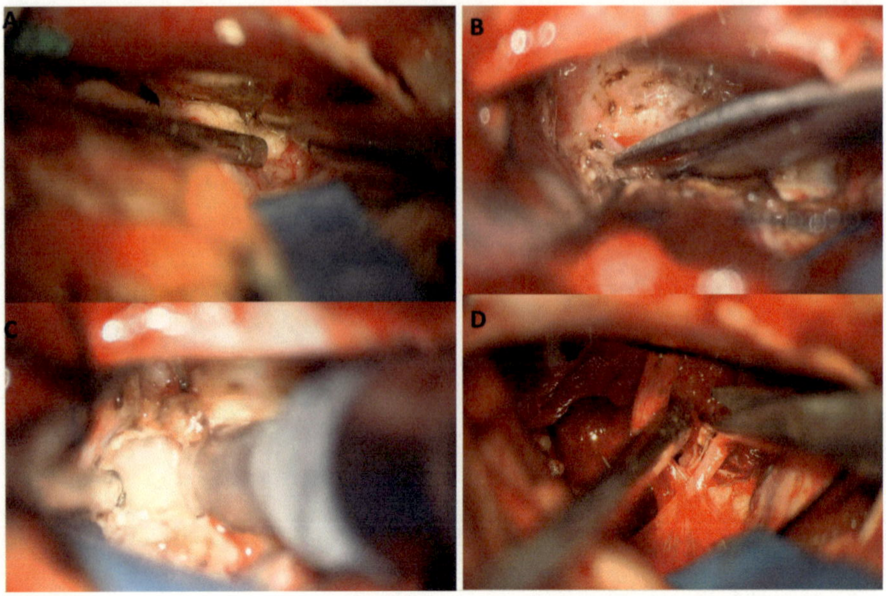

Figure 4.
4Ds-consecutive steps of meningioma surgery, devascularisation, detachment, debulking, and dissection.

3. Use of endoscopy

Endoscopes have facilitated overcoming one of the main limitations of the keyhole approach: illumination. The use of a rigid endoscope, along with the operative microscope, can provide a synergistic effect by significantly enhancing illumination and providing better visualization of blind spots, allowing a more complete tumor resection. A "second look" with the endoscope can ensure gross total resection of tumors, even with a smaller craniotomy. This approach provides enhanced visualization and increases the chances of a complete tumor resection (**Figure 5**).

3.1 Shortcomings of SOKHA approach and their solutions

Supraorbital keyhole approaches have been criticized for their restricted surgical freedom, narrow corridors, blind spots, and associated learning curves (**Figure 6**).

3.2 Narrow surgical corridor

A drawback of the supraorbital approach, which is an inherently limited surgical corridor, can be mitigated by drilling down osseous extensions of the orbital roof providing additional access. Draining CSF from cisternal spaces helps the brain relax, further increases the available workspace. These techniques, combined, expand the surgical corridor and reduce brain retraction. It is also essential to use micro-instruments for keyhole procedures, as they reduce the risk of damage to surrounding structures by offering greater precision and maneuverability without compromising surgical efficacy (**Figure 7**).

3.3 The problem of lighting with the operating microscope

Endoscopic-assisted surgery is a common adjunct and allows for safer dissection compared to a microscope alone since it provides enhanced lighting and visualization. The endoscope's wide field of view is very useful in visualizing far reaches of deep-seated lesions thereby minimizing the risk of any residual tumor (**Figure 8**).

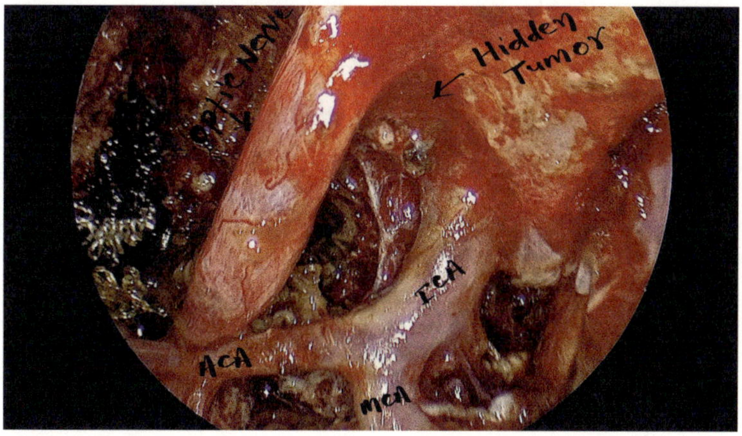

Figure 5.
A "second look" with the endoscope can also improve the gross total resection of tumors with better visualization and feasibility to look in notable blind spots.

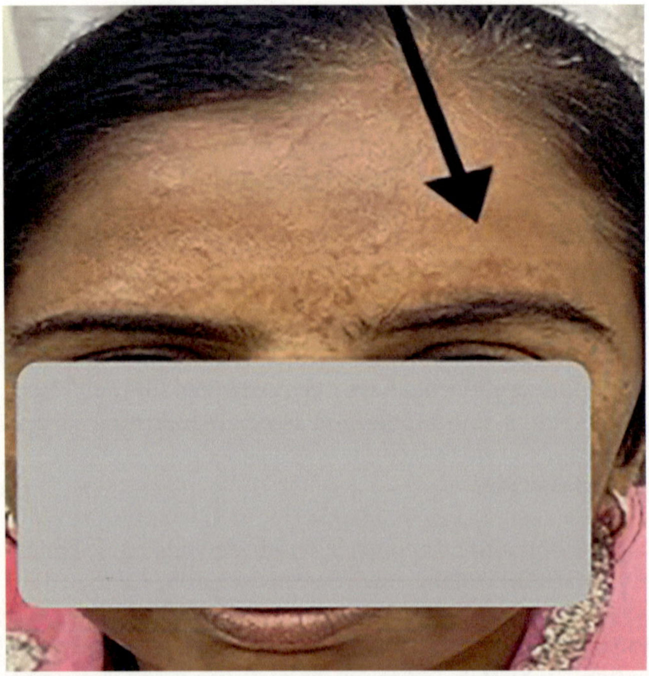

Figure 6.
Cosmetic outcome at 3 months follows up.

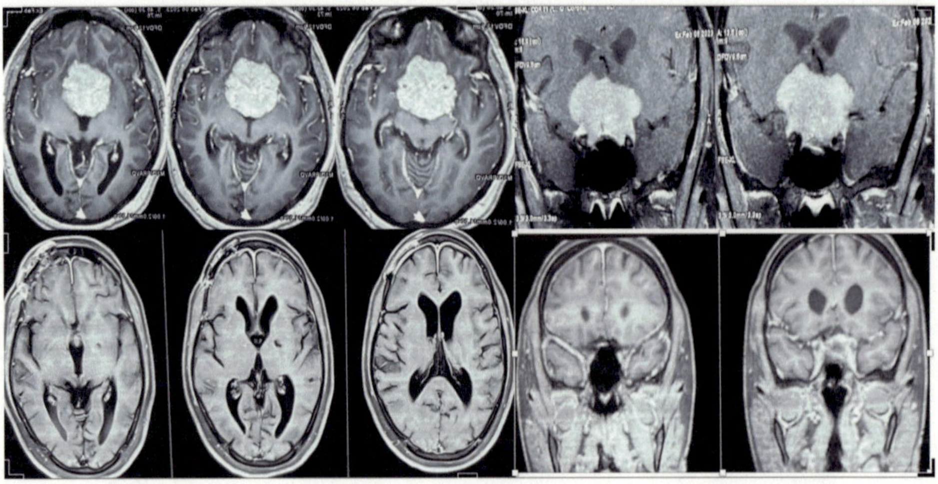

Figure 7.
Preoperative and postoperative MR images of olfactory groove meningioma.

3.4 Frontal sinus complications

The supraorbital keyhole approach can get complicated in cases of a large or laterally extending frontal sinus as its breach can cause postoperative CSF leaks and further lead to infections like meningitis therefore to mitigate these risks the surgeon must assess the size and location of the frontal sinus typically using CT scans or

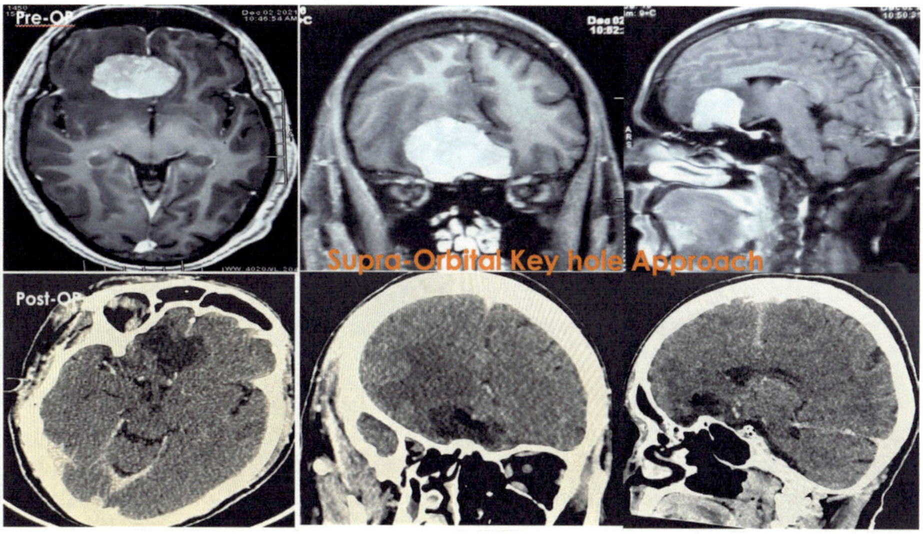

Figure 8.
Preoperative and postoperative images of Planum Sphenoidale meningioma.

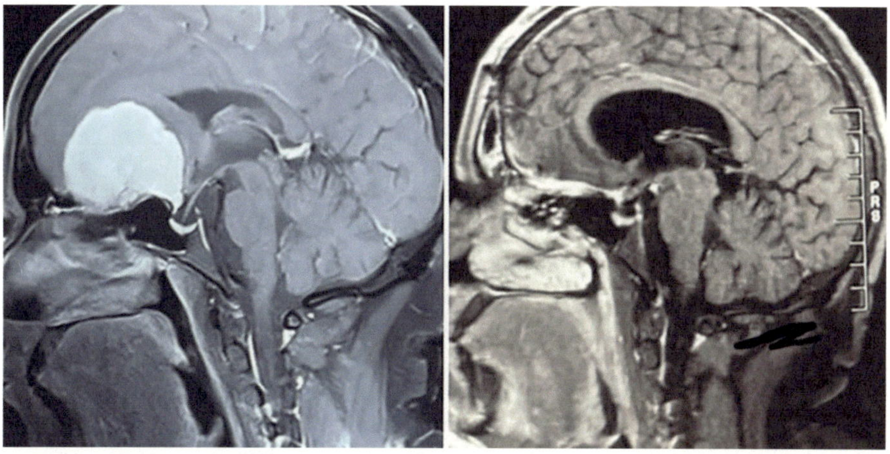

Figure 9.
Preoperative and postoperative contrast-enhanced MR images of large ACF base meningioma.

using techniques like neuro-navigation during craniotomy (**Figure 9**). In certain rare scenarios, if the frontal sinus is considerably large and laterally located then the supraorbital keyhole approach should be avoided due to postoperative complications and alternatives like extended endonasal routes should be opted (**Table 1**).

The fronto-orbital variant of SOKHA (frontal-SOKHA) has also been reported by some authors, who claimed that f-SOKHA provided a larger (60% more) operating corridor (in 75 cases of anterior circulation aneurysm clipping) as compared to the standard supraorbital keyhole approaches while preserving the same degree of minimally invasive nature and cosmetic results [5]. Another large volume Indian centre compared SOKHA (n = 62 vs. n = 104 for pterional approach) for good grade anterior circulation aneurysm [6]. Again, SOKHA appeared to offer the advantage of potential cosmetic benefits with neurological outcomes comparable to those of the traditional approach.

SOKHA	Extended endonasal endoscopic approach
A wider view of the lateral extent of the tumor,	Early devascularization of the tumor,
Avoidance of trauma to the nasal passages	Better visualization of the medial optic canaL
More suitable for tumors with extension lateral to the carotid artery or optic nerve and for tumors with vascular encasement	Removal of all involved bone at the skull base
Avoidance of an infected field	Less manipulation of neurovascular structures

Table 1.
Comparison of SOKHA with extended endoscopic endonasal approach for ACF base meningiomas.

For para-sellar and anterior cranial fossa (ACF) base meningiomas as an indication of this novel technique, gross total resection was achieved in 83.3% of cases in a study [7] of 24 patients (21 females; mean age, 53 + or - 8.6 years) with a Maximal tumor diameter ranged from 1.6 to 6 cm with a nil recurrence at follow-up ranging between 6 and 66 months (mean 31.5 + or - 20.1 months). Some surgeons [8] have even described a contralateral supraorbital eyebrow approach (c-SEA) to address the medial surface of the ipsilateral optic nerve, the often called blind spot of SOKHA in case of tuberculum Sella meningioma excision.

4. Conclusions

The transciliary supraorbital craniotomy (SOKHA) offers a balance of cosmetic outcomes, minimal invasiveness, and surgical efficacy, offering access to deep skull lesions. The addition of endoscopic assistance to the keyhole approach enhances the visualization providing more precise resections. Since this technique is minimally invasive in nature, it has a steep learning curve associated with it; hence, starting with smaller and simpler lesions before progressing to larger lesions is recommended. Optimizing outcomes requires meticulous preoperative planning, careful patient selection, and the use of advanced instruments. The approach should be selected based on tumor anatomy, including aspects such as size and laterality, as well as the surgeon's expertise. SOKHA has consistently shown promising results in terms of tumor resection, along with cosmetic outcomes, when performed correctly after proper training.

Highlights

- The goal of "keyhole" surgery is not merely to perform a small incision and craniotomy but to permit adequate access to skull base lesions while maintaining a minimally invasive approach.

- Take time in the preoperative planning and positioning of the patient.

- The skin incision is placed within an eyebrow for a better cosmetic outcome.

- Attention should be focused on protecting the supraorbital nerve to avoid the risk of frontal numbness.

- Surgeons should avoid opening the frontal sinus while designing the craniotomy. However, when this occurs, a proper repair is essential and recommended.

- After durotomy, open the chiasmatic and carotid artery cisterns to further release cerebrospinal fistula (CSF), relaxing the frontal lobe and providing an optimal trajectory towards the lesion.

Author details

Anil Kumar Sharma[1], Jitender Chaturvedi[2], Mihit Kalawatia[3] and Amit Agarwal[4*]

1 Department of Neurosurgery, All India Institute of Medical Sciences, Raipur, India

2 Department of Neurosurgery, All India Institute of Medical Sciences, Rishikesh, India

3 Rajarshi Chattrapati Shahu Maharaj Government Medical College, Kolhapur, India

4 Department of Neurosurgery, All India Institute of Medical Sciences, Bhopal, Madhya Pradesh, India

*Address all correspondence to: dramitagrawal@gmail.com; dramitagrawal@hotmail.com

References

[1] Robinow ZM, Peterson C, Riestenberg R, Waldau B, Yu N, Shahlaie K. Cosmetic outcomes of supraorbital keyhole craniotomy via eyebrow incision: A systematic review and meta-analysis. Journal of Neurological Surgery Part B: Skull Base. 2022;**84**(5):470-498. DOI: 10.1055/s-0042-1755575

[2] Lan Q, Sughrue M, Hopf NJ, Mori K, Park J, Andrade-Barazarte H, et al. International expert consensus statement about methods and indications for keyhole microneurosurgery from international society on minimally invasive neurosurgery. Neurosurgical Review. 2021;**44**(1):1-17. DOI: 10.1007/s10143-019-01188-z. Epub 2019 Nov 21

[3] Ormond DR, Hadjipanayis CG. The supraorbital keyhole craniotomy through an eyebrow incision: Its origins and evolution. Minimally Invasive Surgery. 2013;**2013**:296469. DOI: 10.1155/2013/296469. Epub 2013 Jul 10

[4] Shahid AH, Butler D, Dyess G, Bassett M, Harris L, Hummel U, et al. Supraorbital keyhole approaches in the first 3 years of practice: Outcomes and lessons learned. Patient series. Journal of Neurosurgery: Case Lessons. 2024;**7**(13):CASE23744. DOI: 10.3171/CASE23744

[5] Chandra PS, Tej M, Sawarkar D, Agarwal M, Doddamani RS. Fronto-orbital variant of supraorbital keyhole approach for clipping ruptured anterior circulation aneurysms (f-Sokha). Neurology India. 2020;**68**(5):1019-1027. DOI: 10.4103/0028-3886.294827

[6] Mehrotra A, Kanjilal S, Kumar BCA, Tataskar P, Verma PK, Bhaisora KS, et al. Comparative analysis of supra-orbital keyhole approach and pterional approach for surgical clipping of intracranial anterior circulation aneurysms in patients with favorable hunt and Hess grades. Clinical Neurology and Neurosurgery. 2024;**239**:108230. DOI: 10.1016/j.clineuro.2024.108230. Epub 2024 Mar 3

[7] Paiva-Neto MA, Tella OI Jr. Supra-orbital keyhole removal of anterior fossa and parasellar meningiomas. Arquivos de Neuro-Psiquiatria. 2010;**68**(3):418-423. DOI: 10.1590/s0004-282x2010000300018

[8] Das KK, Singh K, Mehrotra A, Jaiswal AK. Contralateral supraorbital eyebrow approach for tuberculum sellae meningioma. Acta Neurochirurgica. 2023;**165**(10):2925-2929. DOI: 10.1007/s00701-023-05714-3. Epub 2023 Jul 15

Section 2

Innovations in Spine Surgery

Chapter 5

Locking Lumbar Interbody Cementation: Biomechanics, Manual Reduction, Surgical Techniques, and Long-Term Results

Kung Chia Li, Ching-Hsiang Hsieh, Ting-Hua Liao, Shang-Chih Lin and Yu-Kun Xu

Abstract

Locking lumbar interbody cementation (IBC) involves performing manual reduction to correct lumbar deformities, followed by discectomy and carving grooves in the vertebral bodies above and below the disc. Bone cement was injected into these created grooves, followed by cage insertion to ensure solid bonding. Based on our 20 years of clinical experience with 15,000 cases, IBC has advantages, such as smaller incisions, less blood loss, shorter hospital stay, and significantly fewer complications, both intraoperatively and 30 days after surgery. Compared with traditional screw fixation surgeries, IBC also exhibits fewer adjacent segment diseases. Biomechanical studies have shown that bone-cement fixation effectively reduces disc mobility and achieves stability in the spinal motion unit. Clinically, we categorized IBC bone cement distribution patterns and correlated it with clinical outcomes. As long as the bone cement in the vertebral bodies above and below the treated disc exceeds half of the vertebral height, a long-term follow-up of more than twelve years shows minimal issues with bone cement loosening. The results were excellent even when the bone cement on only one side exceeded half the height. IBC has become a routine procedure, offering advantages over screw fixation surgery in treating lumbar degenerative diseases especially with osteoporosis.

Keywords: locking lumbar interbody cementation, interbody cementation, degenerative scoliosis, degenerative spondylolisthesis, degenerative disc disease, recurrent disc herniation, adjacent segment diseases, biomechanics, manual reduction, posterior instrumentation, cement cage

1. Introduction

Lumbar degenerative diseases, particularly when accompanied by nerve compression and deformity, often disrupt the biomechanics of balance during daily activities and ambulation. Conservative treatment frequently fails to provide relief in such cases, necessitating surgical intervention. However, traditional surgical methods involving pedicle screws are fraught with complications, particularly in patients with concomitant osteoporosis [1]. These complications include vertebral compression fractures, pedicle screw loosening and migration, implant failure, and pseudarthrosis [2, 3]. Even with advancements in minimally invasive surgery, which aim to reduce postoperative complications [4–6], the accurate placement of pedicle screws still carries a risk of failure [7, 8]. Misplacement of screws can lead to damage to the nerves, blood vessels, and internal organs, despite the use of the latest navigation systems [9–11]. Thus, an ideal surgical solution remains elusive.

Historically, there have been attempts to avoid the use of pedicle screws by developing standalone cage techniques. However, a 20-year follow-up study revealed an 11.1% incidence of pseudarthrosis and a 6.6% reoperation rate with this approach, outcomes that are far from satisfactory [12]. Other reports have highlighted that expandable cages used to address adjacent segment disease have resulted in a 21.05% incidence of cage subsidence and a 15.79% incidence of cage backward migration [13]. These findings raise concerns about the safety and clinical efficacy of standalone cage use in the treatment of lumbar degenerative diseases, leading to a decline in its application.

Additionally, for less severe lumbar degenerative disc diseases, percutaneous cement discoplasty has been employed [14–18]. While this procedure offers pain relief, it fails to provide adequate neural decompression or effectively correct spinal deformity [12]. Consequently, its utility is limited, particularly in cases where both neural impairment and spinal deformity are present. Currently, there is no universally accepted method that effectively treats these conditions while also preventing complications. The search for a perfect surgical solution continues.

The mini-open locking lumbar interbody cementation (IBC) without screws has been developed and applied to treat lumbar degenerative diseases, including degenerative lumbar scoliosis (DLS), spondylolisthesis (DLL), degenerative disc disease (DDD), lumbar kyphosis, and recurrent disc herniation [19, 20]. Over the past 20 years of surgical advancements and experience with 15,000 cases, this surgical method has become the standard procedure in our hospital. Its features include a minimal incision, shorter operative time, and reduced blood loss. Most patients can walk within 3 hours after surgery, and 60% can be discharged on the same day, making it a one-day surgery. Additionally, the procedure has low complication rates both intraoperatively and within the first postoperative month. Long-term follow-up over 14 years showed that adjacent segment disease (ASD) occurs much later, with an average onset of 11.5 years, and is significantly less common than in traditional pedicle screw fixation surgeries. There are much less osteoporosis-related complications. Most patients benefit greatly from this surgery and experience improved quality of life.

This chapter provides a detailed introduction to foundational and biomechanical research, manual reduction of lumbar deformities, surgical techniques and indications for IBC, long-term clinical results, and a discussion of the clinical applications of IBC in addressing previously challenging surgical cases.

2. Foundational and biomechanical research of IBC

The current standard treatment for lumbar degenerative diseases is to use a fusion cage to restore disc height and transpedicular screws on both sides to further stabilize the motion unit [21]. The increased rigidity caused by the combined use of fusion and fixation often induces accelerated degeneration of the adjacent segments [22]. Improper placement of transpedicular screws may cause damage to nerves, blood vessels, and facet joints and loosening of implants, increasing the chance of revision surgery [23, 24]. Even if a robotic arm or navigation system is used, in addition to the patient paying a high surgical fee, there is no guarantee that there will be no complications [24]. Therefore, in the past 20 years, experts and clinicians have attempted to develop various techniques to eliminate the need for transpedicular fixation [25].

Many studies have proposed the cage method alone, which involves implantation of a posterior lumbar intervertebral fusion (PLIF) cage separately behind the lumbar spine [26, 27]. However, the 20-year follow-up results after cage-alone surgery showed an 11.1% pseudoarthrosis rate and 6.6% revision rate [12]. The results of adjacent segment degeneration combined with spinal canal stenosis managed with a single expandable intervertebral fusion cage revealed a high complication rate [13].

The cage is characterized by resistance to compression but not tension caused by extension, bending, and twisting. Transpedicular fixation can significantly constrain the occurrence of tension at the cage-vertebrae interfaces. A similar implant (interspinous process distractor: IPD) placed between the interspinous processes to limit extension is also used to enhance the stability of the cage-vertebrae complex [28, 29]. Many biomechanical studies have reported that the flexion-extension ROM of the cage alone can still reach 64% of that of the normal spine [30, 31]. However, the hybrid use of cages and IPD can be limited to only 24.5% of the normal value [32]. This is similar to the 20.4% reduction achieved using cages and pedicle screws [33]. However, the IPD's ability to restrict bending and twisting was not as prominent as that of extension. Furthermore, whether IPD can achieve long-term stability and rigidity with irregular and thin processes has been reported as a potential risk for the hybrid use of cages and IPD [34, 35]. Compared to transpedicular fixation and cage fusion, there is still controversy in the literature regarding the positive and negative views on the bone fusion rate of the cage and IPD combined [36].

Another treatment method that avoids the use of pedicle screws is percutaneous cement discoplasty, which aims to reduce surgical morbidity and complication risks of transpedicular fixation [37]. The bone cement was perfused to fill the empty disc with a vacuum to restore the height of the collapsed motion unit and relieve nerve compression. Cement leakage is a major complication with an incidence rate of up to 30.4%, which does not significantly impact clinical outcomes [38, 39]. Bone cement is further applied to the cage to perfuse the bone cement into the vertebral body, thus forming body and disc cements [19, 20, 22, 40]. It aims to serve as a bridging mechanism for stabilizing the vertebrae–cage complex, avoiding the use of pedicle screws, and strengthening potentially osteoporotic vertebrae.

However, whether perfused cements are sufficient to perform the above functions may be closely related to two factors: the size of the cements within the vertebra and next to the cage [20]. The size of the body cement is related to the diameter of the pre-drilled hole in the vertebra, which is a highly demanding task. The biomechanical mechanism of IBC is schematically shown in **Figure 1**. Using nonlinear lumbosacral finite element analyses (**Figure 2**), six bone cements, two-disc cements, and five bridging cements were simulated in finite element models (**Figures 3–5**). The biomechanical characteristics of the body, disc, and bridging cements were described to gain insight into disc mobility and cement stress after IBC surgery.

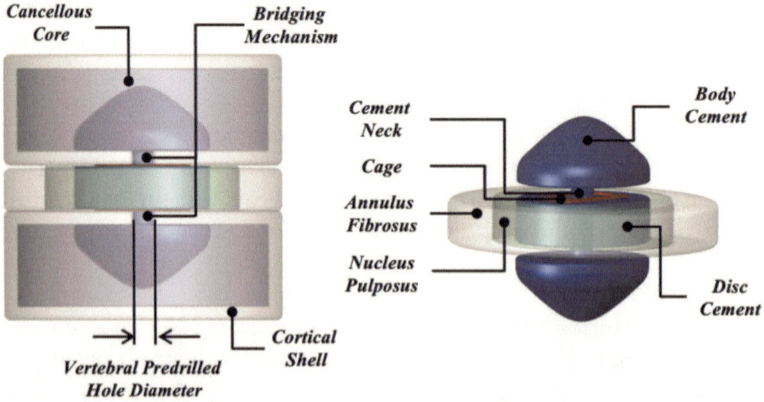

Figure 1.
(A) Satisfactory cement perfusion results in cement covering more than half of the length, width, and height of adjacent vertebrae. (B) and (C) Schematic diagrams showing the complex of vertebrae, cement, cage, and disc.

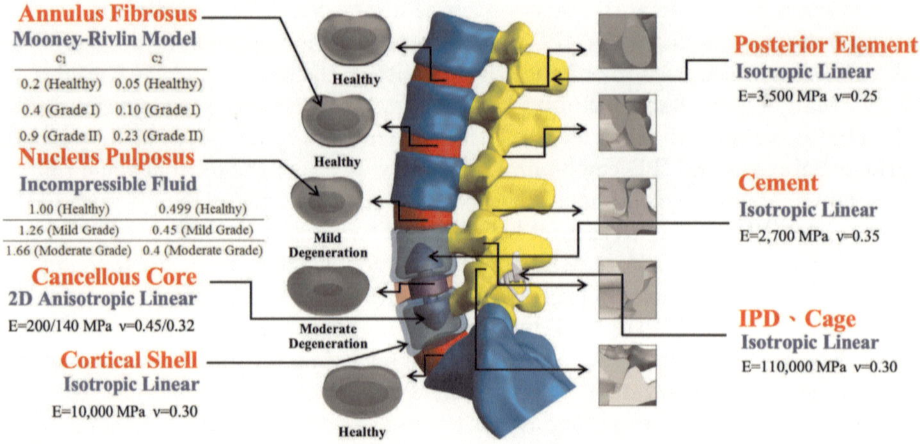

Figure 2.
Lumbosacral finite-element model developed by the current authors with the detailed material and geometric properties of the tissues and implants [25–28].

2.1 Effect of disc cement

The hybrid use of cement and cage aims to perfuse cement into the vertebrae and disc and connect the cage to form a stable complex of the disc, vertebrae, cage, and cement. The body cement was bonded to the cancellous structure in the vertebrae, and the disc cement was integrated into the cage to form a foundation within the disc. The bridging mechanism (i.e., cement neck) is formed between the body and disc cements through pre-drilled holes at the vertebrae–disc interfaces (**Figure 1**).

The effects of the 12 cement sizes on the L4-L5 disc ROM are shown in **Figure 6**. Generally, the higher the height and width of the body cement, the more obvious the decrease in disc ROM. For flexion, extension, bending, and twisting, the height and width ratios were 50% of the body cement, and the decreases in disc ROM were 40.7, 47.6, 49.6, and 70.4%, respectively. In 20% of the cases, the above-mentioned declines

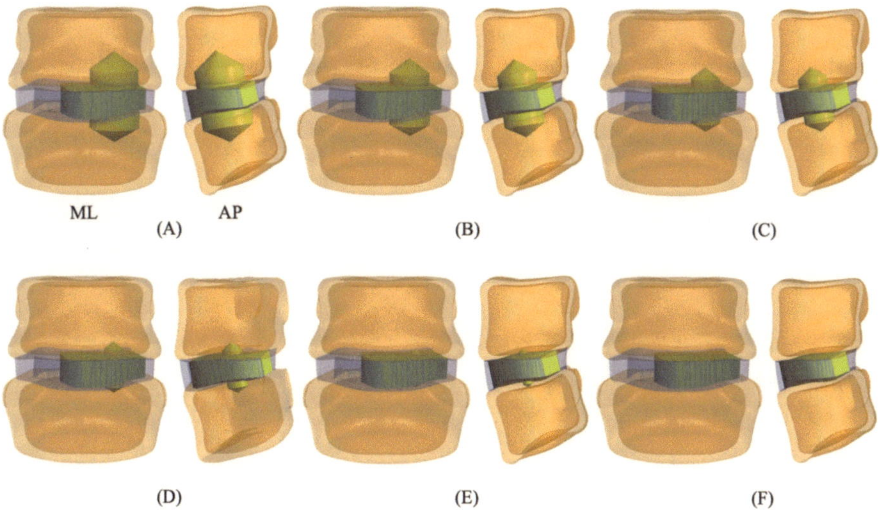

Figure 3.
Six bone cements to simulate the different widths and heights of body cement. The total cement volume within the vertebrae and disc was assumed to be equal among six variations. The ratios of the height and width of the body cement to the height and width of the vertebrae are, respectively, as: (A) 50 and 50%, (B) 40 and 40%, (C) 30 and 30%, (D) 20 and 20%, (E) 10 and 10%, and (F) 0 and 0%.

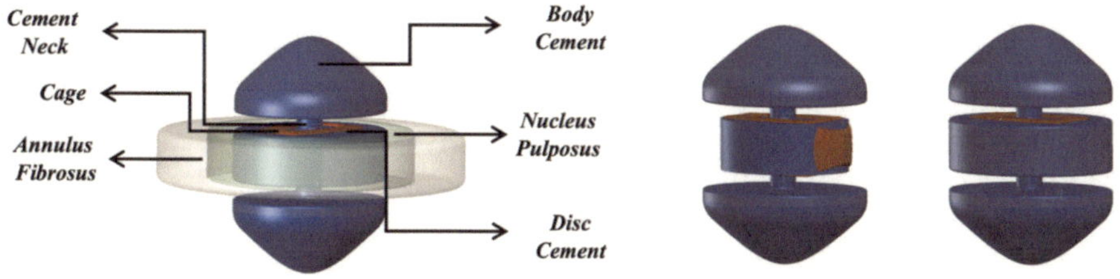

Figure 4.
Two sizes of disc cement covering the cage and surrounding the nucleus pulposus to simulate its effect of stabilizing the cage–cement complex.

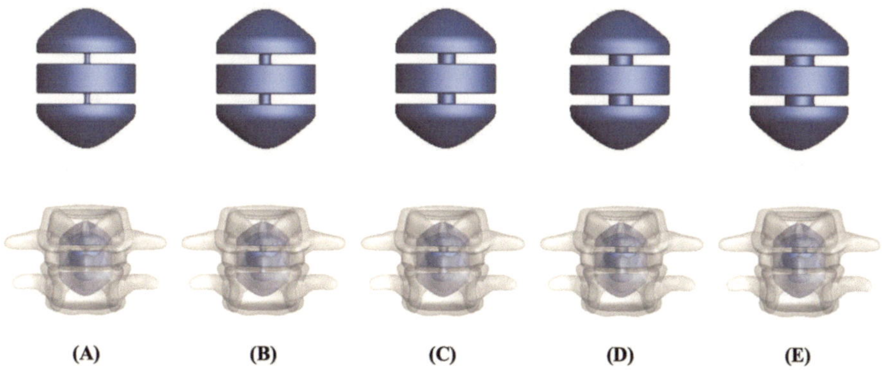

Figure 5.
Five diameters of the cement neck were simulated in the finite-element analysis. From (A) to (E): 2.0, 4.0, 6.0, 8.0, 10.0 mm.

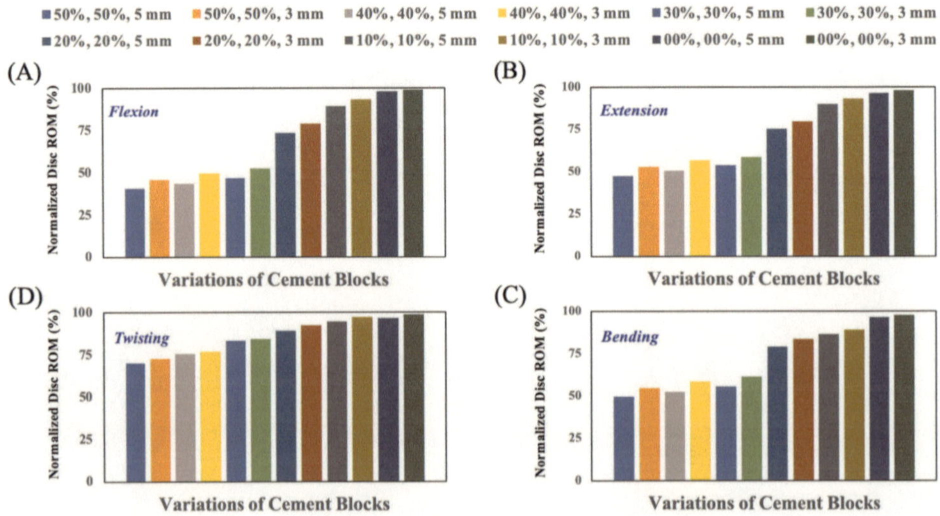

Figure 6.
Normalized disc ROM of the 12 cements relative to the ROM of the healthy disc. (A) Flexion, (B) Extension, (C) Bending, and (D) Twisting.

increased to 73.5, 75.4, 79.4, and 89.3%, respectively. When the height and width ratios were reduced to approximately 20%, the mobility-restricting effect of the body cement was insignificant for all the motions. Compared with the other three motions, the body cement in twisting had significantly less restriction on the mobility of the motion unit. Regardless of the size of the body cement, the ROM of the motion unit can reach almost 70% that of a healthy lumbar region. Additionally, when the height and width ratios of the body cement were approximately 20%, the changes in disc ROM in the four motions exhibited a significant weakening trend. This seems to be an initial reference for intraoperative X-ray image inspection during bone-cement perfusion.

Once the disc cement is perfused and the cage is instrumented into the interior of the disc, the structural rigidity of the originally weak disc is directly strengthened. For sagittal and coronal motions, a larger disc cement acts as a foundation with a larger moment arm, which can effectively reduce the deformation of the unit of motion (**Figure 7A** and **B**). Moreover, the moment arms in the two directions are similar, which shows that the ROM changes of the L4-L5 motion units predicted by the finite-element model have similar trends (**Figure 7A–C**).

For lumbar twisting, the disc cement is only circumscribed by the softer nucleus pulposus and interacts with the disc in a tangential rather than a vertical direction (**Figure 7C**). Consequently, the size of the disc cement did not significantly affect the mobility of the instrumented motor unit (**Figure 7D**). Larger disc cement provides a stable basis for stabilizing the reamed disc. The perfusion of approximately 6-cc of cement into the reamed disc is recommended.

2.2 Effect of body cement

For the first two of the six variations, the normalized disc ROM and concentrated stress of the three pre-drilled hole diameters are shown in **Figure 8**. When the diameter of the bridging cement was reduced from 5.00 mm to 3.75 and 2.50 mm, the mobility restrictions on the movement units were reduced by 39.0 and 66.7%,

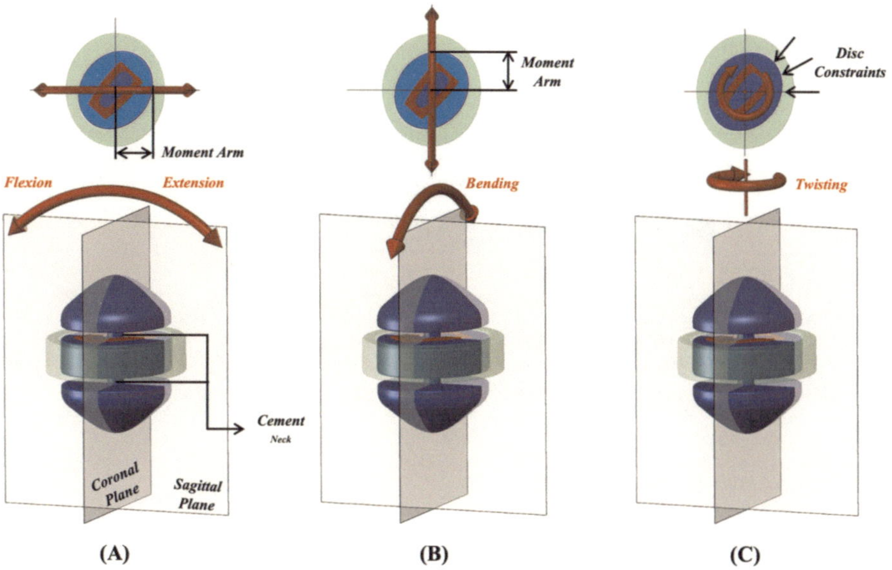

Figure 7.
Schematical diagrams to illustrate the load-transferring mechanism across the complex of the vertebrae, cement, cage, and disc. (A) Sagittal motion. (B) Coronal motion. (C) Transverse motion.

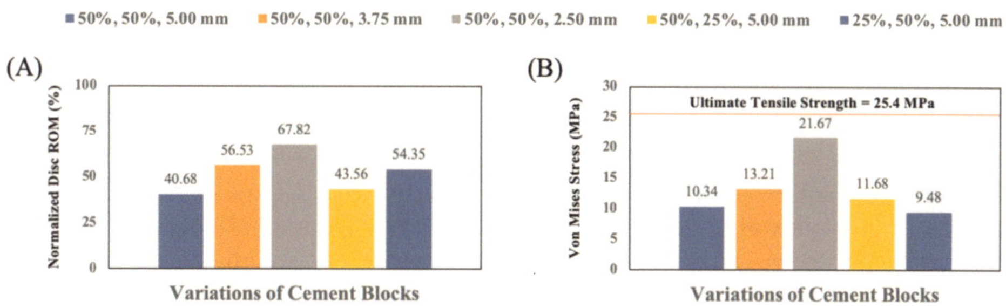

Figure 8.
Predicted results of the five vertebral and bridging cements during lumbar flexion. (A) Normalized disc ROM. (B) Concentrated stress at the bridging cement.

respectively. However, thinner bridging cement led to a significant increase in the concentrated stress at the column. Compared with 5.0-mm diameter columns, the stress of 3.75 and 2.50 mm columns increased by 27.8 and 109.6%, respectively. The ultimate tensile strength (24.5 MPa) of PMMA bone cement was used as a reference for comparison. When the width and height of the body cement were reduced to 25%, the normalized disc ROM increased by 12.4 and 33.6%, respectively, compared with the control group. Regarding the concentrated stress of the bridging cements, the aforementioned changes increased by 7.7% and decreased by 8.3%, respectively. The change in the cement column stress caused by the changes in the size of the body cement was not as obvious as that in the disc ROM.

By systematically varying the height and width of the body cement, the authors provided an evaluation matrix table to evaluate the appropriateness of the cement volume distribution in the tissues (**Table 1**). A cement block with one-half of the vertebral height and width was assumed to have excellent perfusion. Filling the disc with bone cement alone does not create a stable bridging mechanism at the

	Excellent			Good		Fair
w_{L4}/W_{L4}	h_{L4}/H_{L4}					
	50%	**40%**	**30%**	**20%**	**10%**	**0%**
50%	10.0	8.0	6.0	4.0	2.0	0.0
40%	8.0	6.4	4.8	3.2	1.6	0.0
30%	6.0	4.8	3.6	2.4	1.2	0.0
20%	4.0	3.2	2.4	1.6	0.8	0.0
10%	2.0	1.6	1.2	0.8	0.4	0.0
0%	0.0	0.0	0.0	0.0	0.0	0.0

The symbols H_{L4} *and* W_{L4} *denote the effective height and width of the L4 vertebra, respectively.*

Table 1.
Evaluation matrix table of bone cement perfusion.

vertebrae–cage interface. This study assumed that a cement block with one-third of the vertebral height and one-third of the vertebral width is unstable. Based on the ideal and unstable situations, this study divided the matrix table into green, yellow, and red areas that represent the stability of the bridging mechanism formed by the bone cement block as "excellent", "good", and "fair".

2.3 Effect of cement neck

The surgical method of combining bone cement perfusion and intervertebral disc cage to improve cage stability has been considered a feasible way to treat lumbar disc degenerative diseases (DDD) [22, 41–43]. Cement perfusion aims to improve cage stability and possibly eliminate the use of pedicle screws, avoid removing facet joints during transpedicular fixation, and simultaneously reduce foreign body sensation and accelerate adjacent segment degeneration (ASD) [44–46]. However, whether bone cement can establish a stable bridging mechanism at the vertebrae–cage interface is a key factor in the success of this type of surgery [43, 47, 48].

The diameter is determined by the surgical technique and has a significant impact on disc mobility. Disc mobility during extension was affected more by disc cement than by the cement neck. For extension, the thinner cement neck was subjected to the highest stresses approaching the ultimate strength of the cement compared to the other motions. It is recommended that the neck diameter be increased to at least 5 mm during surgery to increase the neck strength. When neck strength is insufficient, IPD may be considered to reduce the risk of fractures that may occur during extension and bending. Neck fractures were initially shown to have little effect on disc mobility; however, more clinical studies are needed to verify this. When cement neck and disc cement perfusion are poor, the use of IPD significantly reduces the risk of neck fracture.

Typical stress distributions of the lumbosacral and cement necks in the stable body and disc cements are shown in **Figure 9**. In addition to the twisting motion, the lumbosacral column exhibited a typical pattern of higher stresses moving downward. On average, disc cement experiences less stress than body cement does. The cement necks in flexion, extension, and bending consistently exhibited highly concentrated stresses at the interfaces of the body and/or the disc cement. The stress concentration

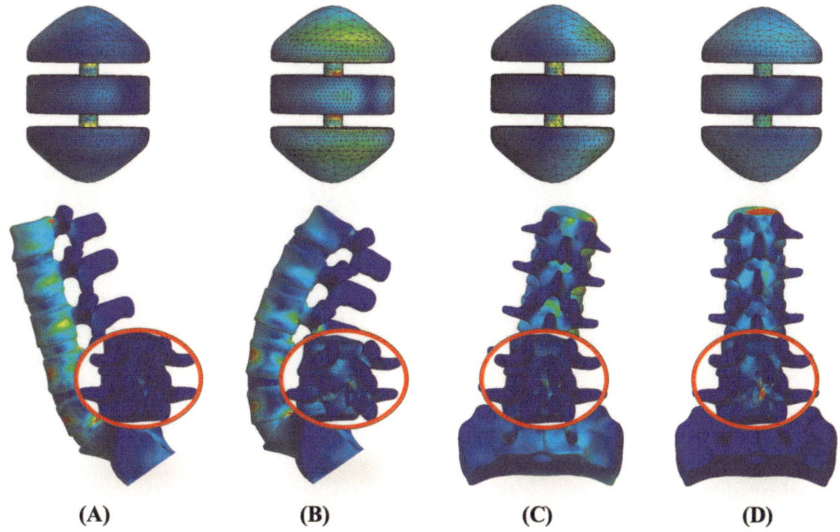

Figure 9.
Typical stress distribution contours of lumbosacral column for four motions. The simulation conditions for this result were stable body and disc cements, and a cement neck diameter of 6.0 mm.

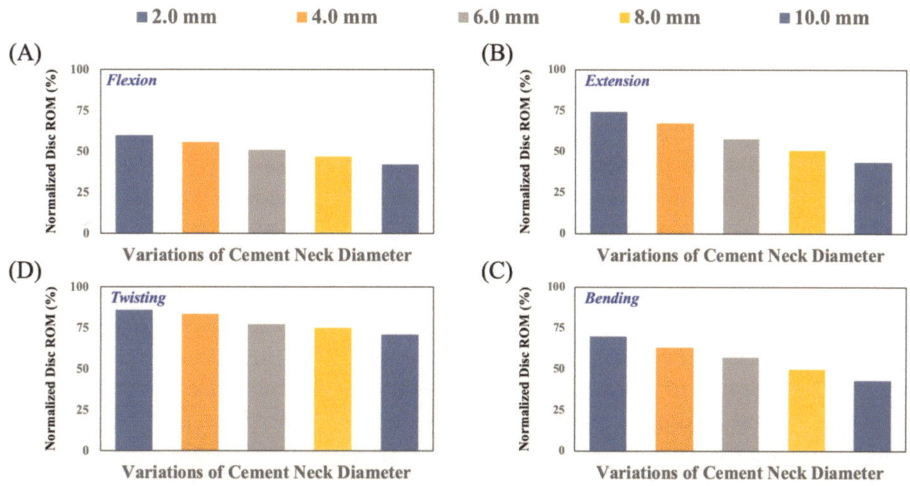

Figure 10.
Normalized disc ROM of the five cement neck diameters relative to the ROM of the healthy disc. (A) Flexion, (B) Extension, (C) Bending, and (D) Twisting.

during extension was much higher than that during the other three motions. However, there was no significant stress concentration on the cement neck during the twisting.

The ROM effects of the five neck diameters on the L4-L5 disc are shown in **Figure 10**. For a 2.0-mm neck diameter, the limiting effect of disc mobility was mainly affected by the size and location of the disc cement. For all motions, the neck diameter had a significant effect on disc ROM. As the neck becomes thicker, the combined effect of the cement neck and disc cement further limits disc mobility. For flexion, extension, bending, and twisting, the normalized disc mobility of the thickest necks increased by 29.9, 41.6, 38.2, and 17.4%, respectively, compared with that of the thinnest necks. Among the four motions, the neck diameter had the greatest and least effect on disc mobility for extension and twisting, respectively.

The cement neck acts as a bridge between the body and disc cement. The diameter is determined by the surgical technique and has a significant impact on disc mobility. Disc mobility during extension was affected more by disc cement than by the cement neck. For extension, the thinner cement neck was subjected to the highest stresses approaching the ultimate strength of the cement compared to the other motions. Neck fractures were initially shown to have little effect on disc mobility; however, more clinical studies are needed to verify this. When cement neck and disc cement perfusion are poor, the use of IPD significantly reduces the risk of neck fracture.

3. Manual reduction for degenerative lumbar deformities

Manual reduction techniques have been applied in spinal surgery for a long time. Biomechanical studies have demonstrated that applying traction to the spine can successfully realign vertebrae and intervertebral discs [49, 50] and is clinically safe and effective [51]. In the early days, when non-surgical treatments were more common, body casts were often used for stabilization, and various types of frames were invented to aid in reduction [52].

In 2003, Li first published the six-member manual reduction technique, which was highly successful in achieving near-complete reduction of acute thoracolumbar burst fractures without complications [53]. Subsequently, this technique was also applied to the reduction of osteoporotic compression fractures and subacute spinal fractures [54–59]. Although later a three-person reduction technique was proposed [60, 61], its effectiveness did not match that of the six-person technique [62].

In this chapter, we will discuss the further evolution and application of the six-member manual reduction technique for the correction of degenerative lumbar deformities. Degenerative lumbar deformities are often associated with osteoporosis. If reduction can be effectively performed before surgery, many intraoperative steps can be avoided, leading to reduced blood loss and shorter surgery time, ultimately minimizing related complications. This technique is now routinely used, and nearly every patient with lumbar degeneration undergoes 6-member manual reduction after anesthesia but before the surgical incision is made. We report our experience with manual reduction for all spinal degenerative deformities, including spondylolytic spondylolisthesis, degenerative spondylolisthesis, disc degenerative disease, and degenerative scoliosis.

3.1 Techniques of 6-member manual reduction for spinal deformities

The techniques associated with the six-member manual reduction method have been previously described in detail [62]. In this section, we will illustrate the differences between performing scoliosis reduction and spondylolisthesis reduction using two diagrams.

Figure 11 demonstrates that during scoliosis reduction, the leg on the concave side of the lumbar spine requires greater force to straighten the spine. Meanwhile, the surgeon needs to apply a pushing force from the convex side of the curve, with both shoulders firmly stabilized by other two assistants. Under the combined forces of traction on the lower limbs and the lateral push, the curved lumbar spine can be straightened. An unfused deformity can be easily and completely reduced.

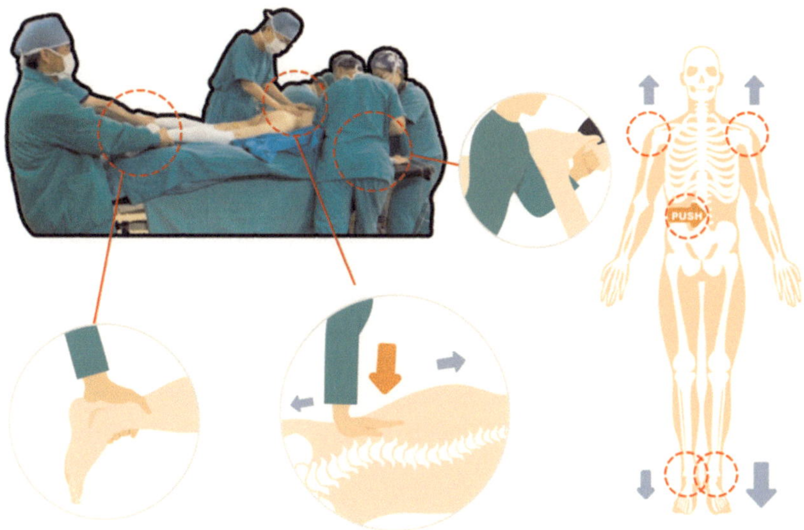

Figure 11.
Diagram showing the detailed techniques of manual reduction for degenerative scoliosis.

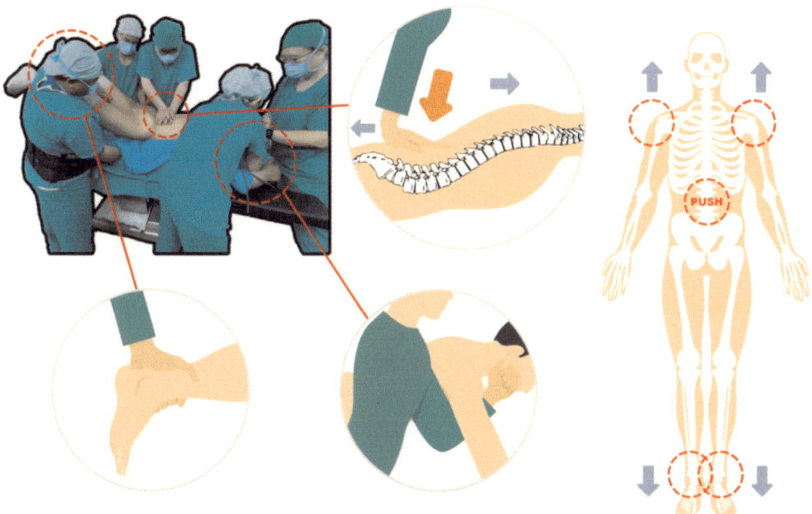

Figure 12.
Diagram showing the detailed techniques of manual reduction for spondylolisthesis and disc degenerative disease.

Figure 12 provides a detailed explanation of lumbar listhesis reduction. For spondylolisthesis reduction, the procedure begins by elevating the hip joint and both legs, followed by applying traction. The surgeon then places both hands on the area of spondylolisthesis and applies downward pressure, with bilateral shoulders stabilized. This maneuver allows for the reduction of the slipped vertebra.

If the reduction is not satisfactory on the first attempt, it can be repeated, even up to two or three times. However, it is crucial not to insist on achieving a perfect reduction. In some cases, the spine may have developed rigid ankylosing bone spurs, making manual reduction alone insufficient. Overzealous attempts can lead to complications, so it is important to proceed with caution.

3.2 Results of manual reduction for lumbar deformities

Fifteen thousand patients with lumbar deformities were included in this study from January 1998 to December 2023. The female-to-male ratio was 10,650: 4350 with average age 66 years (range: 13–102 years). The inclusion criteria for this study were as follows: symptomatic spondylolytic spondylolisthesis (2250 cases), degenerative spondylolisthesis (4650 cases), disc degenerative disease and lumbar kyphosis (3900 cases), and degenerative scoliosis (4200 cases), necessitating surgical intervention.

In reducible cases, lumbar disc height could be restored, and lumbar deformities, including listhesis, kyphosis, and scoliosis, were corrected. All the reduction patterns were categorized below and were presented in **Table 2**.

Type I. Opening of the unfused narrowed intervertebral disc, reduction of subluxated facet joints and listhesis, and enlargement of neuroforamen were achieved. These results lead to indirect decompression of the spinal canal stenosis and neuroforamen root compression. Most lumbar deformities, including spondylolytic spondylolisthesis, degenerative spondylolisthesis, disc degenerative disease, and lumbar kyphosis, can be easily reduced using this mechanism.

Type II. Restoration of the symmetrical disc space and correction of the scoliotic vertebral column were achieved where the stiff annular fibrosa may be released or broken by manual reduction. These forces can open the narrowed and asymmetrical disc space and correct the deformed vertebral column. This mechanism is responsible for the manual reduction of degenerative scoliosis.

Type III. An iatrogenic open-wedge fracture was induced and increased anterior column height, which corresponded to lumbar kyphosis in osteoporotic spine usually accompanied with some scoliosis.

Type IV. Reduction failure was diagnosed when solid interbody fusion was observed in the non-osteoporotic spine. This type can be predicted preoperatively by experienced surgeons.

Type	Description	Effects	Applicable conditions
I	Opening of the unfused disc • Reduction of subluxated facet joints • Stretching the loose annular fibrosa • Enlargement of neuroforamen	• Indirect decompression of canal and neuroforamen stenosis • Reduction of deformity	• Spondylolytic spondylolisthesis • Degenerative spondylolisthesis • Disc degenerative disease • Lumbar kyphosis
II	• Contracted annular fibrosa may be released or broken	• Restoration of the symmetrical disc space • Correction of scoliotic vertebral column	• Degenerative lumbar scoliosis
III	• Latrogenic open wedge fracture	• Increased anterior column height	• Lumbar kyphoscoliosis with osteoporosis
IV	• Failure	• No reduction	• Fused deformity without osteoporosis

Table 2.
Classification of results of manual reduction for lumbar degenerative deformities.

The results of manual reduction may functionally guide subsequent surgery. In Type I, cement discoplasty or percutaneous IBC for DDD, open IBC or posterior instrumentation in situ if spinal instability is found. In type II cases, percutaneous or mini-open IBC, or posterior instrumentation is recommended. In type III cases, vertebroplasty or body augmentation with a body cage is indicated if the manual reduction is successful. In Type IV, open osteotomy or ankylosing spur discontinuities are suggested.

3.3 Discussion

Based on our 20-year experience, manual reduction for correcting lumbar deformities is effective and safe. The learning curve for manual reduction was short and no major complications were observed. The classification of immediate results after manual reduction can guide subsequent operations.

In Type I, manual reduction led to restoration of the disc space, realignment of the vertebral bodies, and induction of indirect decompression. This facilitates decompression procedures and decreases the complications of nerve root injury. Interbody cementation alone can be performed without further reduction in instrumentation. If instrumentation is preferred, instrumentation reduction can be reduced, reducing the possibility of implant loosening.

In type II cases, lumbar degenerative scoliosis is usually partially corrected by manual reduction. Because lumbar degenerative scoliosis has a chronic continuous course, some facet joints and disc spaces are newly involved, and subluxation is not fixed; however, some facet joints and disc spaces have already been bony fused. Manual reduction can only reduce the unfixed motion segments by reducing the subluxation of facet joints and restoring the loosening of the annular fibrosa, or even breaking the stiff annular fibrosa to restore the symmetrical disc space and correct the scoliosis, which can be fixed by simple IBC or instrumentation in situ. The remaining scoliosis segments required open surgery to discontinue the ankylosing spurs or fused facet joints. Manual reduction can alter the treatment modality for lumbar degenerative scoliosis.

In type III, lumbar kyphosis with interbody fusion in the osteoporotic spine, open-wedge fractures can be induced by manual reduction, and the deformity is corrected. However, the degree of osteoporosis should be evaluated first. Success can be predicted when DEXA is <2.5. Theoretically, the force required to create an iatrogenic open-wedge fracture increases with vertebral strength. The ultimate force to prevent vascular complications is the patient's body weight.

In type IV, when the fusion segment is firm and non-osteoporotic, manual force cannot induce iatrogenic fracture, that is, fail to reduce lumbar deformities. In such cases, open procedures are required to discontinue the fixed segment.

3.4 Summary of manual reduction

Manual reduction can reduce lumbar deformities via different mechanisms, leading to a high success rate. The subsequent treatments were related to the results of manual reduction. Since the introduction of manual reduction, new concepts and strategies for the treatment of lumbar deformities have been developed.

4. Long-term clinical results of locking lumbar interbody cementation for degenerative lumbar disease

4.1 Patient population and data collection

Between 2010 and 2012, 240 patients with DLD were treated with IBC, without instrumentation, under general anesthesia. The inclusion criteria were as follows: moderate to severe low back and leg pain (visual analog scale [VAS] score ≥ 6); no response to conservative treatment after a minimum of 6 months; DDD, DLL, or DLS; limiting one motion segment; and moderate-to-severe lumbar stenosis based on the Schizas classification [63]. Patients with active infections or metastases were excluded from this study. Cages were used to ensure construct stability or enlarge the neuroforamen. Finally, 172 patients with 72.8 ± 8.0 years at operation with a mean follow-up of 151 ± 10.4 months, a mean BMI of 22.1 ± 2.9, and female-to-male ratio of 121:51 were included. There were 84 DLL, 50 DLS, and 38 DDD in total. The demographic and surgical data are listed in **Table 3**. Because the demographic data and clinical results were not statistically significant between the IBC with and without cage groups, the following statement focuses on the classification of IBC instead of comparing the two subgroups.

4.2 Preoperative radiological studies

All patients' conventional X-rays, CT scans, and magnetic resonance imaging were integrated into the study. Radiological studies were performed in a standing position (anteroposterior and lateral views). Magnetic resonance imaging of the lumbar spine was performed to analyze the level and severity of the spinal stenosis.

4.3 Operating technique

The detailed procedure for IBC has been previously described [19, 20].

Patients (n = 172)	With cage (n = 79)	Without cage (n = 93)
Females: Males	23: 56	28: 65
Age at surgery	71.9 ± 8.2	73.6 ± 7.5
Body mass index	22.8 ± 3.1	21.5 ± 2.7
Surgical levels		
L3/L4	10	11
L4/L5	56	67
L5/S1	13	15
Indication		
DLL	39	45
DLS	24	26
DDD	16	22

DLL, degenerative lumbar listhesis; DLS, degenerative lumbar scoliosis. DDD: degenerative disc disease.

Table 3.
Summary of demographic and surgical data.

A midline incision was made on the concave side in DLS cases and on the more symptomatic side in the DDD and DLL cases. One incision was approximately 3 cm long to allow the IBC to be used for two continuous discs. The skin and fascia were incised, and the muscles were dissected bluntly. Index facetectomy and discectomy were performed to ensure adequate decompression. Subsequently, the disc space was enlarged in the serial trials until the deformity was corrected as completely as possible. The bony cavities at both vertebrae next to the index disc were created by a 1-cm curette, that is usually easy to complete owing to osteoporosis. All disc pieces and bony fragments were removed. The width × length × height of the trough in each vertebra was approximately 10–15 × 15–20 × 15–20 mm. Polymethylmethacrylate (cement) (Simplex, Stryker USA) with contrast medium in the dough phase was inserted into the disc space and the bony cavities by 3 cc syringe with pressure to make firm bone-cement digital bonding, which was solidified as a three-dimensional interbody fixator. The cage was pushed into the disc space before hardening of the cement to ensure interdigital cement-trabecula bonding. The cement volume for each level was 9 ml (range, 8–12 ml). Because cement-bone bonding is effective in resisting compression stress during spine flexion, but not tensile force during spine extension, the interspinal process device (Rocker, Pao-Nan, Taiwan) was applied to prevent spine extension and enforce the cement-bone structure. **Table 4** summarizes the special characteristic indications and techniques used in this study.

The required cementation standard of body cement (cement in the upper and lower adjacent vertebral bodies) includes body peak cement height and width in the lateral view of more than 50% of the body height and width and body cement width in the anteroposterior view of more than 50% of the body width. Because the cement distribution in the body is similar to that of a dome, a peak cement height of more than 50% of the body height indicates that the average cement height is greater than 20% of the body height. The cement volume within the vertebral body is estimated to be more than 12.5–7.5% (i.e., 50–30% × 50% × 50%) of the body volume, which will provide long-term ultimate fixation power and prevent cement loosening based on our 20-year clinical experience. The required standards for disc cement are 70% of the disc width, 70% of the disc length, and 100% of the disc height. The volume of the disc cement was 49% (70% × 70% × 100%) of the volume of the disc. Final locking interbody cementation can provide three-dimensional fixation to resist spinal motions, including flexion, sliding, lateral bending, rotation, and partial extension. The facet joint is not fixed in this model and allows for some facet motion, as in traditional anterior interbody fusion, which significantly reduces the sensation of stiffness.

4.4 Classification system of IBC

Bone cement is typically easily injected into the intervertebral disc, which is the area with the lowest pressure. Furthermore, as this procedure is an open surgery, any instance of insufficient bone cement in the disc can be immediately addressed by injecting additional cement. Consequently, postoperative radiography did not reveal any cases of insufficient bone cement in intervertebral discs. Therefore, the classification of interbody bone cement is based on the bone cement in the upper and lower vertebral bodies. If the bone cement in both the upper and lower vertebral bodies met the required standard, it was classified as Type A. If only one vertebral body met the standard, whereas the other did not, it was classified as Type B. If the bone cement in both vertebral bodies failed to meet the standard, it was classified as

Item	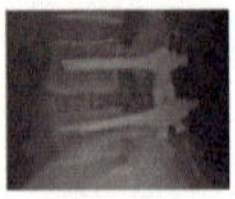 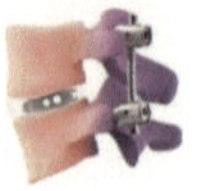	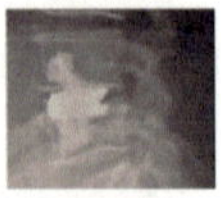 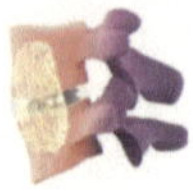	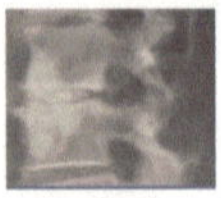 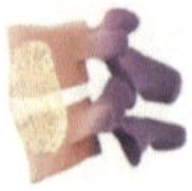	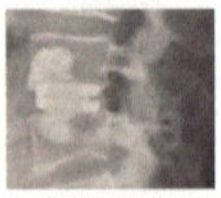 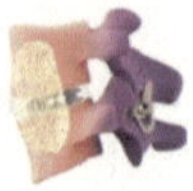	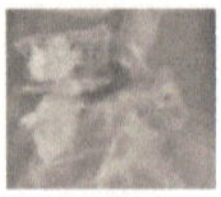 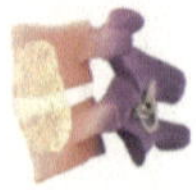
Operation	TPS + Cage +BG	IBC + Cage	IBC alone	IBC + Cage + IPD	IBC + IPD
Listhesis indication	G II-IV	G I-II, DDD, NF stenosis	G I-II, DDD, NF stenosis	G I-II, DDD, NF stenosis, FJA	G I-II, DDD, NF stenosis, FJA
Scoliosis indication	Rigid Translation > 1cm	Concave side, DDD	Concave side, no DDD	Concave side, FJA No DDD	Concave side, FJA
Kyphosis indication	Osteotomy	Disc opening or open wedge fracture by MR	Disc opening or open wedge fracture by MR	Disc opening or open wedge fracture by MR	Disc opening or open wedge fracture by MR
Follow-up interval	Up to 20 years	Up to 15 years	Up to 10 years	Up to 8 years	Up to 8 years
Clinical results	Satisfactory	Satisfactory	Satisfactory	Satisfactory	Satisfactory
Adjacent segment disease	9.9–22% 10-year FU	5.2% 12.6-year FU	No report yet	No report yet	No report yet
Approach	MISS	Mini-open, unilateral	Mini-open, unilateral	Mini-open, unilateral	Mini-open, unilateral
Equipment	O-arm, OR-CT, Navigation system, Robotic system	C-arm	C-arm	C-arm	C-arm

G: grade, FJA: facet joint arthritis, DDD: disc degenerative disease, NF: neuroforamen, O-Arm: arm fluoroscopy, C-Arm: C-arm fluoroscopy.

Table 4.
Summary of characteristic indications for variations in IBC operations.

Type C. **Table 5** presents examples of these three types. Type C closely resembled cement discoplasty.

4.5 Outcome measures

Outcome measures were made preoperatively and postoperatively at 3, 6, 12, and 24 months, and at the final visits. The VAS score (0–10) and Oswestry Disability Index (ODI; 0–100) were used [64, 65]. An excellent grade indicated no back or leg pain, and no medication was required. A good grade indicates occasional back pain after long sitting or working hours and a VAS score equal to or lower than four points. Fair or poor grades were defined as VAS scores higher than 4 points and the occasional or regular need for medicines. For radiological analysis, disc and body cement parameters, cement loosening, disc space narrowing, adjacent compression fractures, and adjacent segment pathologies were evaluated.

IBC types	Schematic diagrams	Without cage	With cages
Type A	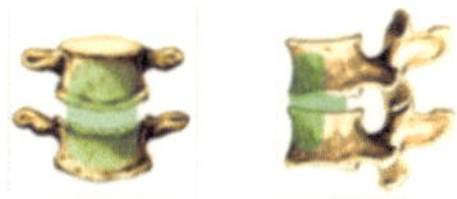	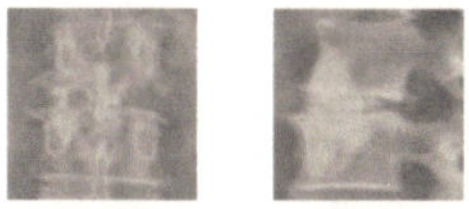	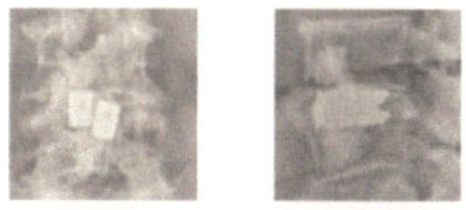
Type B	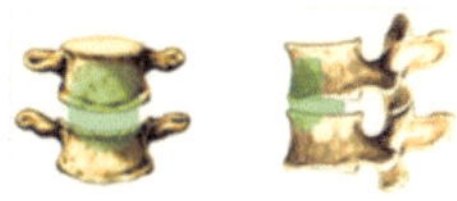	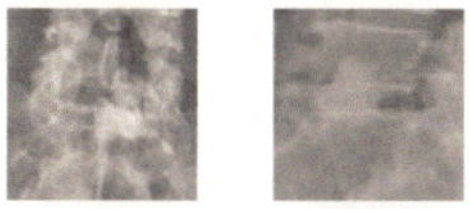	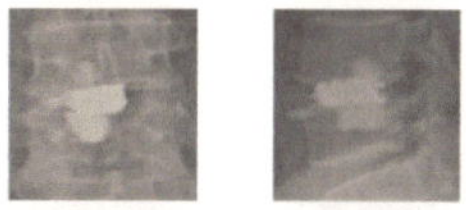
Type C	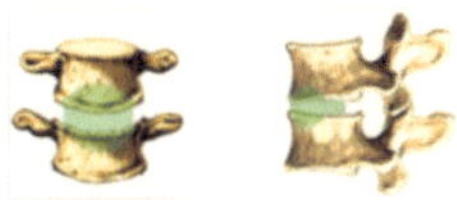	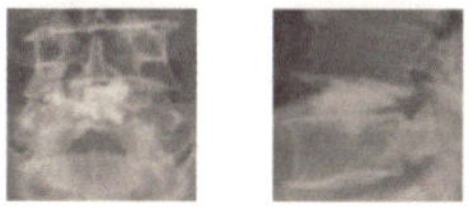	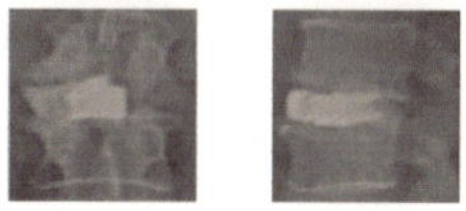

Table 5.
Classification of locking interbody cementation based on cement distribution.

Complications at 30 days were recorded and classified as major or minor using the Glassman classification [66]. The definition of major complications was permanent neural deficits or permanent neural impairment. Minor complications mean temporary postoperative symptoms, which did not lead the subsequent operation.

4.6 Statistical analysis

Categorical variables were described as absolute and relative frequencies with percentages. Quantitative variables are described as mean ± standard deviation. Statistical analyses were performed using Microsoft Excel (Microsoft Office 365, USA).

4.7 Results

The operative time per segment was 26.8 ± 6.4 min with an estimated blood loss of 49.2 ± 18.4 ml. The mean hospitalization was 2.8 ± 1.5 days. All patients were able to walk on the day of surgery.

4.8 Overall clinical result

The preoperative VAS and ODI were 7.7 ± 1.1 and 72.9 ± 8.2, respectively. At the final visit, VAS and ODI were 2.5 ± 1.0 and 24.9 ± 9.6. Significant postoperative improvement was observed.

Twelve (7%) patients experienced at least one complication on post-operative day 30; among them, 10 cases were considered minor, including postoperative radiculopathy (6 cases), superficial skin infection (2), deep vein thrombosis (1 case), and urinary tract infection (1 case). Two patients (1.2%) had symptomatic cement leakage and required revision surgeries.

4.9 Radiological findings and classification of IBC

According to the criteria of the IBC classification, 117 cases were type A (51 cases with cages, 66 without cages), 43 were type B (21 cages, 22 without cages), and 12 were type C (7 cages, 5 without cages) (**Table 6**). At the final visit, types A and B had high clinical satisfaction rates (97.4 and 95.3%) (**Figures 13** and **14**). The satisfaction

Classification	Case number	Excellent	Good	Fair & poor	Satisfaction rate
Type A	117	75 (66.7%)	39 (33.3%)	3 (2.6%)	97.4%
With cage	51	33	17	1	98.0%
Without Cage	66	42	22	2	97.0%
Type B	43	25 (58.1%)	16 (37.2%)	2 (4.7%)	95.3%
With cage	21	12	8	1	95.2%
Without Cage	22	13	8	1	95.4%
Type C	12	4 (33.3%)	5 (41.7%)	3 (25.0%)	75.0%
With cage	7	3	3	1	85.7%
Without Cage	5	1	2	2	60.0%

Table 6.
IBC classification and clinical outcomes.

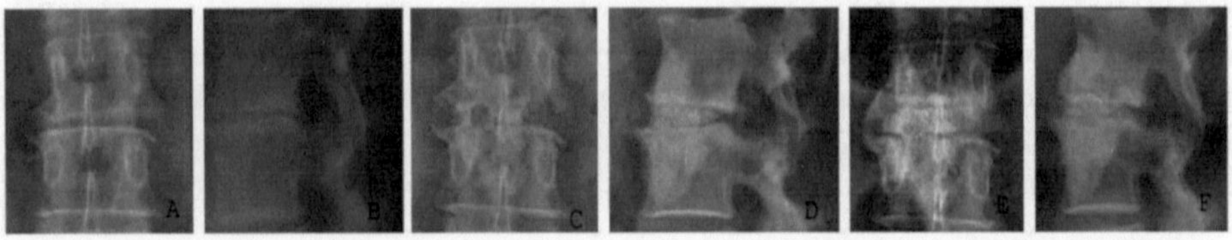

Figure 13.
A 65-year-old female underwent IBC for degenerative scoliosis with DDD (A, B). The initial follow-up was classified as type A cementation (C, D). Ten years after the IBC, ankylosing lateral spurs and no cement loosening were observed (E, F). She lives independently without back symptoms.

rate for Type C (12 cases) was 75% (**Figures 15–17**). Adjacent segment disease (ASD) on radiographic evaluation was noted in 20 patients (11.6%) at the final visit, and 9 patients (5.2%) underwent revision surgery, with an average of 11.5 years after the primary operation (**Figure 18**).

Cement leakage due to breakage of the annular fibrosa during disc distraction was common in 45 patients (26.1%). The cement leaked into the paraspinal space via the annular fibrosa defect, and most patients were asymptomatic. Only 2 patients with cement leakage had nerve root irritation and required revision surgery (1.2%). Asymptomatic cement loosening with a partially localized halo sign in the cemented construct was noted in eleven patients (6.4%) patients without further management. Three type C cases had symptomatic cement loosening with a complete halo sign around the cement block, two were cured with percutaneous vertebroplasty, and one refused further management. Six patients (3.5%) had silent proximal adjacent or remote wedge fractures that were left for observation.

4.10 Discussion

Percutaneous cement discoplasty has shown effectiveness in improving lower back pain but cannot correct listhesis, scoliosis, and coronal imbalance, which may induce disability in patients with DLS [8, 9]. IBC has also been reported to correct spondylolisthesis, scoliosis, and lumbar lordosis with the advantages of a small wound, no bone graft, and no instrumentation [19, 20]. This study classified cement patterns in IBC

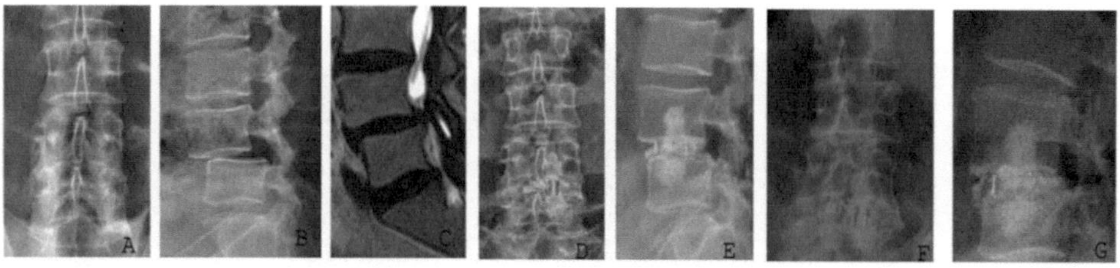

Figure 14.
A 59-year-old male underwent IBC for degenerative listhesis (A, B, and C). The initial follow-up was classified as type A cementation (D, E). Eleven years after IBC, no cement loosening was observed (F, G). He continues to work as a symptom-free stock trader.

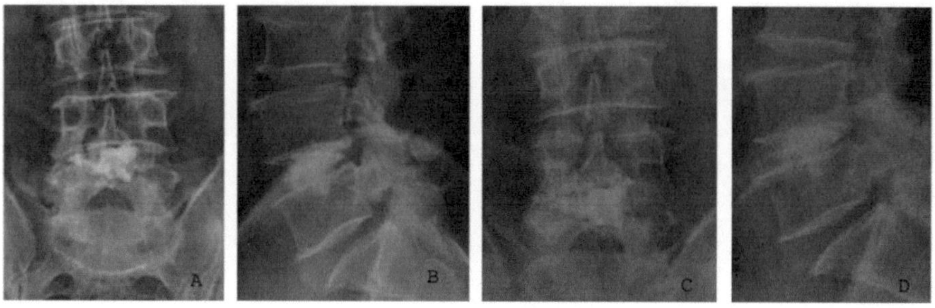

Figure 15.
64 male-year-old received IBC due to degenerative scoliosis with DDD. The initial follow-up is cementation classification type C. (A,B) Nine years after IBC, no cement loosening was noted (CD). He still works as an active farmer without back pain.

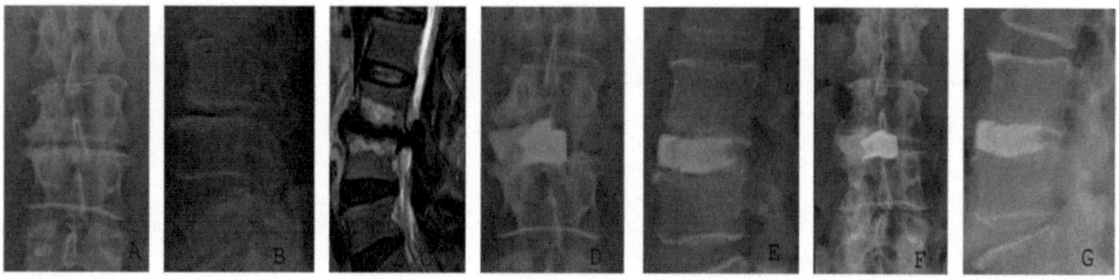

Figure 16.
64 male-year-old received IBC due to degenerative scoliosis with DDD (A, B, C). The initial follow-up was classified as type C cementation (D, E). Thirteen years after the IBC, no cement loosening was noted (F, G). He still worked as a semi-retired farmer without back pain.

and retrospectively correlated the long-term clinical outcomes. This study first established the criteria for standard body and disc cementation in IBC according to the 20-year clinical experiences. Subsequently, the classification system was retrospectively correlated with clinical outcomes. The results showed that disc cement is not a clinical issue because it is always sufficient during the postoperative follow-up. Standard body cementation requires at least one adjacent vertebra to ensure long-term clinical satisfaction and to prevent cement loosening. If both vertebrae above and below do not meet the standard cementation in IBC, symptomatic cement loosening increases, leading to unsatisfactory results.

Compared with the literature on traditional surgery [67–72], the reoperation rate of ASD after IBC was relatively low, and the interval was longer. The reoperation rate

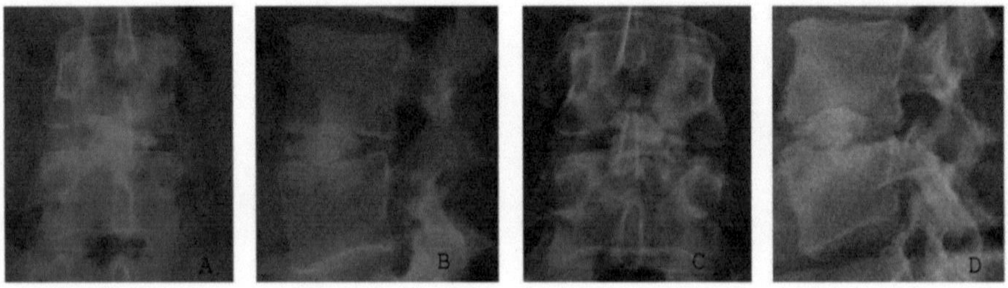

Figure 17.
A 52-year-old female underwent IBC for recurrent HIVD and DDD. The initial follow-up was classified as type C cementation (A, B). Four years after the IBC, a cement loosening sign appeared (C, D). However, she refused vertebroplasty because she was still active in her business with only mild back pain, which could be controlled with painkillers. This case was classified as fair.

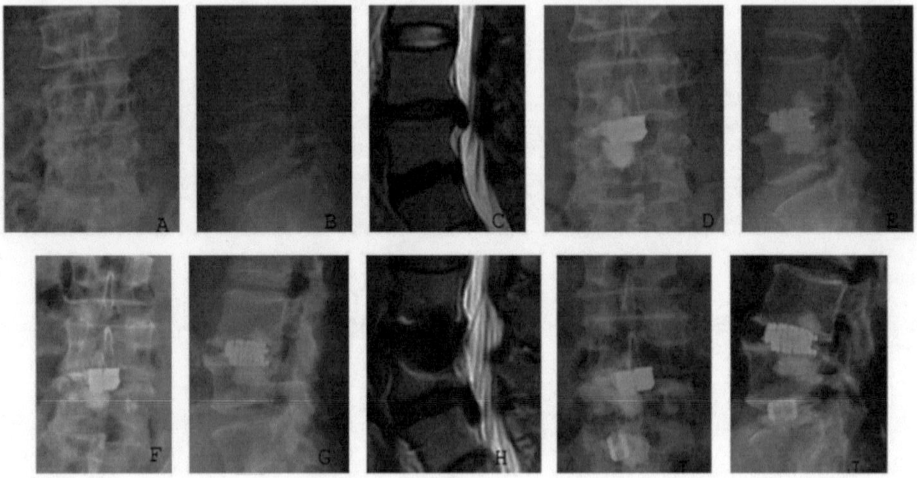

Figure 18.
A 50-year-old male underwent IBC for L4/L5 degenerative scoliosis with a ruptured disc (A, B, C). The initial follow-up was cementation classification type B. (D, E) Twelve years after IBC, an L5/S1 rupture disc was observed (F, G, H). The patient was treated again with IBC. Fourteen years after the primary IBC, no cement loosening was noted (I, J), and the patient continued to engage in farming.

for ASD after spinal fusion ranged from 9.9 to 22.2% at the 10-year follow-up [73–75]. A systematic review revealed that revision surgery rates for ASD were 1.2 and 7.0% in the total disc replacement and fusion groups, respectively, after a maximum of 5 years of follow-up [76]. In the present study, ASD following IBC was noted radiographically in 20 cases (11.6%) at the final visit, and nine cases (5.2%) had received revision surgery, with an average of 11.5 years after the primary operation. The mechanisms of the low ASD rates after IBC may be attributed to two factors. First, the IBC is not as rigid as the posterior instrumentation, and the facet joints in the IBC are not fixed and are allowed to move. Second, cement loosening may replace injuries to adjacent segments during chronic stressful work or acute mechanical overload accidents. Therefore, the reoperation rate of ASD after IBC is relatively low, and the interval is longer than that of classic instrumentation fusion.

Long-term postoperative stability is a major concern after the correction of spinal deformities, and bony fusion is not necessary. In Li's report [20], no patient required revision due to symptomatic cement loosening, with a mean follow-up of 6 years. In the present study, with a mean follow-up of 151 ± 10.4 months, only two type C cases underwent further management for symptomatic cement loosening. The two possible mechanisms proposed by Li et al. [20] are further stabilized by spontaneous ankylosing spur formation, and insensitivity to micromotion caused by cement loosening. In addition, compared to implant failure or ASD after posterior instrumentation, symptomatic cement loosening is a much easier and low-risk issue that can be treated with percutaneous vertebroplasty to re-stabilize the cement construct under local anesthesia.

This procedure is often much simpler than expected if the interbody bone block must be removed. Clinically, if the bone cement is not ideally distributed or if there is a deep bacterial infection, removal of the cement block may become necessary. The process begins with the use of a chisel or awl to crack the visible bone cement, typically on one side of the intervertebral disc space. Because bone cement is hard and brittle, it fractures easily into small pieces. The smaller fragments were extracted individually. The chiseling and removal of pieces were repeated until all easily accessible fragments were removed. If an infection is present, the bone cement located within the vertebral body is usually loose. In such cases, loose cement is first pulled down into the intervertebral disc space and then extracted. If the bone cement in the vertebral body is not loose, removal is considered unnecessary. Compared with deep and long bone cement in the femoral canal of an artificial hip joint [77], removing interbody cement is technically simpler.

Bone cement (Simplex, Stryker USA) is much cheaper ($25 per package) compared with posterior instrumentation ($3000 for one-motion segment fixation) in minimally invasive surgery-transforaminal lumbar interbody fusion (MIS-TLIF) in our country. Based on our clinical findings, the long-term clinical results of IBC are similar to those of posterior instrumentation. ASD and reoperation rates for IBC were lower than for posterior instrumentation. That is, IBC may be a potential option considering the economic factors for people without insurance coverage.

The potential application of IBC is the treatment of ASD after prolonged instrumentation, particularly at the L5/S1 and thoracolumbar junction levels (**Figures 19** and **20**). IBC can not only complete decompression, deformity correction, and fixation at the index level and avoid the removal of previous instrumentation but can also augment the adjacent loosening pedicle screws, which is often noted in ASD

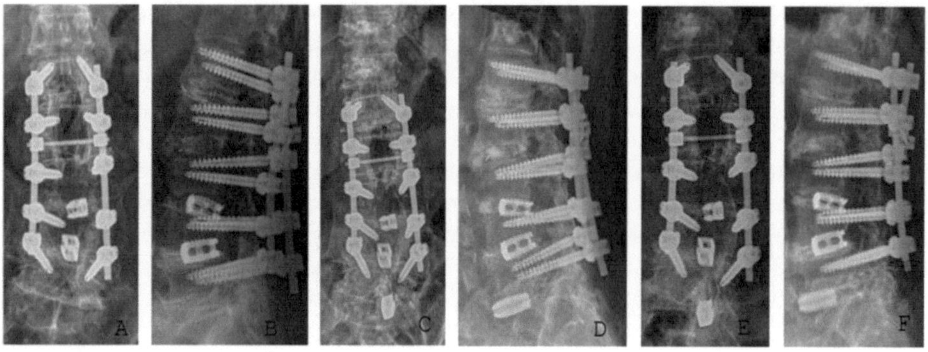

Figure 19.
A 78-year-old female with complicated medical conditions underwent IBC with a cage for L5/S1 adjacent segment disease after L1/L5 instrumentation (A, B). Initial follow-up (C, D) and five-year visit (E, F) showed that cement fixation was adequate.

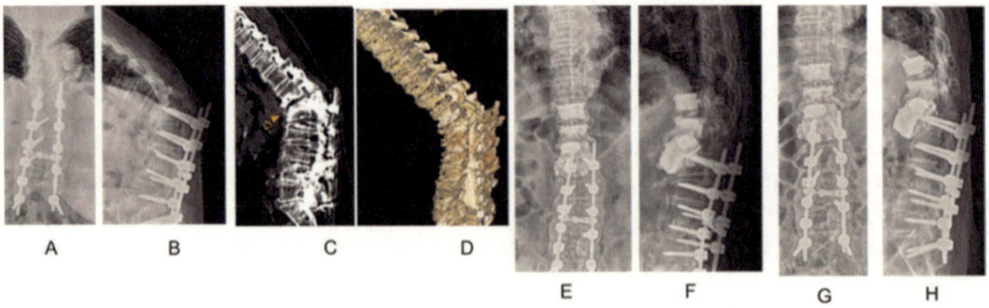

Figure 20.
A 73-year-old female underwent manual reduction and IBC for proximal kyphosis and T12/L1 listhesis 2 years after long segment instrumentation (A-D). The initial (E,F) and one-year (G,H) follow-up showed the well reduction and maintenance.

cases by body cementation while performing IBC. In other words, the two birds were killed using a single stone. IBC has great potential for application in all spinal operations because of its limited exposure, ease of operation, and good long-term results.

This retrospective study has several limitations. First, it was not a random design with selection bias, and the small sample size may have reduced the strength of the study. Second, this was a single-center study. A multicenter, prospective, and long-term studies with larger sample sizes are recommended in the future.

This study demonstrated that IBC led to significant long-term VAS and ODI improvements, a low ASD reoperation rate with a mean 12.6-year follow-up, and few osteoporosis-related complications. The criteria for the standard cementation of IBC have been established, and their clinical correlation is highly significant. At least one standard body cement is required to ensure a high long-term satisfaction rate. If type C fractures were noted during surgery, immediate complementary cementation was recommended.

5. Conclusions

Based on our 20-year clinical experience in treating lumbar degenerative deformities, this chapter covers fundamental and biomechanical studies, surgical techniques, and the long-term clinical results of locking lumbar interbody cementation. The 6-member manual reduction was performed to reduce deformities and induce as much indirect decompression as possible. IBC can directly decompress the spinal cord and reconstruct the deformed vertebra with disc cages and cementation, using a unilateral mini-open approach. The long-term results showed that IBC could maintain the reduction well until the final follow-up, and the correction was further ensured by lateral spontaneous interbody ankylosis. Compared with traditional instrumentation, there were much less osteoporosis-related complications, and adjacent segment disease is much less with longer interval. The long-term results revealed that manual reduction and IBC for lumbar degenerative diseases are safe and fast approaches for lumbar degenerative deformities and lead to good clinical outcomes.

Conflict of interest

The authors declare no conflicts of interest.

Author details

Kung Chia Li[1]*, Ching-Hsiang Hsieh[1], Ting-Hua Liao[1], Shang-Chih Lin[2] and Yu-Kun Xu[3]

1 Yang Ming Hospital, Chiayi, Taiwan

2 Graduate Institute of Biomedical Engineering, National Taiwan University of Science and Technology, Taipei, Taiwan

3 Graduate Institute of Applied Science and Technology, National Taiwan University of Science and Technology, Taipei, Taiwan

*Address all correspondence to: kungchiali@gmail.com

References

[1] Forstein DA, Bernardini C, Cole RE, Harris ST, Singer A. Before the breaking point: Reducing the risk of osteoporotic fracture. The Journal of the American Osteopathic Association. 2013;**113**(2 Suppl. 1):S5-S24

[2] O'Leary PT, Bridwell KH, Lenke LG, et al. Risk factors and outcomes for catastrophic failures at the top of long pedicle screw constructs: A matched cohort analysis performed at a single center. Spine (Phila Pa 1976). 2009;**34**: 2134-2139

[3] Boucas P, Mamdouhi T, Rizzo SE, Megas A. Cement augmentation of pedicle screw instrumentation: A literature review. Asian Spine Journal. 2023;**17**(5):939-948. DOI: 10.31616/asj.2022.0216. Epub 2023 Oct 4

[4] Jain D, Ray WZ, Vaccaro AR. Advances in techniques and technology in minimally invasive lumbar interbody spinal fusion. JBJS Reviews. 2020;**8**:e0171

[5] Kim CH, Easley K, Lee J-S. Comparison of minimally invasive versus open transforaminal interbody lumbar fusion. Global Spine Journal. 2020;**10**:143S-150S

[6] Xu DS, Walker CT, Godzik J. Minimally invasive anterior, lateral, and oblique lumbar interbody fusion: A literature review. Annals of Translational Medicine. 2018;**6**:104

[7] Cheh G, Bridwell KH, Lenke LG. Adjacent segment disease following lumbar/thoracolumbar fusion with pedicle screw instrumentation: A minimum 5-year follow-up. Spine. 2007; **32**:2253-2257

[8] Schwender JD, Holly LT, Rouben DP. Minimally invasive transforaminal lumbar interbody fusion (TLIF): Technical feasibility and initial results. Clinical Spine Surgery. 2005;**18**: S1-S6

[9] Han X, Tian W, Liu Y. Safety and accuracy of robot-assisted versus fluoroscopy-assisted pedicle screw insertion in thoracolumbar spinal surgery: A prospective randomized controlled trial. Journal of Neurosurgery: Spine. 2019;**30**:615-622

[10] Staub BN, Sadrameli SS. The use of robotics in minimally invasive spine surgery. Journal of Spine Surgery. 2019; **5**:S31

[11] Zhang Q, Han X-G, Xu Y-F. Robotic navigation during spine surgery. Expert Review of Medical Devices. 2020;**17**: 27-32

[12] Baeesa SS, Medrano BG, Noriega DC. Long-term outcomes of posterior lumbar interbody fusion using stand-alone ray threaded cage for degenerative disk disease: A 20-year follow-up. Asian Spine Journal. 2016;**10**:1100

[13] Choi WJ, Kim SK, Alaraj M, Kim HS, Lee SC. Stand-alone posterior expandable cage technique for adjacent segment degeneration with lumbar spinal canal stenosis: A retrospective case series. 72 Medicina. 2021;**57**:237

[14] Gaston CW, Gilles N, Nicola B, Gonzalo RK. Percutaneous cement discoplasty for degenerative low back pain with vacuum phenomenon: A multicentric study with a minimum of 2 years of follow up. World Neurosurgery. 2021;**155**:e210-e217

[15] Gaston CW, Kido G, Matias PD, Martin E, et al. Percutaneous cement

Advances in Neurosurgical Procedures – Unveiling New Horizons discoplasty for the treatment of advanced degenerative disc conditions: A case series analysis. Global Spine Journal. 2020;**10**:729-734

[16] Kiss L, Varga PP, Szoverfi Z. Indirect foraminal decompression and improvement in the lumbar alignment after percutaneous cement discoplasty. European Spine Journal. 2019;**28**: 1441-1447

[17] Sola C, Camino Willhuber G, Kido G. Percutaneous cement discoplasty for the treatment of advanced degenerative disk disease in elderly patients. European Spine Journal. 2021;**30**:2200-2208

[18] Yamada K, Nakamae T, Nakanishi K. Long-term outcome of targeted therapy for low back pain in elderly degenerative lumbar scoliosis. European Spine Journal. 2021;**30**:2020-2032

[19] Li KC, Hsieh CH, Liao TH. Cement lumbar interbody fusion (CLIF) for low-grade degenerative spondylolisthesis with minimum 10-year follow-up. Journal of Surgery. 2022;**7**:1691

[20] Li KC, Hsieh CH, Liao TH. Clinical outcome-supported advance of cement lumber interbody fusion for degenerative lumbar scoliosis. Journal of Surgery. 2023;**8**:1697

[21] Chen DJ, Yao C, Song Q, Tang B, Liu X, et al. Unilateral versus bilateral pedicle screw fixation combined with transforaminal lumbar interbody fusion for the treatment of low lumbar degenerative disc diseases: Analysis of clinical and radiographic results. World Neurosurgery. 2018;**115**:e516-e522

[22] Liu CW, Wang LL, Xu YK, Chen CM, Wang JC, et al. Traditional and cortical trajectory screws for static and dynamic lumbar fixation: A finite element study. BMC Musculoskeletal Disorders. 2020;**21**(1):463

[23] Xiao SW, Jiang H, Yang LJ, Xiao ZM. Comparison of unilateral versus bilateral pedicle screw fixation with cage fusion in degenerative lumbar diseases: A meta-analysis. European Spine Journal. 2015; **24**(4):764-774

[24] Wang Y, Kahaer A, Maimaiti A, Guo H, Rexiti P. Complication, fusion, and revision rate in lumbar cortical bone trajectory and pedicle screw fixation techniques: A systematic review and meta-analysis. Journal of Orthopaedic Surgery and Research. 2023;**18**(1):382

[25] Gubian A, Kausch L, Neumann J-O, Kiening K, Ishak B, et al. CT-navigated spinal instrumentations-three-dimensional evaluation of screw placement accuracy in relation to a screw trajectory plan. Medicina (Kaunas, Lithuania). 2022;**58**(9):1200

[26] Sun W, Wang P, Hailiang H, Kong C, Hai Y, et al. Retrospective study on effectiveness of Activ L total disc replacement. Journal of Orthopaedic Surgery and Research. 2021;**16**(1):2

[27] Rathbone J, Rackham M, Nielsen D, Lee SM, Hing W, et al. A systematic review of anterior lumbar interbody fusion (ALIF) versus posterior lumbar interbody fusion (PLIF), transforaminal lumbar interbody fusion (TLIF), posterolateral lumbar fusion (PLF). European Spine Journal. 2023;**32**(6): 1911-1926

[28] Florence TJ, Say I, Patel KS, Unterberger A, Laiwalla A, et al. Neurosurgical management of interspinous device complications: A case series. Frontiers in Surgery. 2022; **16**(9):841134

[29] Meganathan S, Alphin MS. Biomechanical assessment of lumbar stability: Finite element analysis of TLIF with a novel combination of coflex and

pedicle screws. Acta of Bioengineering and Biomechanics. 2024;**25**(4):133-143

[30] Zhang H, Hao D, Sun H, He S, Wang B, et al. Biomechanical effects of direction-changeable cage positions on lumbar spine: A finite element study. American Journal of Translational Research. 2020;**12**(2):389-396

[31] Zhu H, Zhong W, Zhang P, Liu X, Huang J, et al. Biomechanical evaluation of autologous bone-cage in posterior lumbar interbody fusion: A finite element analysis. BMC Musculoskeletal Disorders. 2020;**21**(1):379

[32] Onggo JR, Nambiar M, Maingard JT, Phan K, Marcia S, et al. The use of minimally invasive interspinous process devices for the treatment of lumbar canal stenosis: A narrative literature review. Journal of Spine Surgery. 2021; **7**(3):394-412

[33] Wen J, Shi C, Lei Y, Wang S, Xi Y, et al. Unilateral versus bilateral percutaneous pedicle screw fixation in oblique lumbar interbody fusion. World Neurosurgery. 2020;**134**:e920-e927

[34] Lee CH, Kim YE, Lee HJ, Kim DG, Kim CH. Biomechanical effects of hybrid stabilization on the risk of proximal adjacent-segment degeneration following lumbar spinal fusion using an interspinous device or a pedicle screw-based dynamic fixator. Journal of Neurosurgery. Spine. 2017;**27**(6):643-649

[35] Erbulut DU, Zafarparandeh I, Hassan CR, Lazoglu I, Ozer AF. Determination of the biomechanical effect of an interspinous process device on implanted and adjacent lumbar spinal segments using a hybrid testing protocol: A finite-element study. Journal of Neurosurgery. Spine. 2015;**23**(2): 200-208

[36] Zhu J, Shen H, Cui Y, Fogel GR, Liao Z, et al. Biomechanical evaluation of transforaminal lumbar interbody fusion with coflex-F and pedicle screw fixation: Finite element analysis of static and vibration conditions. Orthopaedic Surgery. 2022;**14**(9):2339-2349

[37] Grewal SS, Hirsch JA, Cancelliere NM, Ghozy S, Mendes V, et al. Pereira efficacy and safety of percutaneous cement discoplasty in the management of degenerative spinal diseases: A systematic review and meta-analysis. The Neuroradiology Journal. 2023;**3**:434-440

[38] Koch K, Szoverfi Z, Jakab G, Varga PP, Hoffer Z, et al. Complication pattern after percutaneous cement discoplasty: Identification of factors influencing reoperation and length of hospital stay. World Neurosurgery. 2023;**178**:e700-e711

[39] Cheng SH, Chou WH, Tsuei YC, Chu W, Chu WC. Assessment of cement leakage in decompressed percutaneous kyphoplasty. Journal of Clinical Medicine. 2024;**13**(2):345

[40] Huang J, Zeng W, Li M, Cheng Z, Huang J, et al. Biomechanical effects of cement discoplasty on the lumbar spinal unit. Frontiers in Surgery. 2022;**9**:951141

[41] Yang L, Kong J, Qiu Z, Shang T, Chen S, et al. Mineralized collagen-modified PMMA cement enhances bone integration and reduces fibrous encapsulation in the treatment of lumbar degenerative disc diseases. Regenerative Biomaterials. 2020;7(2):181-193

[42] Wang QD, Guo LX. Biomechanical role of cement augmentation in the vibration characteristics of the osteoporotic lumbar spine after lumbar interbody fusion. Journal of Materials

Science. Materials in Medicine. 2022;**33**(6):52

[43] Yang F, Yan YC, Ru XL, Qu HB. Effect of acrylic bone cement mixed with calcium sulfate combined with percutaneous kyphoplasty in the treatment of osteoporotic fractures. Zhongguo Gu Shang. 2023;**36**(9):896-900

[44] Barkov O, Tuliakov V, Aplevich V. The use of laboratory criteria in the risk assessment of postoperative complications after transpedicular fixation of the lumbar spine. Orthopaedics Traumatology and Prosthetics. 2024;**1**:19-26

[45] Grin AA, Nikitin AS, Kalandari AA, Asratyan SA, Yundin SV, et al. Rigid transpedicular fusion surgery in the treatment of degenerative lumbar stenosis. Burdenko's Journal of Neurosurgery. 2020;**84**(5):41-49

[46] Wang Q, Dong JF, Fang X, Chen Y. Application and modification of bone cement in vertebroplasty: A literature review. Joint Diseases and Related Surgery 2020;**33**(2):467-478

[47] Cianfoni A, Giamundo M, Pileggi M, Huscher K, Shapiro M, et al. Spinal instrumentation rescue with cement augmentation. AJNR. American Journal of Neuroradiology. 2018;**39**(10):1957-1962

[48] Bereczki F, Turbucz M, Pokorni AJ, Hajnal B, Ronai M, et al. The effect of polymethylmethacrylate augmentation on the primary stability of stand-alone implant construct versus posterior stabilization in oblique lumbar interbody fusion with osteoporotic bone quality- a finite element study. Spine Journal. 2024;**24**(7):1323-1333

[49] Fredrickson BE, Edwards WT, Rauschning W, et al. Vertebral burst fractures: An experimental, morphologic, and radiographic study. Spine. 1992;**17**:1012-1021

[50] Fredrickson BE, Mann KA, Yuan HA, et al. Reduction of the intracanal fragment in experimental burst fractures. Spine. 1988;**12**:267-271

[51] Frankel JL, Hancock DO, Hyslop G, et al. The value of postural reduction in the initial management of closed injuries of the spine with paraplegia and tetraplegia: Part I. Paraplegia. 1969;**7**:179-192

[52] Tropiano P, Huang RC, Louis CA, et al. Functional and radiographic outcome of thoracolumbar and lumbar burst fractures managed by closed orthopaedic reduction and casting. Spine (Phila Pa 1976). 2003;**28**(21):2459-2465

[53] Li KC, Hsieh CH. Pedicle augmenter in treating burst fracture. The Spine Journal. 2003;**3**(Suppl.):148S

[54] Li KC, Wong TU, Kung FC, et al. Staging of Kummell's disease. Journal of Musculoskeletal Research. 2004;**8**:43-55

[55] Li KC, Hsieh CH, Lee CY, Chen TH. Transpedicle body augmenter: A further step in treating burst fractures. Clinical Orthopaedics and Related Research. 2005;**436**:119-125

[56] Li KC, Li AF, Hsieh CH, Liao TH, Chen CH. Another option to treat Kümmell's disease with cord compression. European Spine Journal. 2007;**16**(9):1479-1487

[57] Li KC, Li AF, Hsieh CH, Chen HH. Transpedicle body augmenter in painful osteoporotic compression fractures. European Spine Journal. 2007;**16**(5):589-598

[58] Li KC, Yu SW, Li A, Hsieh CH, Liao TH, Chen JH, et al. Subpedicle decompression and vertebral reconstruction for thoracolumbar Magerl incomplete burst fractures via a minimally invasive method. Spine (Phila Pa 1976). 2014;**39**(5):433-442

[59] Li KC, Hsieh CH, Liao TH, Chen CH. Manual reduction for subacute osteoporotic burst and severe compression thoracolumbar fractures. BioMed. 2024;**4**:136-145

[60] Carlo P, Francesco C. Preoperative manual on-table-traction for the reduction of thoracolumbar burst fractures: A technical note. Journal of Craniovertebral Junction and Spine. 2018;**9**(1):73-75

[61] Li Y, Du Y, Ji A, et al. The clinical effect of manual reduction combined with internal fixation through Wiltse paraspinal approach in the treatment of thoracolumbar fracture. Orthopaedic Surgery. 2021;**13**(8): 2206-2215

[62] Li KC, Hsieh YC, Hsieh CH, Liao CH. Manual reduction, subpedicle approach, and body cages to treat burst fracture [internet]. In: Frontiers in Spinal Neurosurgery. London, UK: IntechOpen; 2023

[63] Schizas C, Theumann N, Burn A, Tansey R, Wardlaw D, Smith FW, et al. Qualitative grading of severity of lumbar spinal stenosis based on the morphology of the dural sac on magnetic resonance images. Spine. 2010;**35**(21):1919-1924

[64] Copay AG, Glassman SD, Subach BR, Berven S, Schuler TC, Carreon LY. Minimum clinically important difference in lumbar spine surgery patients: A choice of methods using the oswestry disability index, medical outcomes study questionnaire short form 36, and pain scales. The Spine Journal. 2008;**8**(6):968-974

[65] Carreon LY, Kelly MP, Crawford CH III, Baldus CR, Glassman SD, Shaffrey CI, et al. SRS-22R minimum clinically important difference and substantial clinical benefit after adult lumbar scoliosis surgery. Spinal Deformity. 2018;**6**(1):79-83

[66] Glassman SD, Hamill CL, Bridwell KH, Schwab FJ, Dimar JR, Lowe TG. The impact of perioperative complications on clinical outcome in adult deformity surgery. Spine. 2007; **32**(24):2764-2770

[67] Zileli M, Dursun E. How to improve outcomes of spine surgery in geriatric patients. World Neurosurgery. 2020; **140**:519-526

[68] Sun W, Lu S, Kong C, Li Z, Wang P, Zhang S. Frailty and post-operative outcomes in the older patients undergoing elective posterior thoracolumbar fusion surgery. Clinical Interventions in Aging. 2020;**15**: 1141-1150

[69] Yuan L, Zeng Y, Chen Z, Li W, Zhang X, Ni J. Risk factors associated with failure to reach minimal clinically important difference after correction surgery in patients with degenerative lumbar scoliosis. Spine. 2020;**45**(24): E1669-E1676

[70] Charosky S, Guigui P, Blamoutier A, Roussouly P, Chopin D. Complications and risk factors of primary adult scoliosis surgery: A multicenter study of 306 patients. Spine. 2012;**37**(8):693-700

[71] Deyo RA. Fusion surgery for lumbar degenerative disc disease: Still more questions than answers. The Spine Journal. 2015;**15**(2):272-274

[72] Carreon LY, Puno RM, Dimar JR, Glassman SD, Johnson JR. Perioperative complications of posterior lumbar decompression and arthrodesis in older adults. The Journal of Bone and Joint Surgery. American Volume. 2003; **85**(11):2089-2092

[73] Sears WR, Sergides IG, Kazemi N, Smith M, White GJ, Osburg B. Incidence and prevalence of surgery at segments adjacent to a previous posterior lumbar arthrodesis. The Spine Journal. 2011;**11**: 11-20

[74] Okuda S, Yamashita T, Matsumoto T, et al. Adjacent segment disease after posterior lumbar interbody fusion: A case series of 1000 patients. Global Spine Journal. 2018;**8**:722-727

[75] Nakashima H, Kawakami N, Tsuji T, et al. Adjacent segment disease after posterior lumbar interbody fusion: Based on cases with a minimum of 10 years of follow-up. Spine (Phila Pa 1976). 2015; **40**:E831-E841

[76] Wang JC, Arnold PM, Hermsmeyer JT, Norvell DC. Do lumbar motion preserving devices reduce the risk of adjacent segment pathology compared with fusion surgery? A systematic review. Spine (Phila Pa 1976). 2012;**37**(Suppl. 22):S133-S143

[77] Tovar-Bazaga M, Sáez-Martínez D, Auñón Á, López-Oliva F, Pardos-Mayo B, Calvo E. Surgical technique of a cement-on-cement removal system for hip and knee arthroplasty revision surgery. Arthroplast Today. 2021;**15**(9): 112-117

Chapter 6

Endoscopic Lumbar Rhizotomy for Facetogenic Pain

Azmi Nasser

Abstract

Chronic lumbar facetogenic pain is a common condition, with broad significance on disability and care costs. Endoscopic rhizotomy (ER) is a minimally invasive surgical procedure that is used to treat chronic spine pain by cutting or destroying the medial branch nerves that supply the facet joints in the spine. The procedure is also known as direct visualized rhizotomy or facet joint denervation. It is more advanced than the typical radiofrequency ablation (RFA) and considered to provide more permanent therapeutic benefit. Endoscopic rhizotomy has the particular advantage of direct visualization of the anatomical structures including the articular capsule, bony landmarks, and the target medial branch nerves. Thus enabling a more accurate neurotomy, and if necessary also a capsulotomy or removal of other pathology such as facet cysts. The goal of this chapter is to introduce the reader to endoscopic spine surgery with regards to rhizotomy, its instruments, and describe the technique.

Keywords: low back pain, lumbar facet joint, medial branch, endoscopic rhizotomy, facet denervation

1. Introduction

Low back pain is acknowledged as one of the most common pain conditions [1] with prevalence increasing [2]. National health survey reviews have recently found that 8.2% of American adults report having chronic severe back pain [3]. It persists as the most common reason for years lived with disability [4], having of course a significant impact on personal and socioeconomic factors. Conservative, interventional, and surgical approaches to treatment have also evolved, helping to identify the many causes of chronic low back pain and elucidate treatments.

Studies have shown the facet (zygapophyseal) joints to be the source of chronic low back pain in approximately 27–40% of patients [5, 6]. While the pain associated with the facet joints is primarily axial, studies have established reproducible radiation patterns into the extremities including distally into the leg [7]. The facet joints are true synovial joints that are richly innervated by the medial branches of the dorsal rami. Thus as with other synovial joints, it is believed that facetogenic pain is due to injury, inflammation, degenerative arthritis, capsular distension, instability, and impinged nerves secondary to osteophytes [8].

While an important aspect to chronic low back pain evaluation, the physical exam and imaging have not been shown to be reliable diagnostic prognosticators of facetogenic pain [9, 10]. Both intra-articular facet joint injections and medial branch blocks have been used to diagnose and confirm facetogenic pain syndromes. Facet joint injections have been shown to have diagnostic value but limited therapeutic benefit [11], and have fallen out of favor due to ease of performance and greater diagnostic value of medial branch blocks. Particularly if progressing to a more therapeutic treatment such as percutaneous medial branch radiofrequency ablation (RFA), also referred to as radiofrequency neurotomy (RFN). While some have argued for one positive block prior to RFA [12], and even studied the cost savings of zero blocks prior to RFA [13], there has been shown to be a higher false positive rate of 27–47% with one block, and both raise ethical concerns of performing RFA in unproven cases. Most current guidelines and insurance programs recommend two separate diagnostic medial branch blocks providing 80% or greater relief for the duration of corresponding anesthetic [14].

In reviews of lumbar facetogenic pain treatments, subsequent RFA had good data [15], and provided sustained clinical relief for 6–12 months [7], with some patients reporting >50% relief at 2 years. Repeat RF procedures were also shown to provide relief for 9–10 months [16]. With RFA the medial branch is not completely interrupted but the axon is coagulated and does regenerate, hence the relative short duration of relief and pain recurrence. The amount of the nerve that is ablated also depends on needle positioning. In addition, initial and repeat ablation procedures do not always provide expected relief even despite diagnostic blocks. Theories of this response include false positive blocks, technique, neuromas [17], and ossified mammillary accessory ligament under which the medial branch courses [18].

2. Endoscopic spine surgery and the advancement to rhizotomy

Endoscopic spine surgery (ESS) has roots tracing back to the 1980s, being first described by Parviz Kambin [19] in treatment of lumbar disc herniations. Developed to provide a less invasive alternative to traditional open or even minimally invasive spine surgery, allowing for reduced tissue damage, shorter recovery times, and less postoperative pain, it has evolved significantly since its inception. Over the years, advancements in imaging technology and instrumentation have further refined ESS, enabling surgeons to perform complex procedures through small incisions. These advancements have solidified ESS as a viable option for many spinal conditions, garnering interest and training among surgeons worldwide.

Endoscopic rhizotomy, also known as direct visualized rhizotomy, or facet joint denervation, applies that evolutionary advancement in ESS for chronic lumbar facetogenic pain as a more definitive treatment option. Instead of relying solely on fluoroscopic guidance it enables direct visualization of the medial branch, and offers more complete denervation of the branch. This procedure also allows the debridement of the facet joint via capsulotomy, and wash out of the articular space, if necessary [20]. Studies have shown the relief to be equal to that of RFA at 1 and 3 months, with better outcomes at 6 and 12 months [21]. And unlike RFA endoscopic rhizotomy provided stable persistent relief at 2 years [22], even up to 5 years [23]. Personal surgical outcomes have corroborated the above results, including the study finding that patients' prior RFAs had no impact on endoscopic rhizotomy results [22].

The technique can be easily mastered by surgeons and interventionalists. Procedure time is typically 45–90 minutes depending on the number of treatment levels, and if unilateral or bilateral. The procedure requires one or more small incisions less than 10 mm, and has minimal rare complications. Bleeding is controlled with irrigation pressure, epinephrine in anesthetic, and endoscopic cauterization. The surgery can be done even with patients awake and local anesthetic only, however light to moderate sedation under monitored anesthesia care is most common. Typical prone patient positioning with gentle lordosis reduction, sterile prep is performed, and special drape to capture endoscopic irrigation runoff. Normal saline irrigation is necessary for visualization and for local thermal control to prevent charring of the bipolar cautery tip, and overheating of nerves/anatomy.

3. Instruments

Since first being utilized endoscopic instruments have undergone further development enhancing endoscopic surgeries capabilities. However some basic instruments remain true. An 18 gauge needle and guidewire are usually separately purchased disposables (**Figure 1**). In the newer surgical trays various working channels and bevel types are usually available (**Figure 2**). Those with wider, flatter working ends and smaller portals may be best for stability and limiting soft tissue encroachment into the visual field. The outside diameter of the working channels are 7.5 mm, with a lumen diameter of 6.5 mm, same as the endoscope outer diameter. Typical optical

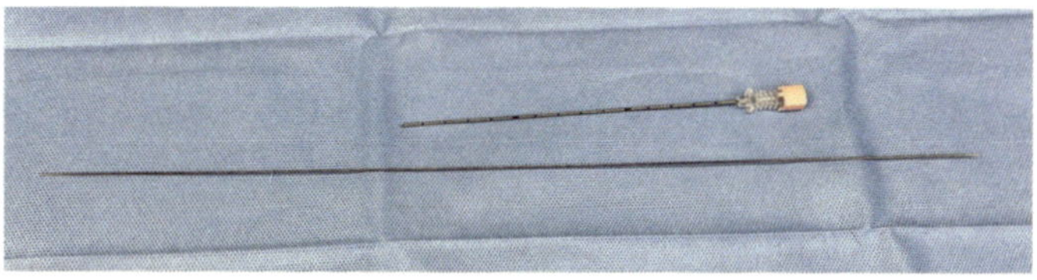

Figure 1.
18 Gauge needle and guidewire.

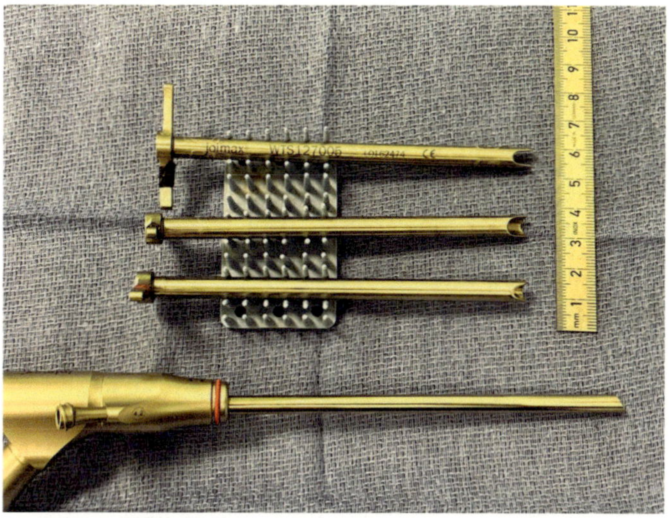

Figure 2.
Examples of JoiMax working channels and endoscope.

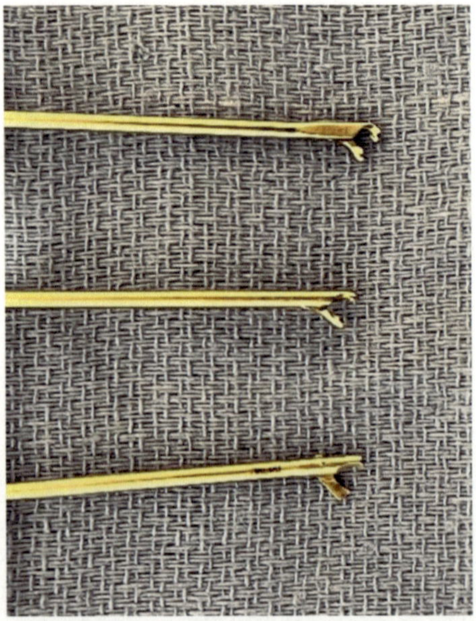

Figure 3.
Examples of JoiMax endoscopic instruments typical endoscopic instruments. TOP: Upbiting Rongeurs. Middle: Straight Rongeurs. Bottom: Scissors.

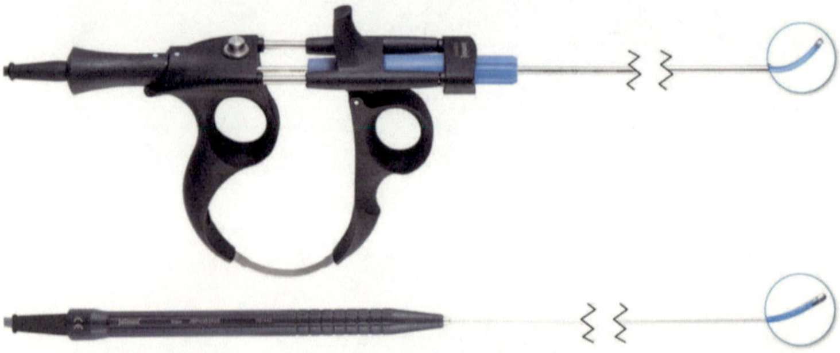

Figure 4.
Example of JoiMax endoscopic electrocautery instruments with disposable, articulating extensions.

angles for the endoscope in rhizotomy is 30 degrees, though other options may be available. Through the endoscopic channel smaller diameter instruments such as forceps, scissors (**Figure 3**) and bipolar electrocautery are used (**Figure 4**).

4. Fluoroscopic guidance

As with spine surgery in general, image guidance is crucial to ER, ensuring accurate needle placement, and minimizing complications intra-operatively. A 20 degree ipsilateral oblique angle has been found to be sufficient to access the target even with facet hypertrophy and help stabilize the working channel at the SAP-TP junction (**Figure 5**). Using fluoroscopy, the target of the medial branch (MB) at the junction of the superior articular process (SAP), and transverse process (TP) or sacral ala, is

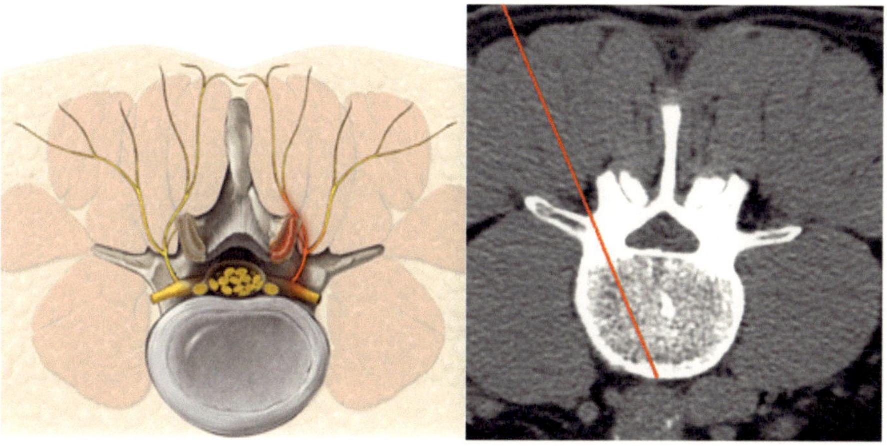

Figure 5.
LEFT-: axial lumbar anatomical depiction including medial branches. RIGHT—axial CT image of lumbar spine with procedural approach angle to the SAP-TP junction.

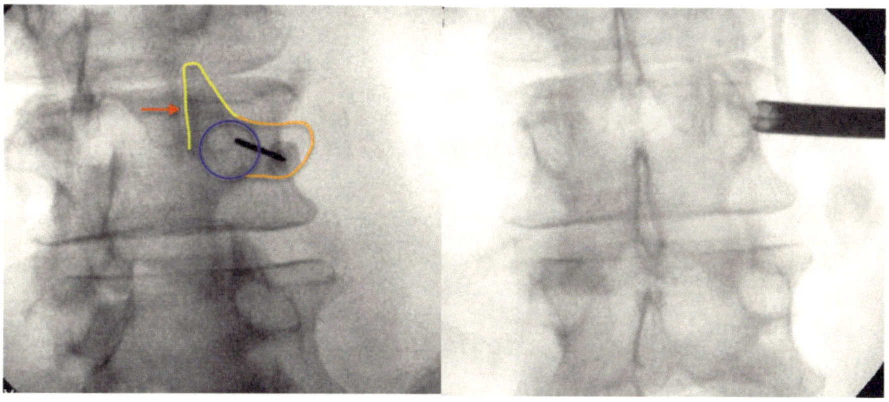

Figure 6.
LEFT—Oblique view of needle to L2 MB at L3 SAP (YELLOW)/TP (ORANGE) junction. Needle docked at the "eye" of the pedicle (BLUE). Red arrow: midportion of facet joint. RIGHT—AP view with beveled working channel and endoscope at L3 VB. Endoscopic bipolar device tip positioned at base of SAP/TP junction.

identified (**Figure 6**). Prominent severe facet hypertrophy still may require a slightly larger oblique approach, that can be determined on fluoroscopy. Thus the endoscope has a 30 degree view angle to optimize medial gaze toward the SAP-TAP junction with the oblique approach.

Proximal MB at levels L1 to L4 (T12 to L3 MBs) are best approached with a separate insertion site for optimal access. Often their respective transverse processes are thinner and more round, and having a direct oblique approach at each level prevents sliding off into the superior or inferior neuroforamen.

However, both the L4 MB and L5 dorsal primary ramus (DPR) can be targeted with one insertion site along the L5 TP, as cephalocaudad tilt is used to direct the instruments caudad to the SAP/ala junction (**Figures 7–9**). Especially in males, the ilium may obstruct access without cephalocaudad approach. The sagittal angle also helps prevent instrument translation over the sacral ala into the L5-S1 foramen.

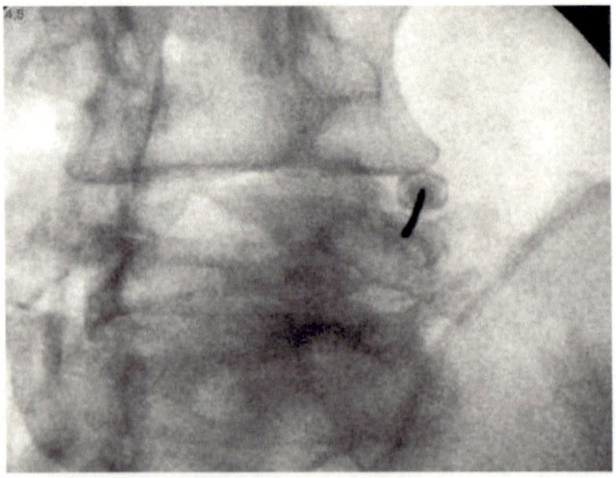

Figure 7.
Oblique view of needle to L4 MB at L5 SAP/TP junction.

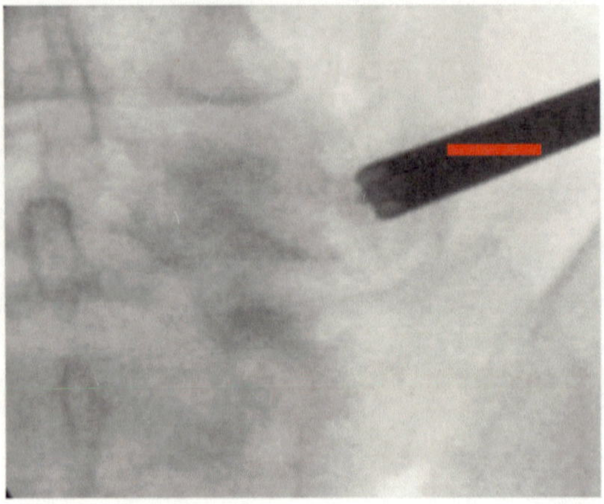

Figure 8.
AP view with working channel and endoscope at L5 VB. Red line: incision at L5 vertebra to target L4 MB.

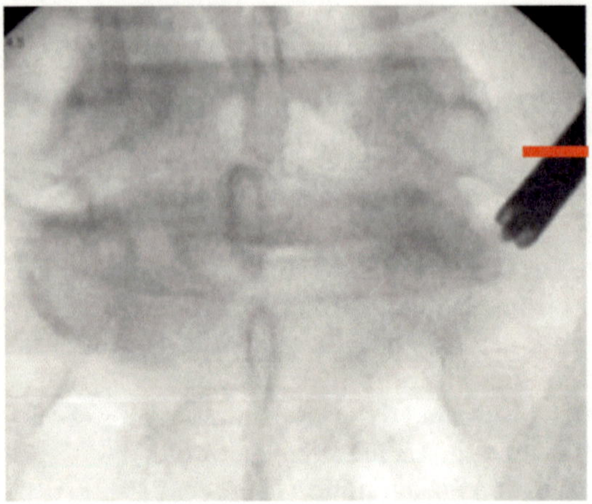

Figure 9.
AP view of working channel and endoscope at L5 DPR target at SAP-sacral ala. Endoscopic scissors can be seen in the working channel. Red line: incision at L5 vertebra with cephalocaudad tilt to target L5 DPR.

5. Technique

The patient is positioned prone with gentle lordotic reversal, prepped and draped in usual sterile fashion, with a special drape for endoscopic irrigation capture. Local anesthetic with epinephrine is injected subcutaneously. Using a draped C-arm, under oblique fluoroscopic guidance, an 18 gauge 15 cm needle is inserted and docked on the SAP-TP junction. One to two milliliters of local anesthetic with epinephrine is instilled at the facet joint to assist in controlling bleeding and for patient comfort especially if awake. The C-arm is rotated to AP position at this time for instrumentational ease. The needle stylet is removed and guidewire inserted. The small <8 mm incision is made over the needle and not the guidewire. However the incision may also be made prior to needle insertion, as positional adjustments requiring a new incision are typically rare. Maintaining the guidewire in place with gentle pressure, the needle is withdrawn. With proper initial approach the guidewire should not skive off the TP. Serial dilators are carefully inserted so as to also not skive off the TP, followed by the working cannula (**Figure 10**). After careful withdrawal of the dilators and guidewire the endoscope with attached irrigation tubing is inserted (**Figure 11**). Intermittent fluoroscopy ensures proper placement is maintained.

Using forceps and bipolar cautery gentle tissue resection is performed to dissect down to the SAP-TP junction. Often in patients with prior RFAs the mammillary-accessory ligament can be disrupted or absent. Once identified, the medial branch (**Figure 12**) nerve is transected with endoscopic scissors (**Figure 13**) and each end cauterized. Alternatively, the bipolar cautery may be used to bisect the nerve(s) (**Figure 13**). After confirming the SAP-TP junction space is cleared attention may be turned to a capsulotomy or other structures if necessary.

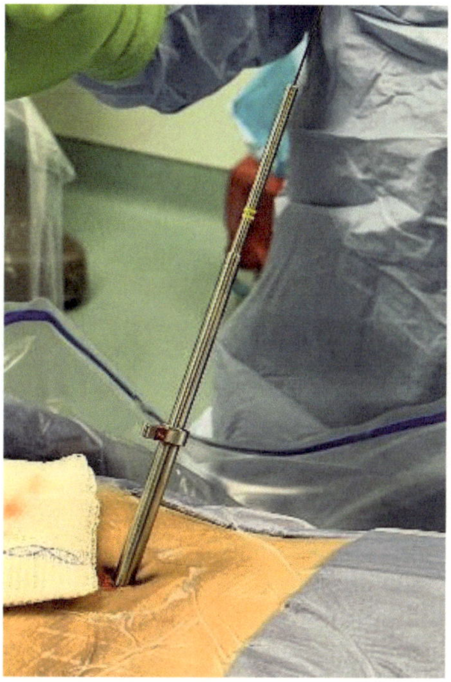

Figure 10.
Guidewire, two serial dilators, and working channel.

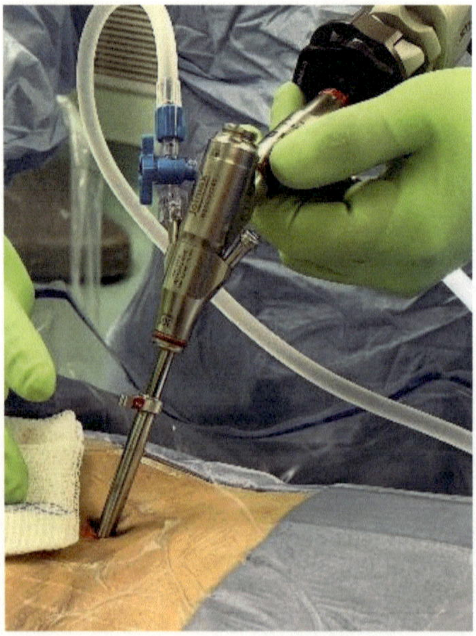

Figure 11.
Endoscope in working channel.

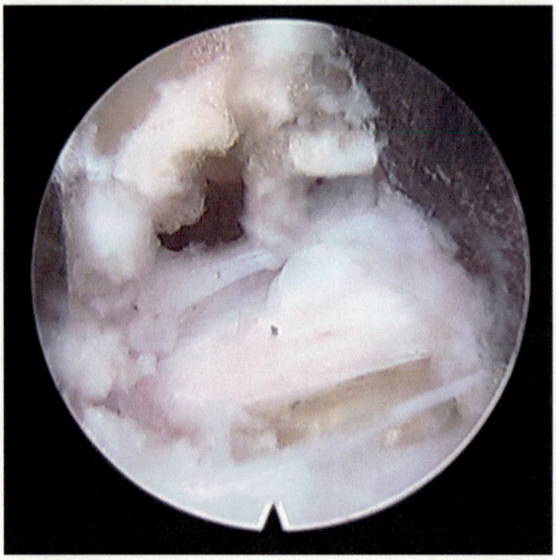

Figure 12.
TOP: SAP and facet capsule. Middle: medial branch traversing left to right. The medial branch is tamped down by the working channel.

It is recommended that the surgeon and C-arm stay on opposite sides of the patient. Thus when performing bilateral ER the OR layout is usually reversed after completing the first side to complete the contralateral side. Simple arrangements can make the process easier, such as positioning the endoscope tower and screen at the foot of the OR table (**Figure 14**).

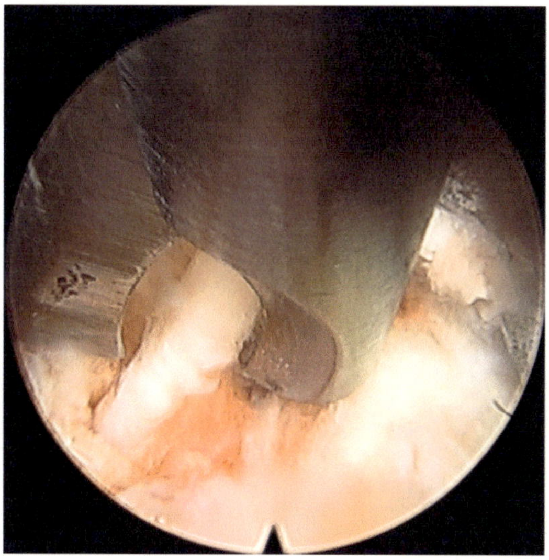

Figure 13.
Endoscopic scissors around medial branch. The endoscope is rotated 60–90 degrees to capture perpendicular view of schissors.

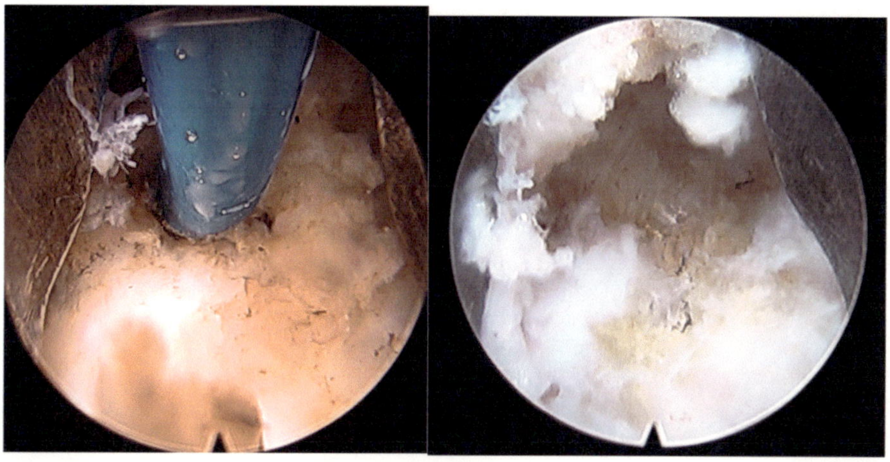

Figure 14.
LEFT—Endoscopic bipolar tip in middle of base of SAP (above bipolar probe) and TP junction (below bipolar probe). RIGHT—The medial branch has been cleared and no other structures are traversing the normal path.

6. Conclusion

Endoscopic rhizotomy represents a significant advancement in pain management techniques, combining the principles of endoscopy with neurosurgical techniques to provide effective long-term relief for chronic lumbar facetogenic pain. It is arguably more effective than traditional radiofrequency ablation, and is a safe procedure with a low complication rate.

Conflict of interest

Azmi Nasser DO is a paid proctor for JoiMax. JoiMax did not pay for or sponsor this chapter.

Author details

Azmi Nasser
Arizona Pain Treatment Centers, Phoenix, AZ, USA

*Address all correspondence to: drazminasser@yahoo.com

References

[1] Hellsing AL, Bryngelsson IL. Predictors of musculoskeletal pain in men: A twenty-year follow-up from examination at enlistment. Spine (Phila Pa 1976). 2000;**25**(23):3080-3086. DOI: 10.1097/00007632-200012010-00016

[2] Freburger JK, Holmes GM, Agans RP, Jackman AM, Darter JD, Wallace AS, et al. The rising prevalence of chronic low back pain. Archives of Internal Medicine. 2009;**169**(3):251-258. DOI: 10.1001/archinternmed.2008.543

[3] Feldman D, Nahin R. Disability among persons with chronic severe back pain: Results from a nationally representative population-based sample. The Journal of Pain. 2022;**23**:2144-2154. DOI: 10.1016/j.jpain.2022.07.016

[4] Murray CJ, Atkinson C, Bhalla K, Birbeck G, Burstein R, Chou D, et al. The state of US health, 1990-2010: Burden of diseases, injuries, and risk factors. Journal of the American Medical Association. 2013;**310**(6):591-608. DOI: 10.1001/jama.2013.13805

[5] Manchikanti L, Boswell MV, Singh V, Pampati V, Damron KS, Beyer CD. Prevalence of facet joint pain in chronic spinal pain of cervical, thoracic, and lumbar regions. BMC Musculoskeletal Disorders. 2004;**5**:15. DOI: 10.1186/1471-2474-5-15

[6] Datta S, Lee M, Falco FJ, Bryce DA, Hayek SM. Systematic assessment of diagnostic accuracy and therapeutic utility of lumbar facet joint interventions. Pain Physician. 2009;**12**(2):437-460

[7] Manchikanti L, Kaye AD, Soin A, Albers SL, Beall D, Latchaw R, et al. Comprehensive evidence-based guidelines for facet joint interventions in the management of chronic spinal pain: American society of interventional pain physicians (ASIPP) guidelines facet joint interventions 2020 guidelines. Pain Physician. 2020;**23**(3S):S1-S127

[8] Peh W. Image-guided facet joint injection. Biomedical Imaging and Intervention Journal. 2011;**7**(1):e4. DOI: 10.2349/biij.7.1.e4. Epub 2011 Jan 1

[9] Bogduk N, McGuirk B. Assessment. In: Bogduk N, McGuirk B, editors. Medical Management of Acute and Chronic Low Back Pain an Evidence-Based Approach: Pain Research and Clinical Management. Vol. 13. Amsterdam: Elsevier Science BV; 2002. pp. 127-138

[10] Bogduk N. Degenerative joint disease of the spine. Radiologic Clinics of North America. 2012;**50**(4):613-628. DOI: 10.1016/j.rcl.2012.04.012

[11] Cohen SP, Doshi TL, Constantinescu OC, Zhao Z, Kurihara C, Larkin TM, et al. Effectiveness of lumbar facet joint blocks and predictive value before radiofrequency denervation: The facet treatment study (FACTS), a randomized, controlled clinical trial. Anesthesiology. 2018;**129**(3):517-535. DOI: 10.1097/ALN.0000000000002274

[12] Derby R, Melnik I, Lee JE, Lee SH. Correlation of lumbar medial branch neurotomy results with diagnostic medial branch block cutoff values to optimize therapeutic outcome. Pain Medicine. 2012;**13**(12):1533-1546. DOI: 10.1111/j.1526-4637.2012.01500.x. Epub 2012 Nov 5

[13] Cohen SP, Williams KA, Kurihara C, et al. Multicenter, randomized,

comparative cost-effectiveness study comparing 0, 1, and 2 diagnostic medial branch (facet joint nerve) block treatment paradigms before lumbar facet radiofrequency denervation. Anesthesiology. 2010;**113**(2):395-405

[14] Centers for Medicare and Medicaid Services. Local Coverage Determination. Facet Joint Interventions for Pain Management. 2024. Available from: https://www.cms.gov/medicare-coverage-database/view/lcd.aspx?LCDId=38803 [Accessed: September 04, 2024]

[15] Falco FJ, Manchikanti L, Datta S, Sehgal N, Geffert S, Onyewu O, et al. An update of the effectiveness of therapeutic lumbar facet joint interventions. Pain Physician. 2012;**15**(6):E909-E953

[16] Son JH, Kim SD, Kim SH, Lim DJ, Park JY. The efficacy of repeated radiofrequency medial branch neurotomy for lumbar facet syndrome. Journal of Korean Neurosurgical Association. 2010;**48**(3):240-243. DOI: 10.3340/jkns.2010.48.3.240. Epub 2010 Sep 30

[17] Yeung A, Gore S. Endoscopically guided foraminal and dorsal rhizotomy for chronic axial back pain based on cadaver and endoscopically visualized anatomic study. International Journal of Spine Surgery. 2014;**8**:23. DOI: 10.14444/1023

[18] Bogduk N. The lumbar mamillo-accessory ligament. Its anatomical and neurosurgical significance. Spine (Phila Pa 1976). 1981;**6**(2):162-167. DOI: 10.1097/00007632-198103000-00010

[19] Kambin P, Sampson S. Posterolateral percutaneous suction-excision of herniated lumbar intervertebral discs. Report of interim results. Clinical Orthopaedics and Related Research. 1986;**207**:37-43. DOI: 10.1097/00003086-198606000-00008

[20] Haufe SM, Mork AR. Endoscopic facet debridement for the treatment of facet arthritic pain--a novel new technique. International Journal of Medical Sciences. 2010;**7**(3):120-123. DOI: 10.7150/ijms.7.120

[21] Xue Y, Ding T, Wang D, Zhao J, Yang H, Gu X, et al. Endoscopic rhizotomy for chronic lumbar zygapophysial joint pain. Journal of Orthopaedic Surgery and Research. 2020;**15**(1):4. DOI: 10.1186/s13018-019-1533-y

[22] Meloncelli S, Germani G, Urti I, Divizia M, Rosciano M, Puntillo F, et al. Endoscopic radiofrequency facet joint treatment in patients with low back pain: Technique and long-term results. A prospective cohort study. Therapeutic Advances in Musculoskeletal Disease. 2020;**12**:1759720X20958979. DOI: 10.1177/1759720X20958979

[23] Hayes VM, Siddiqi FN, Romero JM. Endoscopic rhizotomy. In: Scuderi G, Tria A, editors. Minimally Invasive Surgery in Orthopedics. Cham: Springer; 2015. DOI: DOI. 10.1007/978-3-319-15206-6_110-1

Chapter 7

Anterior Approach to the Cervical Spine: Past, Present, and Future

Max S. Fleisher and Michael K. Rosner

Abstract

This chapter discusses anterior cervical spine surgery and its evolution over time. It is divided into three sections: Past, Present, and Future. The first section reviews the history of this approach, with special attention directed towards its conception, early innovations, and instrumentation that have shaped the techniques used today. Present delves into the questions that remain unanswered today as innovation continues. Topics will include the age old question of fusion versus arthroplasty and the utility of an intraoperative microscope. Expansion of indications in the present day will be covered briefly as well in this section. The final section is a glimpse of future directions. Technical advances on the horizon, including endoscope, exoscope, and intraoperative ultrasound, as they relate to anterior cervical spine surgery, will be explored as opportunities to take the safety and efficacy of this approach to new heights.

Keywords: spine, anterior, cervical, arthroplasty, fusion, history, innovations

1. Introduction

The approach to the anterior cervical spine is still relatively new. In a short amount of time, operations such as anterior cervical discectomy and fusion (ACDF) and cervical disc arthroplasty (CDA) have evolved from theoretical treatment options for degenerative disc disease to common procedures with a rapidly-growing list of indications. In this chapter, the authors describe the people who discovered the approach and facilitated its growing popularity as a safe surgical corridor to the spine, as well as early innovations and early criticisms. The authors discuss pertinent technical questions that have persisted from conception to present day. And finally, the future directions of the operation are explored with special attention to cutting edge technology and adaptations of well-known surgical adjuncts. The anterior approach to cervical spine pathology originated in the 1950s, but the story of its development starts well before this. It emerged from a necessity to address ventral cervical spine pathologies without having to circumnavigate the spinal cord, and in a more direct manner than the already well-established posterior approach. The approach is a byproduct of other procedures that developed over time, namely the cervical discogram. Once a theoretical corridor became reality, early pioneers adapted old instruments and created new ones in order to improve the flow and safety of the operation. The result of their work is the procedure we know today. ACDF and its motion-preserving cousin, CDA, represent common neurosurgical operations used to address cervical degenerative disc disease causing debilitating radiculopathy and myelopathy. The list of pathologies addressed by anterior cervical spine surgery is ever-growing. However the fundamentals of the procedure have largely stood the test of time. Researchers and clinicians alike continue to draw comparisons between ACDF and CDA, the current gold standard versus its increasingly popular alternative, respectively. For both operations, the future is lined with cutting-edge technology, with twin goals of providing better care to these patients and educating the next generation of spine surgeons.

2. Methods

The contents of this chapter are supplemented with Pubmed research. Keywords such as those provided above led to many of the papers used for this writing. Figures and Tables are created by the authors based on their research but are nonetheless original works.

3. Past

To fully appreciate the technical advances and future directions of anterior cervical spine surgery, one must start by looking back to the origins of this approach. All aspects of neurosurgery are still relatively young compared to other surgical fields, and anterior dissection of the neck for cervical fusion or arthroplasty is no exception. Even though just a little over a century has passed since its conception, this approach has rapidly developed into a widely-utilized workhorse of the neurosurgeon's armamentarium, with numerous instruments designed specifically with safety and efficiency of these operations in mind.

An anterior approach to the cervical spine arose out of necessity but also from other existing procedures at the time. Surgeons desired a way to reach cervical spine pathology without having to traverse or retract the spinal cord, as with a posterior approach, and without having to navigate the vertebral arteries, as with a lateral trajectory. Could one adequately decompress neural elements of the cervical spine while simultaneously protecting the vital structures of trachea, esophagus, and carotid sheath contents? And furthermore, could instability of the cervical spine be addressed in this manner as well?

Posterior approaches were described prior to anterior approaches likely due to the palpability of the spinous processes and the more superficial nature of the cervical spine going from that direction. Anterior cervical approaches developed in the late 1800s and early 1900s mostly in the treatment of tuberculosis and bony lesions such as osteoma, not for the purpose of treating degenerative disc disease. Transbuccal and transoral approaches have been described as early as 1896 and 1911, respectively [1]. These approaches were eventually abandoned until the widespread use of perioperative antibiotics. The anterior approach classically used today arose shortly after the growing use of a diagnostic procedure known as provocative discography. Lumbar discograms were first reported by K Lindblom in 1948, and the cervical version was used extensively by Ralph Cloward, who credited Exum Walker with the first cervical discogram in 1955 [2, 3]. Safe passage of a needle between trachea and esophagus medially and the carotid artery laterally was used to inject contrast into the disc to ascertain whether a patient had disc degeneration or protrusion, and furthermore, to classify their pain as discogenic, neurogenic, or cord [3].

This procedure, which developed several years after lumbar provocative discography, demonstrated a theoretical surgical corridor to the cervical spine. With increased use, and the normalization of perioperative antibiotics, variations of the pre-sternocleidomastoid approach were developed. Henry described a retro-carotid retropharyngeal approach in 1957 to access the vertebral artery, transverse foramen, and exiting nerve roots. One year later, Smith and Robinson described the pre-carotid approach used today [4]. That same year, Cloward published a paper describing his technique for this same approach [5]. Similar technical papers were published in the 1960s and 70s [1].

The anterior cervical discectomy and fusion (ACDF) indicated for treatment of cervical spondylosis was first described by Robinson and Smith in 1955. Their technique and first series of cases was further outlined in 1958, the same year as Cloward's technical paper. Robinson and Smith reported on their first 55 cases by 1962. Fusion techniques described by Cloward drew criticism from colleagues, including W.B. Scoville, who showed concern that fusion of two vertebral segments may lead to accelerated degeneration of adjacent levels, a phenomenon known today as adjacent segment disease (ASD) [1]. This topic is still widely debated, and is the main justification for the emergence and rising popularity of cervical disc arthroplasty, a "motion-preserving" operation [6].

Cloward, who played a pivotal role in American history as the sole neurosurgeon in Hawaii during Pearl Harbor, would go on to design over 100 instruments in his career, many of which helped establish the anterior cervical approach as one of the most utilized operations in neurosurgery [7]. He was instrumental in developing a vertebral body spreader for lumbar disc space distraction (1952) and a modification of this instrument for the cervical spine (1971). The handheld retractor commonly used to safely move the trachea and esophagus away from the plane of dissection bear his name. He advocated for leaving a drain at the end of his ACDFs in 1977 and turned his attention to a suitable bone graft, suggesting sterilized cadaver bone, and thereby helping conceptualize one of the first bone banks for iliac crest allografts [8]. His contributions to the origin of the ACDF and his contributions to the field of neurosurgery in general cannot be overstated.

Many of the instruments used in spine surgery, including anterior cervical spine dissection, were designed with these procedures in mind. Many others arose from different fields and were merely adapted or modified slightly for neurosurgical purposes. For example, the Woodson elevator and Freer elevator are instruments originally designed for dentistry, used as spatulas to carry fillers and fill cavities. Woodson was an excellent surgeon, but also a renowned family physician and dentist in Kansas in the late 1800s. The Kerrison rongeur, another staple of the spine surgeon's instrumentation set, was designed by an otologist, Dr. Kerrison. He wanted an instrument that would protect the facial nerve during bony removal, preventing the dreaded complication of facial paralysis. The rongeur was designed to remove bone safely "from inside-out" as opposed to the original method of hammer and chisel. The Kerrison rongeur has been adapted over time to anterior cervical spine surgery for safe decompression of the neural foramina, osteophyte removal, and posterior longitudinal ligament removal. Kerrison noted in his 1904 paper introducing the instrument, and anyone who has assisted in a spine surgery can attest to this, that the rongeur only works effectively if it is cleaned off after every single bite [9].

The self-retaining retractor systems used in the ACDF procedures performed today are largely results of the technical innovations and instrument designs by

Cloward, McCullough, and Caspar. Born in Latvia in the 1930s, Wolfhard Caspar aspired to become a pilot in the air force, but his vision limited him to the life of a neurosurgeon. He designed one the first standardized instrument kit specifically designed for ACDFs. These kits included the Caspar pins and Caspar distractors widely used today for vertebral body distraction. His distraction technique had several advantages over the prior vertebral body spreaders designed by Cloward. First, they docked into the vertebral bodies, rather than into the disc space, allowing greater visualization. And second, they were not limited to one disc space; if the pins were placed in non-adjacent vertebrae, theoretically one could distract over multiple interspaces. And third, the pins could be inserted at acute or obtuse angles for more anterior or posterior distraction based on the demands of the specific case. His kits included the first plating system, as the indications for anterior cervical fusion were expanding to include trauma and tumor [9]. The pioneers of the anterior cervical approach rapidly developed the operation into the one we know today. They described innovative techniques, opening a world of possibilities for the treatment of cervical spine pathology. What was previously inaccessible or limited via a posterior approach, was deemed possible after seeing the development of the cervical discogram procedure. They designed instruments specifically for this purpose, and adapted others to make surgical treatment of the anterior cervical spine safe and effective.

As with all innovations, many criticized the novel idea of the ACDF, despite its technical description by multiple authors and reproducible results. As Cloward had pointed out at the time, "you can always tell a pioneer, he is the one with the arrows in his back" [9]. With Scoville's concern of adjacent segment degeneration in mind, there was a push for an alternative remedy for cervical disc herniation refractory to conservative management. The first cervical disc arthroplasty (CDA), also known today as a total disc replacement (TDR) or total disc arthroplasty, was described in 1966 by Ulf Fernstrom [10]. It involved a ball-bearing implant with stainless steel design, but fell out of favor due to numerous cases of implant migration, subsidence, and adjacent segment hypermobility. New designs would not re-emerge until the conclusion of the 1980s, with the reproducible successes of the ACDF taking precedence as the preferred surgical treatment of cervical spondylosis [11].

4. Present

The techniques used today for the anterior approach to the cervical spine, on a fundamental level, have withstood the test of time. Cloward and Smith and Robinson's papers on ACDF technique mirror the procedure used in the present day. Since then, we have seen further advances in our equipment: monopolar and bipolar electrocautery, surgical loupes and intraoperative microscopes for greater visualization, customizable tool kits to fit surgeons' individual preferences, and increased variability in bone graft delivery (graft material, cage material, cage shapes and sizes, plate length and thickness). However, the steps of the procedure have largely remained the same. Despite the innumerable choices of instrumentation on the market, the road the the anterior surface of the cervical spine still includes an incision well hidden in a natural fold of the neck, appropriately chosen based on localization of the right level with XRay or fluoroscopy, sectioning and careful undermining of the platysma, separating the fascial plane medial to the carotid sheath, protecting the medial structures including trachea and esophagus with your Cloward retractor, dissection of the prevertebral fascia, and localizing once more to ensure you have landed on the intended disc space.

As improvements in visibility and hemostasis and fusion materials progress throughout time, some questions remain unanswered, and new questions emerge. Old questions, such as fusion versus arthroplasty, are still being explored today. When should a patient be offered motion-preserving disc replacement as opposed to fusion, and what are the differences in long-term outcomes for each? Surgeons continue to adapt their techniques to avoid complications. There remains a strong desire to minimize the risks of dysphagia, hoarseness, pain, infection, hematoma, and cerebrospinal fluid leak just as in the past. New questions, often a matter of surgeon preference, emerge, such as the use of intraoperative microscope vs. loupes, or the use of Caspar pins vs. the more antiquated disc space spreader, or whether to use blunt dissection or sharp dissection of the various fascial planes encountered.

A search on PubMed for papers discussing ACDF versus total disc replacement will yield just under 100 results, several of which have follow up data ten years post-operatively. This would suggest that there remains clinical equipoise regarding the appropriate use of the two alternatives. The ongoing issue of adjacent level disease after fusing two or more vertebral bodies together sparked a new lineage of disc arthroplasty devices, despite the shortcomings of the first-generation implants.

With a new line of fusion and arthroplasty devices on the market, and, at its fundamental level, the same safe anterior cervical corridor discovered and used in the 1950s, the stage has been set to determine whether this relatively young technique should lead to placement of a fusion device or a motion-preservation device to aid in the prevention of adjacent level disease. Cervical arthroplasty, as we know from the early adaptations which failed, has drawbacks of its own. Motion-preservation is a moot point in cases of trauma or tumor, where instability needs to be addressed with bony fusion. However, in cases of degenerative disc disease, with primarily ventral decompression necessary, there remains a question of which technique provides the best durable outcome. CDA has rapidly grown in popularity as a viable alternative. An epidemiological review from Brown University 2024 suggests that over the past decade, there has been a 650% increase in utilization of CDA, plateauing in 2019. ACDF had appeared to plateau around 2014, with a much more modest increase in use from 2011 to 2014. This review included over 400,000 patients [12]. However, whether one is superior to the other in complication profile and long term efficacy remains to be seen.

One recent study of 190 patients distributed somewhat evenly into two groups suggests that even patients with symptoms persisting over six months note significant improvement in pain, function, and mental health regardless of treatment modality. These improvements persist beyond six week follow up through final follow up visits [13].

A retrospective study of over 2000 pts. who underwent either ACDF or CDA with similar baseline characteristics suggested no significant differences in surgical or clinical outcomes at two years [14].

Similar comparisons have been made between patients receiving two-level ACDF or two-level CDA. One retrospective study of this nature suggests that the two interventions have similar complication and reoperation rates, regardless of their completion on an inpatient or elective basis. According to one study, sponsored by the device manufacturer, the benefit of CDA over ACDF at the seven year mark became more significant in patients receiving two-level as opposed to single-level surgery, but this finding has yet to be corroborated by other investigators [15, 16].

Another retrospective cohort study of 7450 patients, with surveillance ten years post-operatively, demonstrated no significant difference in "survivability" of the surgery. In other words, whether the patient underwent a single-level ACDF or CDA, the time until a revision surgery (either anterior or posterior approach) was the same in each group. The average time to a second surgery was 6.5 years. Overall revision rate was around 2.5%. There were significantly more patients in the ACDF group, since this modality represents the standard of care, and there were other limitations as well, including significant differences in age, surgical indication, and other demographics between the two cohorts [17].

A recent systematic review with meta-analysis of six comparative studies demonstrated no clinical difference between the two modalities at the ten year mark. There were several statistical differences in the pain and disability scores this far from surgery, but no clinically appreciable difference in those scores. However, the meta-analysis suggested that CDA leads to fewer secondary surgeries over the next ten years, with a statistically significant difference shown between the two groups, but no difference in long-term neurologic outcome [18].

These studies appear to corroborate the claim that total disc replacement has comparable safety and efficacy to ACDF. Many studies are clinically oriented, with outcomes measured with pain and disability indices. Though this is the overarching goal of surgery, there is a relative shortage of studies showing long term radiographic outcomes of each approach. It is implied that an increase in secondary surgery for the ACDF group is attributable to adjacent segment disease, but large studies with long follow-up periods are often unable to demonstrate that the revision surgery was at the adjacent level, or the same level, or a remote level. Also, these large cohort studies and systematic reviews fail to investigate whether the revision was due to failure of fusion, adjacent level disease confirmed with imaging that matches physical exam findings, or due to heterotopic ossification in the case of arthroplasty.

In short, many studies are dedicated to this ongoing question of fusion versus arthroplasty, with an overall trend towards understanding that the two have similar safety and efficacy, with total disc replacement potentially preventing secondary surgery in the long term.

Regardless of implantable device, fusion or arthroplasty, the goal is to address the pathology in the safest and most efficient way possible. The adaptation of the intraoperative microscope to the ACDF by Hankinson and Wilson in 1975 has raised the question of its utility in this approach [19]. The surgery can be done with or without the microscope, according to surgeon preference, but does its implementation affect the clinical outcome? It may aid in teaching, as the learner or observer often has difficulty seeing what the lead surgeon sees through the small opening in the neck without the aid of the microscope. But what is best for the patient? In one study of 140 patients without prior ACDF or confounding comorbidities (rheumatoid arthritis, osteoarthritis, etc.), clinical outcomes and complication rates were compared between those patients whose ACDF surgery included use of an intraoperative microscope and those whose ACDF did not. There was no statistically significant difference in age, BMI or preoperative functional status between the two groups. Post-operative complications and clinical outcomes did not differ significantly between the two groups, at both three month follow up and two year follow up. The only statistically significant difference in outcome was the duration of surgery. The authors also noted that surgical costs rise with use of an intraoperative microscope. These findings mirrored the results of studies on use of the microscope for other surgical specialties [20]. As such, its utilization seems to be non-inferior to using surgical loupes only with regard to clinical outcomes. It may offer better visualization for both the surgeon and assistant and observers, but users should keep in mind the additional OR time and anesthesia time that often result from time needed to adjust the microscope for optimum visualization of the surgical field throughout the case.

Recent innovations have helped optimize the safety of the anterior cervical approach. Even though the microscope may not change short or long term outcomes of ACDF or CDA, it represents the continually evolving landscape of anterior cervical spine surgery, and an attempt to adapt surgical adjuncts to these operations. New implants have replaced autograft painfully extracted from the patient's iliac crest. New materials are used now with improved functionality and a better understanding of biomechanical principles (i.e. Young's modulus of elasticity) in order to prevent complications such as subsidence and pseudoarthrosis. Low-profile plates and stand-alone cages that do not require a plate at all have emerged as popular alternatives to standard cage-and-plate constructs. Self-locking, stand-alone constructs, in comparison to those utilizing a plate, appear to reduce the incidence of postoperative dysphagia, but may not provide the long-term maintenance of cervical lordosis that a plate provides, making them preferable for degenerative cases, but a potential liability for trauma cases and those with a higher level of instability [21]. Bipolar and monopolar cautery, as well as gelatin sponges soaked in thrombin and injectable hemostatic agents minimize blood loss to the point that leaving a drain at the conclusion of the procedure is often superfluous [22].

Regardless of technical nuances employed by various neurosurgeons and orthopedic surgeons, the procedure has progressed to the point where patients often leave the hospital the same day. Technical innovation has allowed surgeons to adapt the approach to more complex operations, including multi-level ACDFs, corpectomy, trauma, deformity correction, tumor resections, and much more [23–26].

5. Future

Technical innovation comes in many forms. Anything from a Cloward handheld retractor to a high-powered intraoperative microscope serves to advance our field in a positive direction. Future directions for anterior cervical spine surgery follow the innovations of past and present. In this section, the authors explore the utility of endoscopic techniques, exoscopic techniques, intraoperative ultrasound, and augmented and virtual reality as they apply to ACDF and CDA.

Endoscopic techniques have been slowly integrated into the world of spinal surgery since the 1990s [27]. The endoscope has been used sporadically since that time with reproducible, successful results as a minimally-invasive approach to lumbar and cervical disc herniations alike. The anterior endoscopic technique for cervical disc herniation management fell out of favor briefly since these patients grew highly susceptible to persistent postoperative pain and kyphotic deformities. Out of this shortcoming came the need for endoscopic ACDF. A retrospective study from China followed 67 patients who underwent fully-endoscopic ACDF with a five year follow-up period. These procedures started with a small transverse incision after localization, and blunt dissection with the surgeon's finger down to the anterior longitudinal ligament, lateral to the trachea and esophagus, and medial to the carotid sheath. Localization was repeated after deploying the first endoscopic dilator. After a series of dilators, the endoscopic system was docked onto the disc space of interest. Discectomy was carried out with a microknife, forceps and curettes, and manual traction was administered before placing an appropriately sized cage made of carbon fiber reinforced polymer, filled with autologous bone graft from the pt's iliac crest. Drains were placed in all cases. All cases were single-level. No cases needed to be converted to open. Mean operative time was 107 minutes and only one patient had a revision six years post-operatively for adjacent segment disease [28].

These patients paved the way for endoscopic ACDF as a potential alternative to conventional ACDF. The potential benefits include smaller incision (2 cm), faster recovery time, faster return to work time, and decreased narcotic use post-operatively. The authors did concede that a potential challenge would be control of intraoperative bleeding, which they rarely encountered in their study. Another would be the limitation of manual distraction. Endoscopic approach to the anterior cervical spine does not yet allow for placement of a vertebral body distractor or Caspar pins. Staff had to pull up on the patient's head and down on their shoulders while they are asleep, making neuromonitoring even more imperative during these cases where a focal distraction cannot be achieved. Nevertheless, endoscopic surgery for mild to moderate cervical spondylosis causing myelopathy or radiculopathy has been studied on multiple occasions as a safe and efficacious alternative to conventional ACDF, with no significant difference in clinical outcomes or complication profiles, but a tendency to increase duration of the operation [28, 29]. Like the intraoperative microscope, the endoscope utility for ACDF and CDA may be for a select patient cohort that values minimal scarring and in the academic setting where observers and lead surgeons alike have increased visualization to aid in education. Whether or not its routine use will benefit clinical outcomes, reduce harm, or speed recovery time still needs further delineation.

As endoscopic spine surgery continues to gain traction, another technical innovation has raised questions regarding its own utility. The exoscope, as its name would imply, is a device for enhanced visualization that hovers outside the surgical field, in opposition to the endoscope, which goes inside the body. Its utilization in cranial operations and other surgical subspecialties continues to expand, but its adaptation to the anterior cervical spine remains a relatively novel endeavor.

The use of the exoscope in neurosurgical procedures dates back as far as the 1990's, however the most recent generation of this technology has been applied to anterior cervical spine surgery only within the last decade [30]. In theory, the exoscope allows the same advantages as the use of an intraoperative microscope. Though it may take extra time for setup and setting adjustments throughout the case, it would allow better illumination and magnification, and enhanced visualization especially for an observer. The putative advantages of exoscope over microscope are numerous. The exoscope has increased maneuverability and does not interfere with certain instruments that are long and can potentially bump into the microscope during their use. Second, the exoscope allows for multiple learners or assistants to watch on the screen with 3D viewing glasses, as opposed to the intraoperative microscope which really only allows for one observer to comfortably get the same viewing experience as the primary surgeon.

One of the first reports of its use for ACDF appeared in 2019. Two patients in Italy underwent a two-level ACDF with good results using the exoscope for enhanced teaching purposes [31]. Further comparisons to operative microscope use for dozens of ACDF patients suggested that the visualization for the operator may be slightly inferior with the exoscope, although visualization for the observers was rated as superior. All in all, the exoscope seems to provide better visualization for the assistants and observers, worse visualization for the lead surgeon, and increased comfort level from an ergonomic standpoint for the surgeon when compared to the operative microscope [32, 33]. In addition, a recent study suggested no difference in operative time, length of hospital stay, or complication rates, but did suggest decreased estimated blood loss with use of exoscope [34].

The use of an exoscope for ACDF was not significantly different than the use of surgical loupes or intraoperative microscope in terms of intraoperative costs, with the exception of consumables, such as drapes required for the device. However, there tends to be an exceptionally high upfront cost for an exoscope, ranging from $200,000 to $1.5 million, making it inaccessible for many institutions [35]. Nevertheless, the exoscope appears to be a reasonable alternative to the operative microscope for use in ACDF and TDR. It offers increased visualization compared to surgical loupes, less interference with long instruments compared to the microscope, and better visualization for learners and assistants to the primary surgeon. The shortcomings of upfront cost and decreased visualization compared to microscopy (for the main operator) may be overcome in the near future to make it an irreplaceable education tool during anterior cervical spine surgery. Like the microscope, the exoscope does not appear in early comparisons to increase the safety or efficacy of ACDF, but seems to serve as a useful educational tool for others present in these cases. **Table 1** provides a brief overview of the technological innovations adapted to ACDF/CDA, and comparison of their strengths and weaknesses in relation to the use of surgical loupes.

Table 1 represents a side-by-side comparison of microscope, endoscope, and exoscope, in terms of advancing safety, efficacy, and educational value during anterior cervical spine surgery. Arrows indicate a relative increase or decrease of the variable compared to use of surgical loupes only. Relative cost is indicated by the number of "$" symbols.

New instrumentation designed with a specific task in mind represents one aspect of technical innovation. Far more commonly, however, innovators find novel ways to repurpose old instruments. The microscope, endoscope, exoscope, and many other surgical adjuncts were not designed for the anterior approach to the cervical spine. There are very few Caspars and Clowards of the world today, who design a set of instruments for a specific operation, and put these together in a kit. Innovators now look to the past, and see what can be repurposed for an operation with set kits that have withstood the test of time.

Another surgical adjunct adapted for the future of ACDF is the ultrasound. The design of smaller and smaller transducers allows surgeons to obtain intraoperative images in hard to reach places. The anterior cervical spine is no exception. In August 2024, a proof of concept study demonstrated the feasibility of using a minimally-invasive ultrasound probe on the anterior cervical spine to visualize the neural

	Magnification	**Ergonomics**	**Visualization for operator**	**Visualization for others (Educational value)**	**EBL**	**Duration of surgery**	**Upfront cost**
Microscope	↑↑	↓	↑↑	↑	↓	↑	$$
Endoscope	↑	↑	↑	↑	↓↓	↑	$
Exoscope	↑	↑↑	↑	↑↑	↓↓	↑	$$

Table 1.
Comparison of technological adjuncts for anterior cervical dissection.

elements. The small probe successfully identified central and foraminal stenosis after discectomy was completed, without having to remove distraction pins (Caspar pins), and was influential in directing further decompression in around half of the reported cases. When an absence of CSF pulsatility around the spinal cord or relevant nerve root was noted, further decompression was warranted. Whether or not the use of intraoperative ultrasound affects patient outcomes, operative duration, and complication rates remains to be seen [36].

Virtual reality has been integrated into multiple cranial and spinal neurosurgical procedures from a patient education standpoint, but also as an educational tool and even an adjunct to surgery in order to facilitate incisional planning, craniotomy planning, and screw trajectories during fusion procedures. Its utility in ACDF procedure remains limited at this point. It has been used mostly as an educational tool where residents and students alike have opportunities to practice the procedure in a virtual environment [37].

6. Conclusion

The anterior approach to the cervical spine dates back to the 1950s, an epiphany arising from the cervical discogram. The techniques and instruments used today remain relatively unchanged from their conception, corroborating the brilliance of those who designed it and created the tools necessary to make it safe, effective, and reproducible by others. The timelines provided show the rapid development of the operation and the technology used in a brief period of time (**Figures 1** and 2). The early innovators and early adopters of the ACDF adapted technology from other specialties and designed several tools and kits of their own. This trend continues on today, as surgeons and researchers continue to develop new equipment, and adapt old instrumentation for novel purposes. The age-old question of fusion versus a motion-preserving arthroplasty procedure remains in the present day. Ongoing discussions of ideal surgical candidates for each and whether one reliably produces a better, more durable, clinical outcome permeates the current literature. The approach is the same for each, and the differences in pain and function outcome measures are often imperceptible according to most studies. With ACDF, stability is gained at the risk of

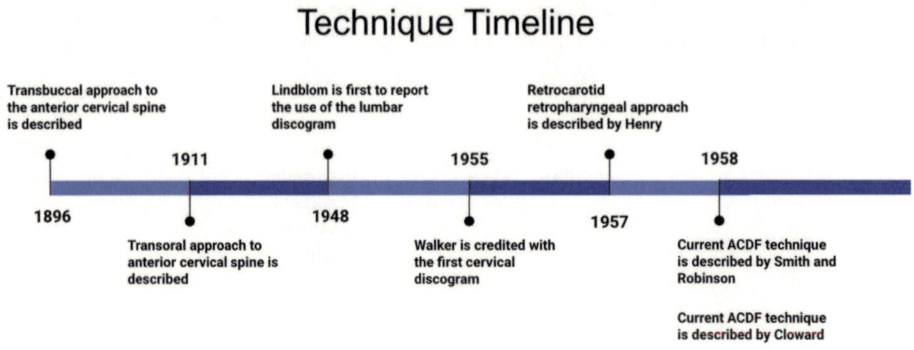

Figure 1.
*Technique timeline. **Figure 1** demonstrates the stepwise progression of techniques used to address anterior cervical spine pathology, culminating in the current approach for ACDF and TDR, outlined by Cloward as well as Smith and Robinson in 1958.*

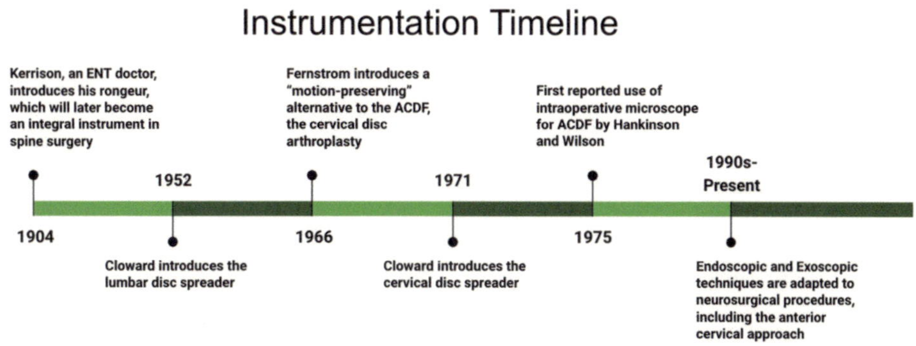

Figure 2.
Instrumentation timeline. ***Figure 2*** *provides a similar visual, but this time shows the innovative devices designed for anterior cervical spine surgery, and those adapted from other specialties.*

adjacent segment disease later on. With CDA, motion is preserved at the expense of stability, and eventual fusion in the form of heterotopic ossification still looms years down the road. Patient selection remains key, avoiding patients with relative contra-indications for each. Risk profiles appear equivalent, but some studies suggest CDA may prevent secondary surgeries over a ten year follow up period. ACDF remains the gold standard today, but we are already beginning to see a future where both options are equally viable in the right patient population. The future is lined with new (and old) modalities to further educate the next generation of surgeons. The intraoperative microscope, ultrasound, exoscope, endoscope, as well as augmented reality, all serve as means to aid both the operator and those who wish to learn the techniques put into practice by our common ancestors not long ago.

Acknowledgements

The authors of this chapter would like to thank the editors, publishers and all those who helped make this book possible, and who invited us to contribute. They would like to acknowledge the physicians who paved the way for the techniques discussed.

Conflict of interest

The authors declare no conflict of interest.

Author details

Max S. Fleisher* and Michael K. Rosner
Department of Neurosurgery, George Washington University Hospital,
Washington, DC, USA

*Address all correspondence to: maxsfleisher@gwu.edu

References

[1] Denaro V, Di Martino A. Cervical spine surgery: An historical perspective. Clinical Orthopaedics and Related Research. 2011;**469**(3):639-648. DOI: 10.1007/s11999-010-1752-3

[2] Lindblom K. Diagnostic puncture of intervertebral disks in sciatica. Acta Orthopaedica Scandinavica. 1948;**17**(3-4):231-239. DOI: 10.3109/17453674808988943

[3] Klafta LA Jr, Collis JS Jr. The diagnostic inaccuracy of the pain response in cervical discography. Cleveland Clinic Quarterly. 1969;**36**(1):35-39. DOI: 10.3949/ccjm.36.1.35

[4] Smith GW, Robinson RA. The treatment of certain cervical-spine disorders by anterior removal of the intervertebral disc and interbody fusion. The Journal of Bone and Joint Surgery. American Volume. 1958;**40-A**(3):607-624

[5] Cloward RB. The anterior approach for removal of ruptured cervical disks. Journal of Neurosurgery. 1958;**15**(6):602-617. DOI: 10.3171/jns.1958.15.6.0602

[6] Denaro V, Papalia R, Denaro L, Di Martino A, Maffulli N. Cervical spinal disc replacement. Journal of Bone and Joint Surgery. British Volume (London). 2009;**91**(6):713-719. DOI: 10.1302/0301-620X.91B6.22025

[7] Sherrod BA, Wilkerson CG, Rolston JD, Bisson EF, Mazur MD, Couldwell WT, et al. Neurosurgery at Pearl Harbor: Ralph Cloward's legacy. Neurosurgical Focus. 2022;**53**(3):E14. DOI: 10.3171/2022.6.FOCUS22127

[8] Maiti TK, Konar SK, Bir SC, Kalakoti P, Nanda A. Ralph Bingham Cloward (1908-2000): Spine polymath. World Neurosurgery. 2016;**89**:562-567. DOI: 10.1016/j.wneu.2015.06.061

[9] Buraimoh M, Basheer A, Taliaferro K, Shaw JH, Haider S, Graziano G, et al. Origins of eponymous instruments in spine surgery. Journal of Neurosurgery. Spine. 2018;**29**(6):696-703. DOI: 10.3171/2018.5.SPINE17981

[10] Fernström U. Arthroplasty with intercorporal endoprothesis in herniated disc and in painful disc. Acta Chirurgica Scandinavica. Supplementum. 1966;**357**:154-159

[11] Derman PB, Zigler JE. Cervical disc arthroplasty: Rationale and history. International Journal of Spine Surgery. 2020;**14**(s2):S5-S13. DOI: 10.14444/7086

[12] Singh M, Balmaceno-Criss M, Anderson G, Parhar K, Daher M, Gregorczyk J, et al. Anterior cervical discectomy and fusion versus cervical disc arthroplasty: An epidemiological review of 433,660 surgical patients from 2011 to 2021. The Spine Journal. 2024;**24**(8):1342-1351. DOI: 10.1016/j.spinee.2024.02.016

[13] Hartman TJ, Nie JW, Khosla I, Oyetayo OO, MacGregor KR, Zheng E, et al. Cervical disk replacement versus anterior cervical Diskectomy and fusion: Effect of procedural variant on patients with a prolonged preoperative duration of symptoms from disk herniation. The Journal of the American Academy of Orthopaedic Surgeons. 2024;**32**(12):558-562. DOI: 10.5435/JAAOS-D-23-00655

[14] Miller AK, Zakko P, Park DK, Chang VW, Schultz L, Springer K, et al. Cervical disc arthroplasty versus anterior cervical discectomy and fusion: An

analysis of the Michigan spine surgery improvement collaborative database. The Spine Journal. 2024;**24**(5):791-799. DOI: 10.1016/j.spinee.2023.12.004

[15] Doan MK, Chung AS, Makovicka JL, Hassebrock JD, Polveroni TM, Patel KA. Comparison of two-level cervical disc replacement versus two-level anterior cervical discectomy and fusion in the outpatient setting. Spine. 2021;**46**(10):658-664. DOI: 10.1097/BRS.0000000000003871

[16] Radcliff K, Davis RJ, Hisey MS, Nunley PD, Hoffman GA, Jackson RJ, et al. Long-term evaluation of cervical disc arthroplasty with the Mobi-C© cervical disc: A randomized, prospective, Multicenter clinical trial with seven-year follow-up. International Journal of Spine Surgery. 2017;**11**(4):31. DOI: 10.14444/4031

[17] Paek S, Zelenty WD, Dodo Y, Sarin M, Shue J, Soffin EM, et al. Up to 10-year surveillance comparison of survivability in single-level cervical disc replacement versus anterior cervical discectomy and fusion in New York. Journal of Neurosurgery. Spine. 2023;**39**(2):206-215. DOI: 10.3171/2023.3.SPINE221377

[18] Quinto ES Jr, Paisner ND, Huish EG Jr, Senegor M. Ten-year outcomes of cervical disc arthroplasty versus anterior cervical discectomy and fusion: A systematic review with meta-analysis. Spine. 2024;**49**(7):463-469. DOI: 10.1097/BRS.0000000000004887

[19] Hankinson HL, Wilson CB. Use of the operating microscope in anterior cervical discectomy without fusion. Journal of Neurosurgery. 1975;**43**(4):452-456. DOI: 10.3171/jns.1975.43.4.0452

[20] Adogwa O, Elsamadicy A, Reiser E, Ziegler C, Freischlag K, Cheng J, et al. Comparison of surgical outcomes after anterior cervical discectomy and fusion: Does the intra-operative use of a microscope improve surgical outcomes. Journal of Spine Surgery. 2016;**2**(1):25-30. DOI: 10.21037/jss.2016.01.04

[21] Zhang Y, Ju J, Wu J. Self-locking stand-alone cage versus cage-plate fixation in monosegmental anterior cervical discectomy and fusion with a minimum 2-year follow-up: A systematic review and meta-analysis. Journal of Orthopaedic Surgery and Research. 2023;**18**(1):403. DOI: 10.1186/s13018-023-03885-4

[22] Battistelli M, Polli FM, D'Alessandris QG, D'Ercole M, Izzo A, Rapisarda A, et al. An overview of recent advances in anterior cervical decompression and fusion surgery. Surgical Technology International. 2023;**43**:sti43/1732. DOI: 10.52198/23.STI.43.NS1732

[23] Angevine PD, Kellner C, Haque RM, McCormick PC. Surgical management of ventral intradural spinal lesions. Journal of Neurosurgery. Spine. 2011;**15**(1):28-37. DOI: 10.3171/2011.3.SPINE1095

[24] Lau D, Ziewacz JE, Le H, Wadhwa R, Mummaneni PV. A controlled anterior sequential interbody dilation technique for correction of cervical kyphosis. Journal of Neurosurgery. Spine. 2015;**23**(3):263-273. DOI: 10.3171/2014.12.SPINE14178

[25] Russo VM, Graziano F, Russo A, Albanese E, Ulm AJ. High anterior cervical approach to the clivus and foramen magnum: A microsurgical anatomy study. Neurosurgery. 2011;**69**(1 Suppl Operative):s103, s115-s114, s116. DOI: 10.1227/NEU.0b013e31821664a6

[26] Chang HK, Huang WC, Wu JC, Tu TH, Fay LY, Chang PY, et al.

Cervical arthroplasty for traumatic disc herniation: An age- and sex-matched comparison with anterior cervical discectomy and fusion. BMC Musculoskeletal Disorders. 2015;**16**:228. DOI: 10.1186/s12891-015-0692-1

[27] Fontanella A. Endoscopic microsurgery in herniated cervical discs. Neurological Research. 1999;**21**(1):31-38. DOI: 10.1080/01616412.1999.11740888

[28] Yao N, Wang C, Wang W, Wang L. Full-endoscopic technique for anterior cervical discectomy and interbody fusion: 5-year follow-up results of 67 cases. European Spine Journal. 2011;**20**(6):899-904. DOI: 10.1007/s00586-010-1642-0

[29] Tan J, Zheng Y, Gong L, Liu X, Li J, Du W. Anterior cervical discectomy and interbody fusion by endoscopic approach: A preliminary report. Journal of Neurosurgery. Spine. 2008;**8**(1):17-21. DOI: 10.3171/SPI-08/01/017

[30] Wu ZP, Wei ZY, Song XL. Comparison of efficacy between endoscope-assisted anterior cervical discectomy and fusion (ACDF) and open ACDF in the treatment of single-segment cervical spondylotic myelopathy. Journal of Orthopaedic Surgery and Research. 2024;**19**(1):35. DOI: 10.1186/s13018-023-04514-w

[31] Barbagallo GMV, Certo F. Three-dimensional, high-definition Exoscopic anterior cervical discectomy and fusion: A valid alternative to microscope-assisted surgery. World Neurosurgery. 2019;**130**:e244-e250. DOI: 10.1016/j.wneu.2019.06.049

[32] Lin H, Chen F, Mo J, Lin T, Wang Z, Liu W. Cervical spine microsurgery with the high-definition 3D exoscope: Advantages and disadvantages. World Neurosurgery. 2022;**161**:e1-e7. DOI: 10.1016/j.wneu.2021.07.033

[33] Siller S, Zoellner C, Fuetsch M, Trabold R, Tonn JC, Zausinger S. A high-definition 3D exoscope as an alternative to the operating microscope in spinal microsurgery. Journal of Neurosurgery. Spine. 2020;**33**(5):705-714. DOI: 10.3171/2020.4.SPINE20374

[34] Encarnacion Ramirez M, Peralta Baez I, Nurmukhametov R, Goncharov E, Efe IE, Sufianov A, et al. Comparative survey study of the use of a low cost exoscope vs. microscope for anterior cervical discectomy and fusion (ACDF). Frontiers in Medical Technology. 2023;**4**:1055189. DOI: 10.3389/fmedt.2022.1055189

[35] Sarikonda A, Leibold A, Ali DM, Thalheimer S, Heller J, Prasad S, et al. What is the marginal intraoperative cost of using an exoscope or operative microscope for anterior cervical discectomy and fusion? A time-driven activity-based cost analysis. World Neurosurgery. 2024;**181**:e3-e10. DOI: 10.1016/j.wneu.2023.11.069

[36] Chryssikos T, Tawil ME, Ambati VS, Macki M, DiGiorgio AM, Mummaneni PV, et al. Real-time intraoperative ultrasound using a minimally invasive transducer during anterior cervical spine surgery. Operative Neurosurgery. 2024;**27**(2):213-219. DOI: 10.1227/ons.0000000000001065

[37] Ledwos N, Mirchi N, Bissonnette V, Winkler-Schwartz A, Yilmaz R, Del Maestro RF. Virtual reality anterior cervical discectomy and fusion simulation on the novel Sim-Ortho platform: Validation studies. Oper Neurosurg (Hagerstown). 2020;**20**(1):74-82. DOI: 10.1093/ons/opaa269

Chapter 8

Lumbar Disc Surgery: Advances in the Last Few Decades

Ahmed Shawky Abdelgawaad

Abstract

Surgery for lumbar disc herniation is a widely used spinal procedure. In the last three decades, advancements in surgical magnification and illumination have changed the standard procedure from open discectomy to microsurgical discectomy, minimally invasive trans-tubular microdiscectomy, and endoscopic discectomy. The shift from more to less invasiveness was associated with less approach-related surgical trauma, less intraoperative blood loss, reduced postoperative analgesic demand, shorter hospital stays, and rapid ambulation, rehabilitation, and return to work. Subsequently, surgery-related and hospital expenditures are reduced. Long-term outcomes did not prove the superiority of one surgical procedure over the others. This chapter will highlight the commonly used procedures, focusing on the indications, technical steps, advantages, and complications. It will also highlight the future perspectives of treating lumbar disc herniations.

Keywords: lumbar disc herniation, lumbar disc disease, disc prolapse, minimally invasive discectomy, endoscopic discectomy, trans-tubular discectomy

1. Introduction

Lumbar disc herniation is the main cause of discogenic low back pain. Almost 60–80% of people will suffer back pain during their lifetime [1]. Patients commonly present with low back pain and symptoms related to nerve root compression (**Figure 1**). Pain, sensory, and motor deficits distribution depends on the anatomical level affected and the site of herniation [1].

Mixter and Barr first described the surgical treatment of lumbar disc herniation through open discectomy in 1934 [2]. In 1977, Caspar [3] and Yasargil [4] popularized a less invasive microscopic discectomy. Several modifications of the microsurgical technique were reported. Foley popularized the minimally invasive trans-tubular discectomy in 1997. Over the past two decades, different corridors were described to approach different anatomical sites of disc herniations, including postero-lateral, cranially migrated, foraminal and extraforaminal herniations (**Figure 2**) [5, 6]. Kampin was the first to approach the intervertebral disc using an endoscope [7].

In the last three decades, the main highlight of the surgical procedures to treat lumbar disc herniations has been the shift from open traditional surgery to less and minimally invasive procedures with less approach-related collateral tissue injury and

IntechOpen

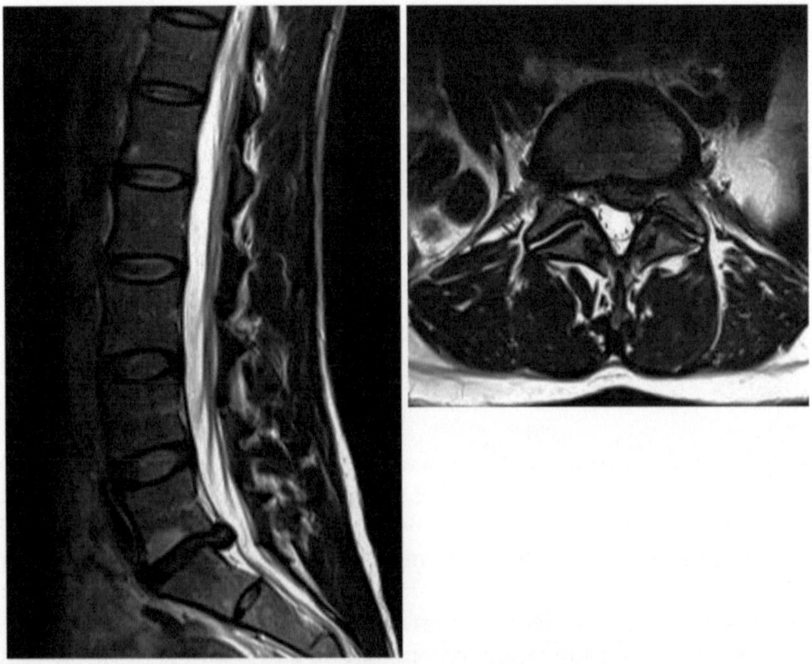

Figure 1.
Sagittal and axial T2 MRI images of a postero-lateral lumbar disc herniation at L5/S1 level.

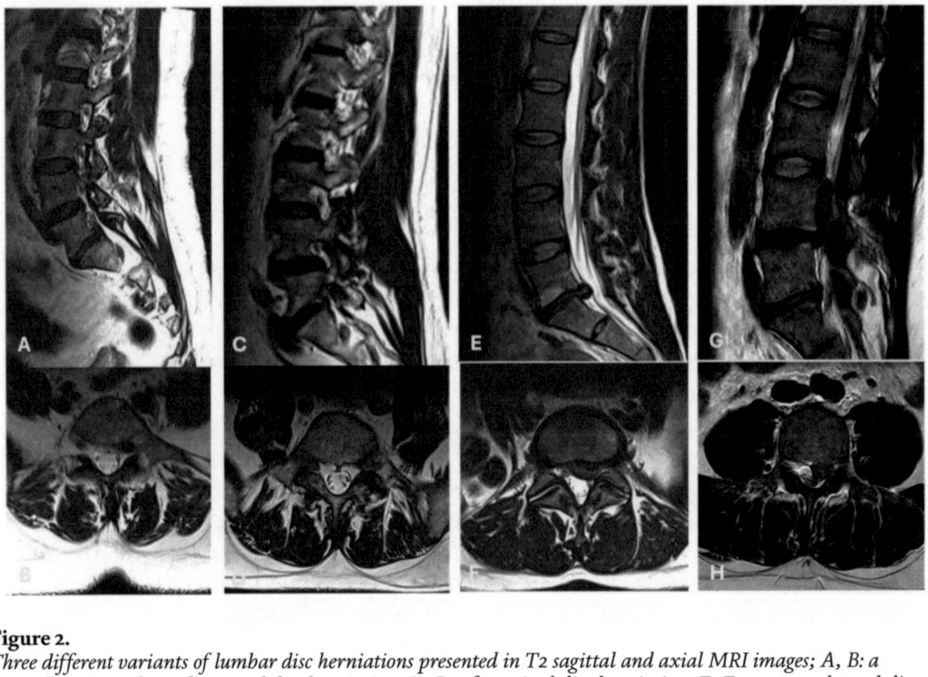

Figure 2.
Three different variants of lumbar disc herniations presented in T2 sagittal and axial MRI images; A, B: a cranially migrated pre-foraminal disc herniation. B, C: a foraminal disc herniation. E, F: a postero-lateral disc herniation. G, H: huge cranially migrated disc herniation.

subsequently improved early postoperative outcomes. Less approach-related muscle injury and collateral tissue trauma have also been objectively proven [8, 9]. Tools and techniques to perform lumbar discectomy have evolved so that surgeons can perform these procedures with limited operative exposures. Furthermore, moving the point of anatomic perspective into the patient's body and closer to the surgical site increases the area and quality of visualization. This improvement in anatomic perspective during surgery minimizes surgical dissection and may allow for reduced requirements for inpatient care, lower surgical expenditures, and expedited recovery [10].

Currently, there is global adoption of endoscopic techniques to lumbar-disc herniations. Many surgeons are shifting from microscopic- to endoscopic-assisted procedures. This shift has its demands related to infrastructure and learning curve [11].

2. Surgical techniques

Several surgical techniques are currently available to manage lumbar disc herniations. This chapter focuses on surgical techniques and does not include pain and interventional techniques, such as infiltration of local anesthetics and steroids or radiofrequency procedures.

The currently available techniques include (**Figure 3**): (1) open surgical discectomy, (2) microsurgical discectomy, (3) trans-tubular microscopic discectomy, (4) uni-portal endoscopic discectomy, (5) bi-portal endoscopic discectomy and (6) micro-endoscopic discectomy. Selecting a specific technique primarily depends on surgical training, available infrastructure, and patient characteristics. In the last three decades, a trend toward minimally invasive techniques is gaining more acceptance. Technological improvements in surgical instruments, magnification, and visualization support this trend. Furthermore, patients' access to media, the internet, and social media platforms impacts the selection of their treating surgeons. This pushes institutions and surgeons to introduce more recent procedures to cope with market demands [12, 13].

The techniques mentioned above have been modified, and different anatomical approaches have been used to access the herniated disc fragment (**Figure 4**).

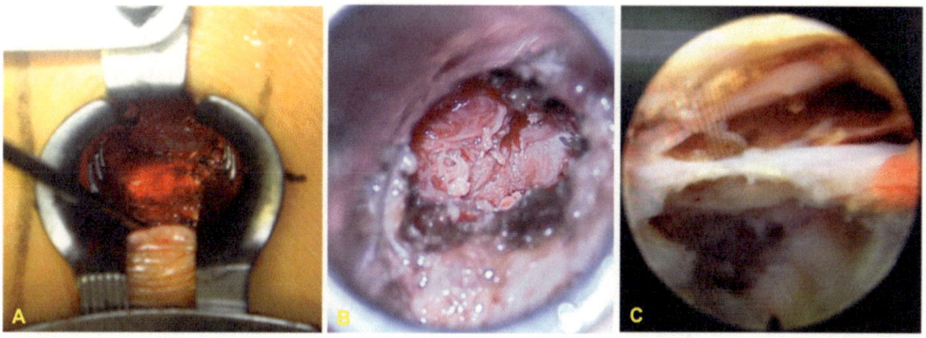

Figure 3.
The different surgical views: A: micro-surgical approach, B: microscopic trans-tubular approach, C: endoscopic approach.

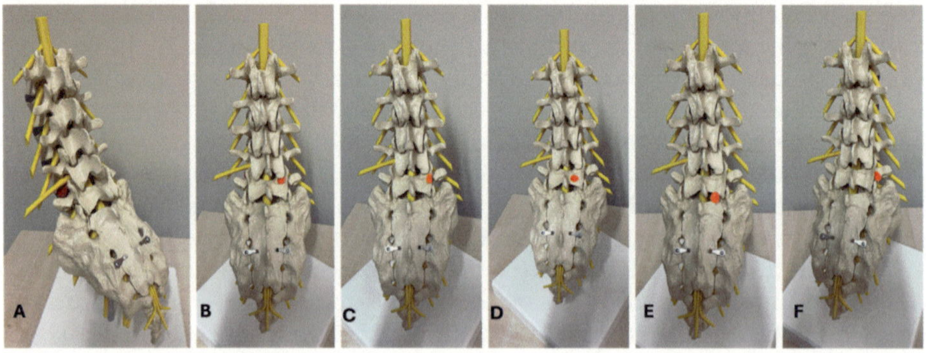

Figure 4.
Different surgical anatomical corridors (windows) to access the disc herniation. A: Extra-foraminal disc herniation. B: Trans-pars window. C: Lateral to the lamina (pars) window. D: Trans-laminar window. E: interlaminar window (the most common). F: Extra-foraminal window.

2.1 Open microsurgical discectomy

The term "microsurgical discectomy" describes removing herniated parts of lumbar intervertebral discs via a posterior approach utilizing a surgical microscope and microsurgical instruments. It applies the general microsurgery principles and accesses the anatomical target area through a small skin incision [14].

For median, postero-lateral, and foraminal disc herniations, the pathology is approached via a median or paramedian incision (approximately 5 mm lateral to the spinous process on the symptomatic side). The interlaminar window is accessed after the incision of the dorso-lumbar fascia and blunt retraction of the muscles without dissection of any insertions. The ligamentum flavum is opened laterally, and the nerve root is exposed and mobilized from lateral to medial, starting at the shoulder of the nerve root. The prolapsed part of the lumbar disc is removed. It is controversial to remove the rest of the nucleus pulposus from the intervertebral disc space, assuming a decrease in the risk of recurrent herniations. The skin incision is 3–5 cm lateral to the midline in cases of extraforaminal disc herniations. The dorso-lumbar fascia is opened, and the space between the cranial and caudal transverse processes is approached using blunt trans-muscular dissection. The inter-transverse ligament and muscle are excised lateral to the facet joint, exposing the dorsal root ganglion. The nerve root is mobilized if necessary to expose the herniated disc, which typically compresses the nerve root against the lower border of the cranial pedicle. The herniated disc is removed, and in most cases, there is no need to remove nucleus pulposus material from the disc space. There is no need to open the spinal canal [14].

2.2 Microdiscectomy *versus* sequestrectomy

Thomé et al. [15], in a randomized prospective study, compared microdiscectomy, which removes disc material from the intervertebral disc to sequestrectomy, which removes only the extruded disc fragment. They concluded that sequestrectomy does not entail a higher rate of early recurrences than microdiscectomy, which involves the removal of the nucleus pulposus from the intervertebral disc space. Early results demonstrated a trend toward better outcomes when sequestrectomy is performed. However, long-term follow-up data are necessary; sequestrectomy may represent a good alternative to standard microdiscectomy.

A recent systematic review and meta-analysis compared discectomy to sequestrectomy regarding the risk of re-herniation, reoperation rate, complications, pain, satisfaction, and perioperative outcomes (operative time, blood loss, length of stay). Based on the current evidence, discectomy and sequestrectomy do not significantly differ regarding the risk of re-herniation, reoperation rate, and postoperative complications. There was a slightly higher improvement in pain, better satisfaction outcomes, and a shorter operative time in patients treated with sequestrectomy. However, the clinical relevance of these differences needs to be validated in larger, prospective, randomized studies [16].

2.3 Trans-tubular microscopic-assisted percutaneous nucleotomy (MAPN)

The operation is performed under general anesthesia with the patient positioned prone [17]. The herniated disc level is identified using a K-wire inserted paravertebral on the contralateral side. A lateral fluoroscopic image is taken to confirm the level. A skin incision of 1.4 cm longitudinal and about 1 cm lateral to the midline is made. Muscle dilators are then applied sequentially. The 14-mm working channel is then docked and its docking position is checked by fluoroscopy and a holding arm is used to secure it to the operating table. The current tubular retractor systems provide different diameters of the tubes. In cases of facet joint hypertrophy, docking of a larger tube to the inter-laminar window may be difficult. The following steps are done using the surgical microscope. The interlaminar fenster is then identified. The ligamentum flavum is then opened and partially resected to expose the dura and the traversing nerve root. Using a high-speed burr or Kerrison rongeurs, the medial part of the facet joint, the caudal part of the cranial lamina, or the cranial part of the caudal lamina is resected according to the exact position of the herniated fragment. The dural sac and the nerve root are then mobilized to expose the herniated disc. The herniated disc is then mobilized and removed. After removing the herniated disc, a ball-pointed hooks of different lengths are used to check that the nerve root is freed and no other fragments are left. Hemostasis is then performed using bipolar coagulation or hemostatic agents. The working channel (tube) is removed under microscopic vision, and bleeding control is achieved throughout the approach. The fascia and subcutaneous layer are closed without a local drain. Postoperatively, there is no need for lumbar support, and mobilization can begin once patients adequately recover from anesthesia and are able to move (**Figure 5**) [5].

According to the site of the sequestrated fragment, different anatomical corridors were used to access the disc prolapse. Trans-laminar and trans-pars techniques were used to approach cranially migrated fragments. Extra-laminar and extra-foraminal approaches (**Figure 6**) were also described to access foraminal and extraforaminal herniations [18].

For cranially migrated disc herniations, the docking site of the working tube is at the cranial lamina. A 4 mm diamond burr is utilized to create a hole into the hemi-lamina, just cranial and medial to the facet joint. As the ligamentum flavum is deficient beneath the upper half of the lamina, the epidural space is accessed directly. A 3 mm bone rim in all directions should be preserved to prevent iatrogenic pars interarticularis fractures. Mobilization of the dural sac begins at its lateral border to explore the disc herniation. Bayonet-shaped instruments are preferably used as they do not obstruct the surgical field.

Further careful dissection is directed toward the herniated disc fragment. Finally, the fragment is mobilized and removed using hooks and discectomy forceps. After cautious epidural hemostasis, the working tube is removed [6].

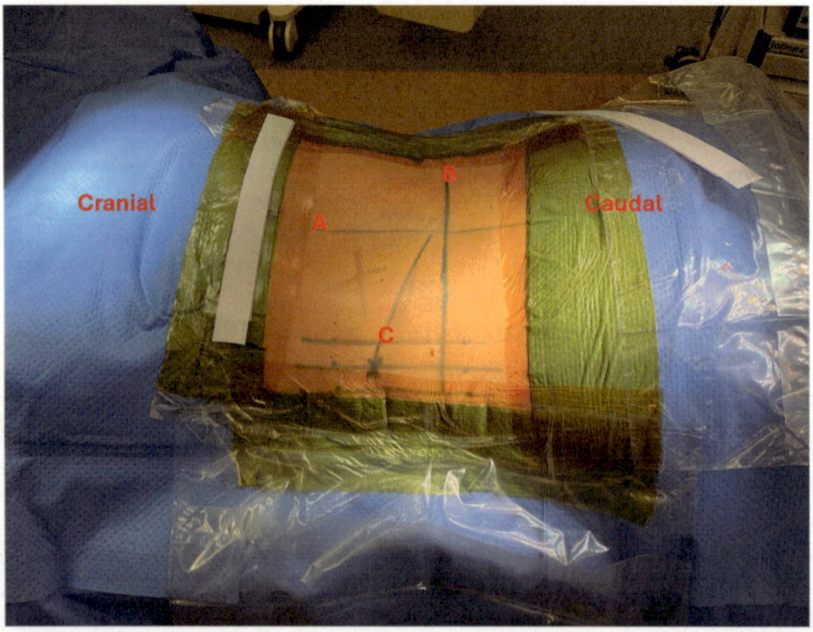

Figure 5.
Intraoperative images showing the different steps of tran-tubular discectomy. A: localizing the level under fluoroscopy. B: skin incision (about 14 mm). C- H: sequential dilatation until inserting the working tube.

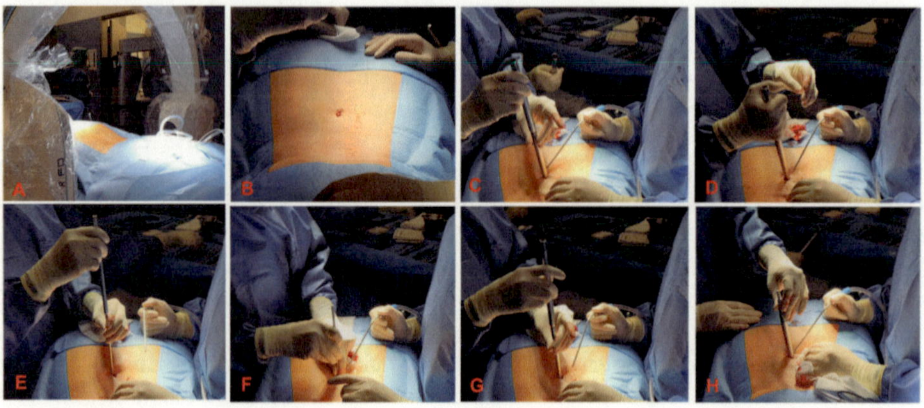

Figure 6.
Extraforaminal microscopic assisted percutaneous nucleotomy for foraminal and extraforaminal lumbar disc herniations. Yellow is the nerve root, red is the herniated fragment, and blue is the surgical field inside the tube.

In the case of foraminal and extraforaminal disc herniations, the skin incision is about 4–6 cm from the midline to allow inclination of the working tube toward the foramen and resection of the sequestrated fragment without violating the facet joint [5]. Preoperative planning on CT and/or MRI is important to consider. The site of skin incision and trajectory of the working channel will differ according to the distance from the skin incision to the docking site and subsequently the herniated fragment.

Tubular discectomy has many advantages. It is entirely a muscle-splitting approach, and sequential dilators do not include dissection or disinsertion of the paravertebral muscles. The muscle fibers restore their position once the working channel is removed and the approach corridor is closed. Blood loss is minimal, the demand for post-operative analgesics decreases, and the hospital stay is short [17, 19].

Tubular microdiscectomy has its learning curve. Technical skills like triangulation, ambidexterity, and the ability to operate with the surgical instruments parallel or with minimal angulation without obstructing the surgical field are required [20]. The more proximal the affected level, the smaller the interlaminar window. Also, in cases of severe degenerative changes with facet joint hypertrophy, the exact docking of the tube may be difficult. The use of a smaller diameter tube or partial medial facetectomy using a high-speed burr is often helpful. Furthermore, the management of incidental durotomies through a tube is challenging.

2.4 Endoscopic discectomy

An endoscope is a visualization device that is inserted into the body. Although, it is mainly a visualization tool, integration of a working channel provides a surgical corridor for surgical instruments to manipulate, ablate, and resect tissues. "full endoscopic" describes procedures performed with a working channel endoscope, while "endoscope assisted" describes operations where tools are passed through trajectories separate from the endoscope [21]. Endoscopic spine surgery is now being adopted globally for treating lumbar spine herniations, with a growing body of internationally developed literature demonstrating its efficacy and safety (**Figure** 7) [22–24].

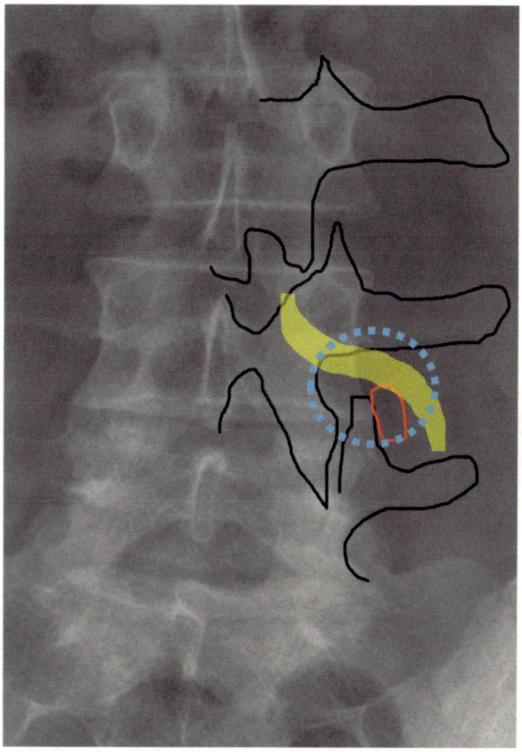

Figure 7.
Intraoperative photo showing the prone position and the preoperative planning for a transforaminal endoscopic lumbar discectomy. Line A represents the midline; Line B represents the disc level (L3/4). Line C represents the trajectory of the endoscope in the coronal plane. The three parallel lines laterally are the 10, 12, and 14 cm lines from the midline.

Endoscopic techniques have evolved over the last few years due to advances in endoscopes and imaging technologies. Different approaches were described, including interlaminar and transforaminal approaches [25, 26]. Also, uniportal and biportal approaches were described [26, 27]. Many endoscopic techniques can be utilized in the treatment of spine disorders. The different types of spinal endoscopy are categorized according to the sizes and the number of working channels. The various systems' capabilities and inherent advantages and disadvantages depend on size and number of working channels. The three most commonly used techniques include full endoscopy, microendoscopy, and biportal endoscopy (**Figure 8**) [28].

Recently, the AOSpine published a consensus paper outlining nomenclature and terminology to standardize terms in endoscopic procedures. This enables the development, uniformity of procedures, teaching, and global acceptance of full-endoscopic spinal procedures [21].

Endoscopic discectomy whether using a full endoscopic procedure or a biportal endoscopic procedure has a long and steep learning curve. Different studies have addressed the issue of the learning curve of endoscopic discectomy. The average number of cases required to improve operative time and minimize complications ranges from 30 to 50 cases [11, 29, 30]. Recently, the use of virtual reality and simulators may provide a suitable platform for learning spinal endoscopy in a shorter time and with less *in vivo* complications [31].

2.4.1 Full-endoscopic lumbar discectomy

Full-endoscopic or percutaneous endoscopic lumbar discectomy is the most commonly used endoscopic surgery. This technique is characterized by applying a working channel endoscope that includes an optic system and a working channel in a thin tubular device. The endoscope is introduced percutaneously via a stab incision. The technique is a uni-portal procedure performed under constant saline irrigation [32]. For lumbar spine procedures, there are interlaminar and transforaminal approaches to full-endoscopic discectomy. Transforaminal full-endoscopic lumbar discectomy has been developed as a representative endoscopic spine surgery. Different terms are used to describe this procedure. The AOSpine group proposed the standard term

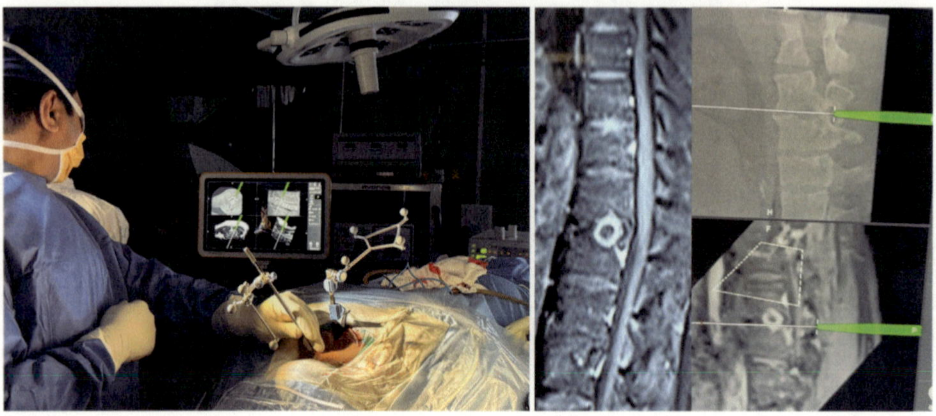

Figure 8.
Example of AI software that combines CT and MRI images with real-time intraoperative navigation. The pathology shown in this example is a spondylodiscitis case.

"transforaminal endoscopic lumbar discectomy" (TELD) [21]. The main disadvantages of full-endoscopic procedures are that they do not allow independent movement of the camera and the surgical instrument, and the working channel allows only the use of one instrument at a time. The use of implants like interbody fusion cages is also limited by the small diameter of the working channel. The use of implants, such as interbody fusion cages, is limited by the narrow diameter of the working channel. However, a beveled working channel can compensate for the absence of retractors by helping to protect neural tissues [28].

Endoscopic lumbar discectomy can be performed in a prone or lateral position. The lateral decubitus position is more comfortable for the surgeon, as gravity assists in secure positioning of the working channel and minimizes fatigue of the surgeon's hand holding the endoscope. Other surgeons prefer the prone position, as it is the one they are more familiar with. The surgeon can operate while sitting.

Percutaneous endoscopic discectomy is a novel technique for removing lumbar disc herniations via a posterolateral approach. It employs specially designed instruments that integrate rigid, straight, angled, and flexible forceps with automated high-power suction shaver and cutter systems. This allows access to the dorsal parts of the intervertebral space where the disc herniation is situated. The procedure is monitored using a 30° angled endoscope connected to a television and video unit. It is conducted with the patient under local or general anesthesia [33]. Surgical outcomes of endoscopic procedures are comparable to or even superior to those of traditional open surgery [34–36].

Different types of anesthesia can also be used, including general, local, and epidural [37]. Local anesthesia remains the most common method in full-endoscopic lumbar discectomy and serves as the comparison standard for other anesthesia techniques due to its high safety profile. Although epidural anesthesia offers better intraoperative pain control and equivalent safety thanks to ropivacaine's motor preservation and pain-blocking properties, it is less frequently used in full-endoscopic lumbar discectomy compared to local anesthesia. While general anesthesia can provide complete pain relief during surgery, the risk of nerve injury must not be overlooked, although intraoperative neuromonitoring can help mitigate this concern. Deep relaxation should be avoided in the case of using general anesthesia. Regional anesthesia is uncommon, yet it has been associated with improved anesthesia outcomes during surgery while maintaining similar safety levels. The selection of anesthesia methods for full-endoscopic lumbar discectomy is guided by patient-specific factors, surgical considerations, and the anesthesiologist's assessment to ensure a satisfactory anesthesia experience and a successful surgical outcome [37].

2.4.1.1 Transforaminal endoscopic lumbar discectomy

The most widely used endoscopic spinal surgery technique is the transforaminal endoscopic approach to the lumbar spine. It allows the endoscopic spine surgeon to address most herniated discs in the lumbar spine [38].

Patients are positioned prone on a radiolucent operating table and maintained under conscious sedation to monitor for adverse events or if not fully relaxed in case of general anesthesia. The skin entry is determined according to the location of the targeted sequestrated fragment and planned on the preoperative MRI or CT scan. It is also influenced by the patient's body size, foraminal dimensions, and the target landing point on the disc surface. The procedure is performed under intraoperative fluoroscopic imaging according to the preoperative plan on MRI (magnetic resonance imaging) images. The typical entry point is approximately 8–14 cm paramedian.

Local anesthetic infiltration of the skin and the proposed trajectory of the endoscope is performed. An 18-gauge needle is inserted under fluoroscopic guidance. The needle tip is placed between the medial and lateral pedicular borders on the anteroposterior fluoroscopic view and the posterior vertebral line on the lateral view. Many surgeons use discography to identify the pathologically herniated disc material. This discography facilitates the precise removal of prolapsed disc fragments. A guidewire is then introduced through the needle and the needle is removed. A 5 mm stab skin incision is performed for port insertion. The cannulated obturator can slide over the guidewire and inserted into the disc via the foramen. Sequential dilators of different sizes are used before insertion of the final port to decrease approach-related pain. Pain may occur due to irritation of the exiting nerve root or any inflamed epidural tissues. A beveled working sheath is finally introduced over the obturator.

After the working sheath is securely positioned against the disc, the final position is confirmed with a fluoroscopic image. Then, a rigid ellipsoidal endoscope with an eccentrically positioned working channel and two irrigation channels is inserted. For aminoplasty, the use of shavers to expand the bony neuroforamen to access a cranially or caudally migrated disc fragment is described. Initial sub-annular decompression can be performed using rongeurs and radiofrequency ablation, enabling the surgeon to confirm better anatomical orientation. Anatomical layers can be identified, including the dura, nerve root, surrounding epidural fat, annulus, and herniated nucleus. It is essential to differentiate the herniated disc fragments and pathological soft tissues from compressed neural tissues through the endoscopic view. Different hooks are used to mobilize and separate the herniated disc from the surrounding neural structures, specifically the exiting nerve root and the dural sac.

After removing the herniated disc, the surgeon can identify the decompressed neural tissues. The endpoint of the procedure can be determined by checking for a strong dural pulsation and free mobilization of the nerve root. Finally, the endoscope is removed; subcutaneous closure, steri-strips, and a sterile dressing are applied. The patients can be discharged on the same day after checking for postoperative complications [32].

2.4.1.2 Interlaminar endoscopic lumbar discectomy

Postero-lateral lumbar disc herniations are traditionally approached via the interlaminar window. Reported endoscope-assisted techniques via tubular retractors include posterior endoscopic discectomy, endoscopic lumbar discectomy, or microendoscopic discectomy (MED) [21].

The patient's anesthesia and positioning are similar to those of the transforaminal approach. The endoscope's docking site is the interlaminar space. To reach the epidural space, the ligamentum flavum must be resected. The dural sac is mobilized from lateral to medial. The postero-lateral herniated disc fragment is then mobilized and removed [39].

2.4.2 Microendoscopic procedures

Microendoscopy is performed through a single working channel. The size of the channel is large enough to allow the use of multiple instruments, one of them is the endoscope itself. It allows slight independent angulation of the endoscope and the surgical instrument used. The large size of the portal allows insertion of implants such as interbody cages and so allows performing endoscopic spinal fusion. The main disadvantage is the slightly larger size of the incision and possibly soft tissue trauma. The procedure is also done in a dry medium, without the use of fluid that aids tissue delineation and dissection [28].

2.4.3 Biportal endoscopic procedures

This techniques utilizes two working channels; one for the endoscope and the other for surgical instruments. It allows independence angulation, movement of the endoscope and surgical instruments. It is similar to the technique used in shoulder and knee arthroscopy. It uses fluid environment, which helps tissue delineation and dissection. The two portals add to the approach-related tissue trauma [28].

3. Future perspectives

3.1 Navigation

Navigation systems that utilize real-time images enhance surgical accuracy. A high-quality computed tomography scan can be performed using the O-arm. By integrating it with a real-time anatomical tracking tool, surgeons can conduct intra-operative three-dimensional anatomical mapping in real-time. Spine surgeons initially employed navigation systems for percutaneous pedicle screw fixation, but currently, navigation is also used to improve safety and accuracy in endoscopic spinal discectomy [22]. In endoscopic spinal discectomy, a navigation system can assist operators in calculating an optimal trajectory, identifying docking sites, determining ideal incision points in the early stages of surgery, and confirming the exact locations of surgical instruments during uniportal and full endoscopic discectomy procedures [40].

3.2 Image quality (ultraresolution (4K) and 3-dimensional and ultraresolution endoscope applications)

Advances in resolution and image quality have improved intraoperative endoscopic imaging. The advantage of higher resolutions lies in their ability to delineate patient tissues precisely. Additionally, the available 2-dimensional endoscopic spine systems lack depth perception, leading to unfamiliarity with surgical anatomy and potentially resulting in adverse events [40]. Three-dimensional endoscopic equipment offers clear views of surgical anatomy, including the dura and nerve root exposure, and provides better depth perception. With a 4K ultra-resolution endoscope, structures like foraminal ligaments, which are challenging to observe with conventional microscopes, can be easily identified. Moreover, accurately perceiving the severity of spinal canal compromise and disc protrusion through 3D visualization could improve surgical confidence, leading to better decompression of neural structures and improved surgical outcomes [22].

3.3 Augmented reality and virtual reality

Augmented reality (AR) is an interactive experience that enhances the real world with computer-generated perception. Digital content is overlaid in a real-life surgical environment using software, applications, and VR glasses. AR systems primarily function as navigation tools in operating rooms. One of the main limitations of standard navigation systems is simultaneous visualization, whereas head-mounted displays allow visualization of both the surgical field and navigation data simultaneously. AR reduces radiation exposure, shortens operation time, and enhances safety and precision. AR assistants can be employed to determine the ideal endoscopic trajectory and entry points, similar to standard navigation systems used in endoscopic spine surgery [40].

Virtual reality (VR) is a highly advanced technology that allows surgeons to experience surgery in a virtual world created by a computer. VR simulators are gaining attention in education and preoperative planning. VR preoperative planning system for full endoscopic spine surgery could significantly improve accuracy and reduce operation times [41]. Since endoscopic spine surgery is performed with a monitor, it is ideal for VR education, which could help overcome the steep learning curve.

Recently, a high simulation training system based on the combination of VR/AR and magneto-optical navigation for spinal full-endoscopic surgery was presented. The model may be used by surgeons starting with spinal endoscopy and can be considered a comparable and sufficiently realistic tool to train key operation steps to reduce the learning curve [31].

3.4 Robot-assisted surgery

Robot-assisted spine surgery is commonly performed for pedicle screw fixation, and recent studies suggest that higher accuracy, shorter hospital stay, and lower radiation exposure can be achieved with robot-assisted screw fixation compared to traditional surgery. Robots place pedicle screws in precisely, and robot-assisted spine surgery shares overlapping features with navigation systems. Robots provide exact physical guidance to perform preoperatively customized surgical plans. Therefore, endoscopic spine surgery could also apply robot assistance to position endoscopes at ideal locations accurately. Wang et al. [42] applied robot assistance in full endoscopic lumbar discectomy and concluded that robot assistance systems was safe, effective, and less invasive than conventional fluoroscopic-guided endoscopic procedures. The robot system used provided real-time guidance to facilitate the placement of punctures. Robot-assisted endoscopic spine surgery is also expected to help overcome steep learning curves by helping to put the endoscope in the correct position.

3.5 Artificial intelligence and deep learning applications

Recent studies have indicated promising artificial intelligence (AI) integration into healthcare, particularly in medical imaging analysis. Deep learning's self-learning capabilities and ability to extract key features from large datasets [43] have demonstrated remarkable clinical diagnosis and treatment performance. Given the critical need to minimize complications, such as dural tears and neural tissue injuries, developing and implementing deep learning algorithms for neural tissue recognition in spinal endoscopy is necessary.

Qualitative evaluations demonstrated the excellent identification of neural tissue features. A U-Net-based model robustly performed neural tissue segmentation. This potentially supports spine surgeons, especially those with less experience, and improves surgical outcomes during the learning curve of endoscopic procedures. Therefore, further advancements may enhance the clinical applicability of this technique [44]. Recently, AI has been used to combine CT and MRI images in real-time navigation. This enables surgeons to perform endoscopic procedures with accurate trajectory localization while visualizing the pathology in a high-quality MRI image [45].

3.6 Mechano-protection against intervertebral disc degeneration

Recent studies aim to define inflammatory triggers that lead to intervertebral disc extracellular matrix (ECM) degeneration. They seek to determine the impact of a proinflammatory microenvironment on cell mechanobiology and subsequently develop drugs that exhibit mechano-protective effects. The continued development of cell contractility-modulating therapeutics will enhance our understanding of the cross-talk between mechanobiological and inflammatory signaling and facilitate the creation of effective treatments for disc degeneration [46].

4. Conclusion

The management of lumbar disc herniations has evolved over the last few decades. Advancements in techniques and technology have allowed minimally invasive spinal procedures to expand its capabilities and success. Standard treatment has evolved from open discectomy, microsurgical discectomy, trans-tubular percutaneous discectomy, and endoscopic discectomies. Nowadays, the most commonly used surgical procedures are microsurgical and endoscopic discectomies. There is an increasing global adoption of endoscopic techniques in the past few years. Also, the bulk of published literature over the past two decades confirms the efficacy, safety, reproducibility and comparable outcomes to microsurgical techniques.

Recent advances in image quality, magnification, 3D visualization, and virtual and augmented reality have improved the precision, accuracy, and safety of minimally invasive spinal procedures. The introduction of robot-assisted surgery and AI and ML software modules is expected to further improve accuracy, reduce complications, and improve the education of young surgeons.

The data supporting clinical outcomes and cost-effectiveness enhances ongoing implementation in the operating room. Many challenges still confront this constantly advancing area, but technological innovations and surgeon education will promote its growth. As the drive to improve the cost and quality of patient care persists, innovations will advance this expanding field.

Conflict of interest

The author declares no conflict of interest.

Author details

Ahmed Shawky Abdelgawaad[1,2]

1 Department of Spinal Deformities, Helios Hospitals Erfurt, Germany

2 Assiut University Hospitals, Egypt

*Address all correspondence to: ahsh313@yahoo.com

References

[1] Chang X, Chen B, Li HY, Han XB, Zhou Y, Li CQ. The safety and efficacy of minimally invasive discectomy: A meta-analysis of prospective randomised controlled trials. International Orthopaedics. 2014;**38**(6):1225-1234

[2] Mixter WJ, Barr JS. Rupture of the intervertebral disc with involvement of the Spinal Canal. New England Journal of Medicine. 1934;**211**(5):210-215

[3] Caspar W. A new surgical procedure for lumbar disc herniation causing less tissue damage through a microsurgical approach. In: Wullenweber RBM, Hamer J, et al., editors. Advances in Neurosurgery. Berlin: Springer-Verlag; 1977. pp. 74-80

[4] Yasrgil MG. Microsurgical operation of herniated lumbar disc. In: Wullenweber RBM, Hamer J, et al., editors. Advances in Neurosurgery. Berlin: Springer-Verlag; 1977. p. 81

[5] Shawky Abdelgawaad A, Babic D, Siam AE, Ezzati A. Extraforaminal microscopic assisted percutaneous nucleotomy for foraminal and extraforaminal lumbar disc herniations. The Spine Journal. 2018;**18**(4):620-625

[6] Abdelrahman H, Seyed-Emadaldin S, Krajnovic B, Ezzati A, Abdelgawaad AS. Trans-tubular translaminar microscopic-assisted nucleotomy for lumbar disc herniations in the hidden zone. Global Spine Journal. 2022;**12**(7):1420-1427

[7] Kambin P, Casey K, O'Brien E, Zhou L. Transforaminal arthroscopic decompression of lateral recess stenosis. Journal of Neurosurgery. 1996;**84**(3):462-467

[8] Sasaoka R, Nakamura H, Konishi S, Nagayama R, Suzuki E, Terai H, et al. Objective assessment of reduced invasiveness in MED. Compared with conventional one-level laminotomy. European Spine Journal. 2006;**15**(5):577-582

[9] Shin DA, Kim KN, Shin HC, Yoon DH. The efficacy of microendoscopic discectomy in reducing iatrogenic muscle injury. Journal of Neurosurgery. Spine. 2008;**8**(1):39-43

[10] Pranata R, Lim MA, Vania R, July J. Biportal endoscopic spinal surgery versus microscopic decompression for lumbar spinal stenosis: A systematic review and meta-analysis. World Neurosurgery. 2020;**138**:e450-e4e8

[11] Olinger C, Coffman A, Campion C, Thompson K, Gardocki R. Initial learning curve after switching to uniportal endoscopic discectomy for lumbar disc herniations. European Spine Journal. 2023;**32**(8):2694-2699

[12] Smailhodzic E, Hooijsma W, Boonstra A, Langley DJ. Social media use in healthcare: A systematic review of effects on patients and on their relationship with healthcare professionals. BMC Health Services Research. 2016;**16**(1):442

[13] Benetoli A, Chen TF, Aslani P. How patients' use of social media impacts their interactions with healthcare professionals. Patient Education and Counseling. 2018;**101**(3):439-444

[14] Mayer HM. Principles of microsurgical discectomy in lumbar disc herniations. In: Mayer HM, editor. Minimally Invasive Spine Surgery: A Surgical Manual. Berlin, Heidelberg: Springer; 2000. pp. 73-77

[15] Thomé C, Barth M, Scharf J, Schmiedek P. Outcome after lumbar sequestrectomy compared with microdiscectomy: A prospective randomized study. Journal of Neurosurgery. Spine. 2005;**2**(3):271-278

[16] Ambrosio L, Vadalà G, de Rinaldis E, Muthu S, Ćorluka S, Buser Z, et al. Discectomy versus sequestrectomy in the treatment of lumbar disc herniation: A systematic review and meta-analysis. The Spine Journal. 2025;**25**(2):211-226

[17] Greiner-Perth R, Bohm H, El Saghir H. Microscopically assisted percutaneous nucleotomy, an alternative minimally invasive procedure for the operative treatment of lumbar disc herniation: Preliminary results. Neurosurgical Review. 2002;**25**(4):225-227

[18] Alhashash M, Gendy H, Shousha M. Extra-laminar microscopic-assisted percutaneous nucleotomy (EL-MAPN) for the treatment of foraminal lumbar disc prolapse, a modified minimally invasive approach. Archives of Orthopaedic and Trauma Surgery. 2022;**142**(10):2405-2411

[19] Franke J, Greiner-Perth R, Boehm H, Mahlfeld K, Grasshoff H, Allam Y, et al. Comparison of a minimally invasive procedure versus standard microscopic discotomy: A prospective randomised controlled clinical trial. European Spine Journal. 2009;**18**(7):992-1000

[20] Jain S, Merchant Z, Kire N, Patel J, Patel A, Kundnani V. Learning curve of microendoscopic discectomy in single-level prolapsed intervertebral disc in 120 patients. Global Spine Journal. 2020;**10**(5):571-577

[21] Hofstetter CP, Ahn Y, Choi G, Gibson JNA, Ruetten S, Zhou Y, et al. AOSpine consensus paper on nomenclature for working-channel endoscopic spinal procedures. Global Spine Journal. 2020;**10** (Suppl. 2):111s-121s

[22] Gunjotikar S, Pestonji M, Tanaka M, Komatsubara T, Ekade SJ, Heydar AM, et al. Evolution, current trends, and latest advances of endoscopic spine surgery. Journal of Clinical Medicine. 2024;**13**(11):3208

[23] Liu Y, Kotheeranurak V, Quillo-Olvera J, Facundo VI, Sharma S, Suvithayasiri S, et al. A 30-year worldwide research productivity of scientific publication in full-endoscopic decompression spine surgery: Quantitative and qualitative analysis. Neurospine. 2023;**20**(1):374-389

[24] Zhao T, Shen J, Zheng B, Huang Y, Jin M, Morizane K, et al. The 100 Most-cited publications in endoscopic spine surgery research. Global Spine Journal. 2021;**11**(4):587-596

[25] Ahn Y. Transforaminal percutaneous endoscopic lumbar discectomy: Technical tips to prevent complications. Expert Review of Medical Devices. 2012;**9**(4):361-366

[26] Yin J, Gao G, Chen S, Ma T, Nong L. Comparative study between unilateral biportal endoscopic discectomy and percutaneous interlaminar endoscopic discectomy for the treatment of L5/S1 disc herniation. World Neurosurgery. 2024;**194**:123526

[27] Ahn Y, Lee S. Uniportal versus biportal endoscopic spine surgery: A comprehensive review. Expert Review of Medical Devices. 2023;**20**(7):549-556

[28] Simpson AK, HMT L, Xiong GX, Crawford AM, Minamide A, Schoenfeld AJ. Spinal endoscopy:

evidence, techniques, global trends, and future projections. The Spine Journal. 2022;**22**(1):64-74

[29] Liu Y, Li X, Tan H, Hao X, Zhu B, Yang Y, et al. Learning curve of uniportal compared with biportal endoscopic techniques for the treatment of lumbar disc herniation. Orthopaedic Surgery. 2025;**17**(2):513-524

[30] Peng J, Lin R, Fang D, He Z, Zhao Q, Li Q. Learning curve insights in unilateral biportal endoscopic (UBE) spinal procedures: Proficiency cutoffs and the impact on efficiency and complications. European Spine Journal. 2025;**34**:954-973

[31] Fan T, Shi L, Peng X, Wu M, Yu L, Zhu B. High simulation training system for spinal full-endoscopic surgery, based on the combination of VR/AR and magneto-optical navigation technology. Orthopaedic Surgery. 2025;**17**(4):1243-1254

[32] Lee SG, Ahn Y. Transforaminal endoscopic lumbar discectomy: Basic concepts and technical keys to clinical success. International Journal of Spine Surgery. 2021;**15**(suppl. 3):S38-s46

[33] Mayer HM, Brock M. Percutaneous endoscopic discectomy: Surgical technique and preliminary results compared to microsurgical discectomy. Journal of Neurosurgery. 1993;**78**(2):216-225

[34] Li XC, Zhong CF, Deng GB, Liang RW, Huang CM. Full-endoscopic procedures versus traditional discectomy surgery for discectomy: A systematic review and meta-analysis of current global clinical trials. Pain Physician. 2016;**19**(3):103-118

[35] Righesso O, Falavigna A, Avanzi O. Comparison of open discectomy with microendoscopic discectomy in lumbar disc herniations: Results of a randomized controlled trial. Neurosurgery. 2007;**61**(3):545-549; discussion 9

[36] Ruetten S, Komp M, Godolias G. An extreme lateral access for the surgery of lumbar disc herniations inside the spinal canal using the full-endoscopic uniportal transforaminal approach-technique and prospective results of 463 patients. Spine (Phila Pa 1976). 2005;**30**(22):2570-2578

[37] Zheng B, Guo C, Xu S, Li H, Wu Y, Liu H. Anesthesia methods for full-endoscopic lumbar discectomy: A review. Frontiers in Medicine (Lausanne). 2023;**10**:1193311

[38] Lewandrowski KU, Lorio MP. Determination of work related to endoscopic decompression of lumbar spinal stenosis. Journal of Personalized Medicine. 2023;**13**(4):614

[39] Nazwar TA, Bal'afif F, Wardhana DW, Panjaitan C. A comparative study of transforaminal and interlaminar approaches in percutaneous endoscopic lumbar discectomy for L5-S1 disc herniation: Systematic review. Journal of Clinical Neuroscience. 2025;**133**:111022

[40] Kwon H, Park JY. The role and future of endoscopic spine surgery: A narrative review. Neurospine. 2023;**20**(1):43-55

[41] Zheng C, Li J, Zeng G, Ye W, Sun J, Hong J, et al. Development of a virtual reality preoperative planning system for postlateral endoscopic lumbar discectomy surgery and its clinical application. World Neurosurgery. 2019;**123**:e1-e8

[42] Wang Z, Tan Y, Fu K, Meng Z, Wang L. Minimally invasive trans-superior articular process percutaneous endoscopic lumbar discectomy with robot assistance. BMC Musculoskeletal Disorders. 2022;**23**(1):1144

[43] Ryu K, Kitaguchi D, Nakajima K, Ishikawa Y, Harai Y, Yamada A, et al. Deep learning-based vessel automatic recognition for laparoscopic right hemicolectomy. Surgical Endoscopy. 2024;**38**(1):171-178

[44] Lee HR, Rhee W, Chang SY, Chang BS, Kim H. Deep learning in spinal endoscopy: U-net models for neural tissue detection. Bioengineering (Basel). 2024;**11**(11):1082

[45] Yang H. Artificial intelligence and minimally invasive spine surgery. In: Ahn Y, Park J-K, Park C-K, editors. Core Techniques of Minimally Invasive Spine Surgery. Singapore: Springer Nature Singapore; 2023. pp. 411-417

[46] Hernandez PA, Jacobsen TD, Chahine NO. Actomyosin contractility confers mechanoprotection against TNFalpha-induced disruption of the intervertebral disc. Science Advances. 2020;**6**(34):eaba2368

Chapter 9

Lumbar Fusion for Spondylosis: Indications and Techniques for Interbody Fusion, Comparing TLIF, PLIF, Extreme Lateral, ALIF and Oblique/Approach

Bhoresh Dhamija and Steven Tominey

Abstract

Advances in medicine have resulted in an aging population with improved survival for a wide spectrum of pathology. With this, there is an increased incidence of degenerative disc disease, facet joint disease, central, lateral and foraminal stenosis. The biomechanical stresses on the lumbar spine producing back pain with a combination of radicular and claudicant symptoms. It is well recognized that lumbar interbody fusion can help to provide mechanical stability, to produce an indirect decompression of neural structures with an improvement in back and leg pain, restoration of lumbar lordosis with deformity correction. The current study aims to review the literature to produce a comprehensive analysis of the common techniques used, Transforaminal Lumbar Interbody Fusion (TLIF), Posterior Lumbar Interbody Fusion (PLIF), Extreme Lateral Interbody Fusion (XLIF), Oblique/Anterior To Psoas and Anterior Lumbar Interbody Fusion. We review the indications, the nuances in surgical technique with the risks and benefits of each.

Keywords: lumbar fusion, spondylosis, TLIF, PLIF, ALIF, XLIF, ATP, OLIF

1. Introduction

Lumbar fusion of the spine is commonly performed to address conditions such as spinal instability and deformity. During lumbar fusion, two or more vertebrae are fused together to stabilize the spine. Different techniques, such as bone grafting and the use of instrumentation including screws and rods, may be employed to facilitate the fusion process. Lumbar fusion is typically considered for patients who have not responded to conservative treatments and have persistent symptoms that impact their daily activities.

The preservation of load-bearing capacity, restoration of disc height, and stabilization of all three spinal columns through additional fixation are key drivers behind the choice to opt for lumbar fusion. It can facilitate compressive loading on the bone, restore sagittal alignment, and provide biomechanical stabilization.

Spondylosis is a degenerative condition of the spine that typically occurs with age. It involves the wear and tear of the spinal discs, facet joints, and other structures in the spine, leading to symptoms such as pain, stiffness, and reduced mobility. Spondylosis can result in the formation of bone spurs, disc herniation, and spinal stenosis, impacting the overall function of the spine and causing pain.

1.1 Non-surgical treatment modalities

Prior to operative intervention, patients will often complete a trial of conservative management through lifestyle interventions, analgesia and physical therapy. Nonsteroidal anti-inflammatory drugs (NSAIDs) are frequently prescribed to reduce pain and inflammation, while opioid analgesics and muscle relaxants may also be used to further alleviate discomfort and spasms, respectively [1].

Physiotherapy can be another effective conservative treatment for spondylosis. By focusing on strengthening muscles, enhancing flexibility, and promoting better posture, physical therapy aims to reduce pain and improve overall function. Various therapeutic exercises and modalities, such as heat or ice therapy, may be incorporated into the treatment plan.

Lifestyle modifications are encouraged to complement medical interventions. Weight management, regular exercise, and correct ergonomics can help alleviate spinal stress and minimize symptom exacerbation. Individuals are advised to avoid activities that may worsen their condition, such as heavy lifting or prolonged sitting.

Additional non-surgical approaches used include alternative therapies like acupuncture, chiropractic care, and massage therapy, which may offer relief for some patients. Transcutaneous electrical nerve stimulation (TENS) units can also be used to help control pain. In certain cases, corticosteroid injections directly into the affected area may provide temporary relief from pain and inflammation [1].

1.2 Surgical treatment options

For individuals with severe symptoms intractable to conservative management or progressive spinal deformity, surgical intervention is often considered. Decompressive procedures, such as laminectomy or discectomy, aim to alleviate nerve compression resulting from spinal stenosis. However, spinal fusion surgery may be

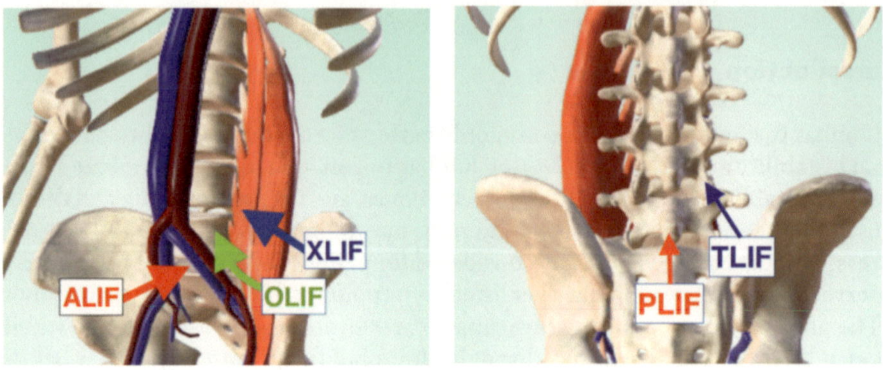

Figure 1.
The various approaches used to achieve lumbar fusion.

recommended to mechanically stabilize the spine and reduce pain in cases of significant instability or deformity.

This chapter aims to provide an in-depth exploration of the various techniques available for stabilizing the lumbar spine in the context of spondylosis. By examining and comparing different stabilization methods, including but not limited to posterior, anterior, and lateral fusion approaches, this text seeks to offer a succinct yet comprehensive understanding of the considerations, advantages, and limitations associated with each technique. Additionally, through appraisal of the evidence base and clinical outcomes, readers will gain insight into the optimal selection of stabilization techniques tailored to individual patient needs in the management of lumbar spondylosis (**Figure 1**).

2. Posterior lumbar interbody fusion (PLIF)

Posterior Lumbar Interbody Fusion (PLIF), first described by Briggs and Milligan in 1944 [2] and later popularized by Cloward in the 1950s [3], has evolved significantly over the decades. PLIF can be performed alongside pedicle screw fixation and posterolateral fusion, which together establish a comprehensive circumferential fusion that bolsters spinal stability. The procedure is primarily applicable to the L3-S1 vertebral segments, as the necessary dural retraction can pose serious risks if attempted at higher levels, potentially damaging the conus medullaris, cauda equina, or nerve roots [4].

The surgical approach involves accessing the intervertebral disc from a posterior perspective, with the patient positioned prone. Surgeons may employ either an open midline technique with bilateral muscle dissection or a minimally invasive approach to reach the posterior vertebral body. After identifying the spinous processes and laminae, a laminotomy is performed medial to the facet joint. This facilitates dural retraction and provides access to the disc space allowing for the preparation of the endplates for the insertion of interbody grafts or spacers when deemed suitable.

The procedure is designed to maintain the integrity of the facet joints but requires nerve root retraction to enable comprehensive discectomy and the placement of interbody grafts or cages. The surgical process includes thorough decompression, an extensive discectomy, and fusion, which can be augmented by instrumented stabilization. Various materials, including iliac crest autograft, allograft, or cages filled with bone graft, may be utilized for fusion [5].

A significant advantage of PLIF is the extensive visualization it provides, facilitating the thorough decompression of neural structures without necessitating a separate incision. This procedure allows for fusion under compression, further enhancing spinal stability.

Nonetheless, PLIF is associated with certain risks, including epidural bleeding and fibrosis secondary to retraction, cage migration (particularly in the absence of instrumentation), cage subsidence, and adjacent segment degeneration.

3. Transforaminal lumbar interbody fusion (TLIF)

Transforaminal Lumbar Interbody Fusion (TLIF) emerged in 1982, initially introduced by Blume and Rojas [6] and later refined by Harms [7]. TLIF confers benefit partially due to its minimally invasive nature, which reduces the retraction of surrounding tissues, theoretically resulting in reduced scarring and blood loss. The

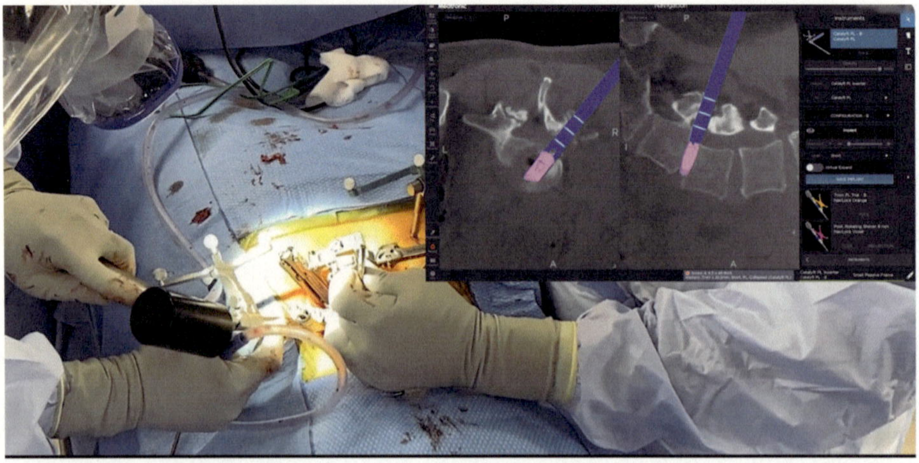

Figure 2.
Navigation assisted insertion of a TLIF cage.

technique is applicable at various spinal levels, without the limitations associated with sometimes a more excessive retraction when performing a PLIF. However, the procedure often achieves a less extensive discectomy compared to alternative methods, relying most commonly on a unilateral cage that may result in reduced stability and lesser surface area for fusion compared to a bilateral approach.

The TLIF procedure (**Figure 2**) involves accessing the intervertebral disc through the posterolateral aspect of the vertebral foramen, employing pedicle screw fixation to distract the disc space and restore lumbar lordosis with an interbody spacer. This is achieved through a unilateral laminectomy and inferior facetectomy, while preserving the contralateral facet joint. The discectomy and preparation of the endplates are performed through a lateral entry, which minimizes traction on the dura and adjacent nerve roots, a significant advantage over traditional posterior lumbar interbody fusion. Moreover, TLIF preserves the interlaminar surface on the contralateral side, providing additional grafting surface area and reducing the risk of neural damage.

The technique can be executed using either an open method or a minimally invasive "mini-open" approach [4]. With the patient positioned prone, a midline or bilateral paramedian incision is made to access the disc space from L1 to S1, allowing for effective placement of bone grafts. The technique primarily targets the ipsilateral neural foramen, however, bilateral decompression is possible.

The most common complications include postoperative hematoma, superficial infections, nerve root lesions, and dural tears. Rarely, intraoperative pneumothorax can occur.

4. Anterior lumbar interbody fusion (ALIF)

Anterior lumbar interbody fusion (ALIF) was first introduced by Lane and Moore in 1948 [8]. This method is particularly effective for accessing the L5-S1 intervertebral disc space, its utility diminishes at higher lumbar levels due to anatomical limitations.

ALIF effectively addresses discogenic disease by providing direct access to the anterior spine, facilitating the removal of increased diseased disc material, restoration of disc height, and simplified placement of interbody implants for spinal stabilization. The ALIF procedure involves discectomy and preparation of the endplates before evaluating the disc space for suitable coverage, height, and lordotic angle prior to the insertion of a cage or graft. Surgeons can utilize either a retroperitoneal or transperitoneal approaches to reach the disc. The transperitoneal route is generally limited to levels below L4, while the retroperitoneal approach is more frequently preferred as it allows access to all lumbar vertebrae from L1 to the sacrum. In certain cases, such as in significantly obese patients or following previous retroperitoneal exposure, the transperitoneal technique may still be viable.

The advantages of ALIF include direct visualization and efficient access to the anterior spinal column, which improves the extent of clearance achieved in discectomy. This technique promotes distraction of the disc space, thereby increasing neuroforaminal volume and allowing for the use of larger interbody devices. ALIF has been associated with elevated fusion rates and minimized damage to adjacent musculature, nerves, and bony structures. It is effective in restoring lumbar lordosis and maintaining coronal and sagittal balance while reducing anterolisthesis. The placement of the graft under compression against a larger osseous surface, coupled with a theoretically improved vascular supply, further enhances the likelihood of successful fusion. Additionally, ALIF preserves posterior spinal muscles and the anterolateral psoas muscles, which may contribute to reduced postoperative pain and faster recovery (**Figure 3**).

Despite its benefits, ALIF is not without the risk of complications, many of which stem from the surgical approach itself. These include the risks of postoperative hernias, bowel obstruction, iliac venous thrombosis, and urological injuries. There is also a significant risk of retrograde ejaculation in 45% of males as result of damage to the hypogastric plexus [9]. Major vascular complications occurring in approximately 0.5 to 4.3% of cases [10, 11].

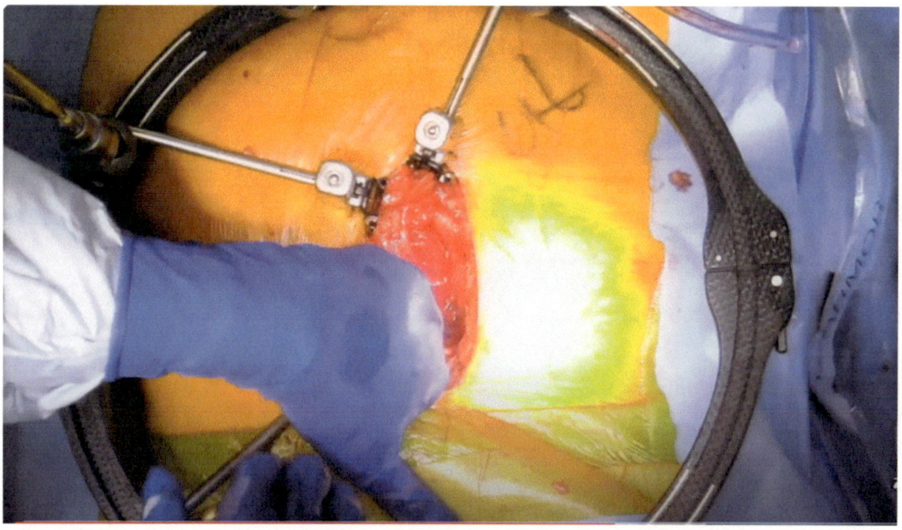

Figure 3.
ALIF with application of the Synframe retraction system along with soft tissue / muscle retractors.

While the technique entails certain risks, including vascular injury during the anterior approach and extended operative times, its application remains suitable for various conditions, particularly at the L4-L5 and L5-S1 levels, with a preference for the latter due to vascular considerations. However, its use at L2-3 and L3-4 levels is limited due to the need for significant peritoneal retraction and the rare risk of superior mesenteric artery thrombosis [4]. Contraindications for ALIF include significant prior abdominal surgery resulting in adhesions, unfavorable vascular anatomy, severe peripheral vascular disease, and presence of a solitary kidney on the surgical side. High-grade degenerative spondylolisthesis and isthmic spondylolisthesis at L5-S1 are considered a relative contraindication, often necessitating posterior stabilization in conjunction. Many surgeons choosing to augment the anterior fusion in all cases with posterior stabilization using a minimally invasive (e.g. percutaneous) or open technique.

5. Extreme lateral lumbar interbody fusion (XLIF/LLIF)

The extreme lateral interbody fusion (XLIF) technique, first introduced in 2006 [12] facilitates access to the intervertebral disc space through a lateral retroperitoneal and trans-psoas corridor. This approach is effective for treating various pathology at disc levels ranging from T12/L1 to L4/L5, however, it is not a feasible option at the L5/S1 level due to obstruction from the iliac crest. Additionally, the anterior positioning of the lumbar plexus and the lateral location of the iliac vessels at lower lumbar levels can heighten the risk of injury during the procedure.

In the XLIF procedure, the patient is positioned laterally, with the side selected based on the surgeon's preference and the specific anatomical considerations. A small incision, typically around 3–4 cm, is made, guided by imaging to ascertain the optimal positioning and angulation of the disc. The procedure involves three primary stages: lateral flank access, retroperitoneal dissection, and transpsoas navigation. The initial stage entails navigating through the abdominal muscles using a blunt, muscle-sparing technique. The subsequent stage requires meticulous dissection around important structures, including the subcostal and ilioinguinal nerves, while the final stage encounters the lumbar plexus, which exists between the L1/2 and L4/5 disc spaces (**Figure 4**).

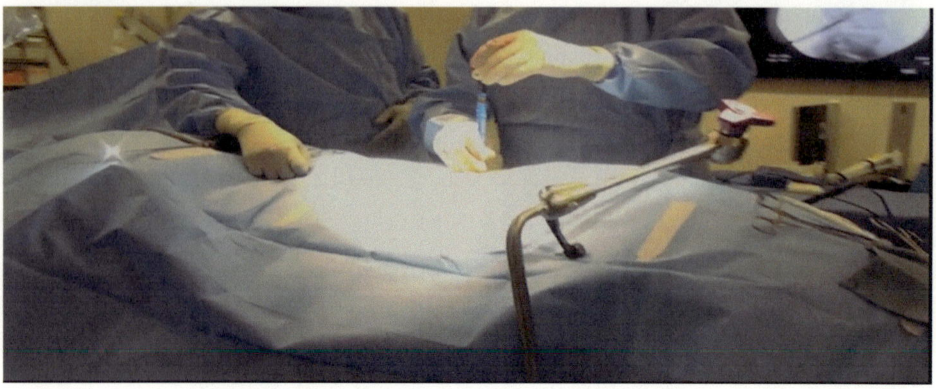

Figure 4.
XLIF with sequential dilation through the psoas.

XLIF is particularly effective for correcting sagittal and coronal deformities, such as lumbar degenerative scoliosis with lateral listhesis. The technique provides several advantages, including minimally invasive access that promotes faster post-operative recovery, effective deformity correction, high fusion rates, and thorough disc space clearance. Furthermore, the lateral positioning of the patient utilizes gravity to facilitate access while preserving posterior musculature and longitudinal ligaments, thus avoiding direct trauma to abdominal organs and major vascular structures.

It may not be suitable for patients with severe central canal stenosis, and anatomical variations can complicate access at the L4-5 level. Additionally, direct penetration of the psoas muscle may lead to postoperative hip flexion weakness, and there is a risk of thigh and groin pain if the genitofemoral nerve is stretched or injured. In addition, there are risks to the lumbar plexus and gastrointestinal structures.

Clinical outcomes associated with XLIF indicate that fusion rates are comparable to those achieved with traditional anterior and posterior approaches. Common postoperative symptoms include thigh-related paraesthesia, numbness, and weakness, affecting approximately one in five patients. Most of these sensory and motor deficits are transient, with recovery rates of about 50% at 3 months and 90% by 1 year [13].

6. Oblique/anterior to psoas lumbar interbody fusion

The oblique lateral interbody fusion (OLIF), also referred to as the anterior to psoas (ATP) approach, was first introduced in 1976 by Mayer [14], primarily for the revision of posterior non-unions. This minimally invasive technique allows access to the intervertebral disc space through a retroperitoneal corridor situated anterior to the psoas muscle and major abdominal vessels. Unlike the extreme lateral lumbar interbody fusion (XLIF), which faces limitations at the L5–S1 level due to obstruction from the iliac crests, the OLIF approach avoids the need for dissection or splitting of the psoas muscle, resulting in decreased postoperative pain and faster recovery. It confers the advantage that by passing anterior to the iliac crest, remaining in a retroperitoneal corridor it eliminates the need for neuro-monitoring by staying entirely anterior to the psoas muscle.

During the procedure, the patient is again positioned laterally, with the surgeon selecting either the left or right side based on accessibility. Most commonly though the patient is in the right lateral decubitus position with the left side up. A left sided incision is the frequent approach, as the vena cava on the right side either hinders access to or is close to the OLIF corridor. An incision is made laterally, guided by imaging to ascertain the position and angulation of the disc (**Figure 5**).

The OLIF approach offers several advantages, including efficient disc space clearance, and the ability to place larger interbody devices, which enhances foraminal decompression and potential for high fusion rates. Additionally, the oblique trajectory provides a unique view of the epidural space, facilitating the removal of ventral osteophytes and disc herniations.

In some cases, if the retroperitoneal corridor is narrow, additional retraction of the psoas may be necessary, increasing the likelihood of related neurological

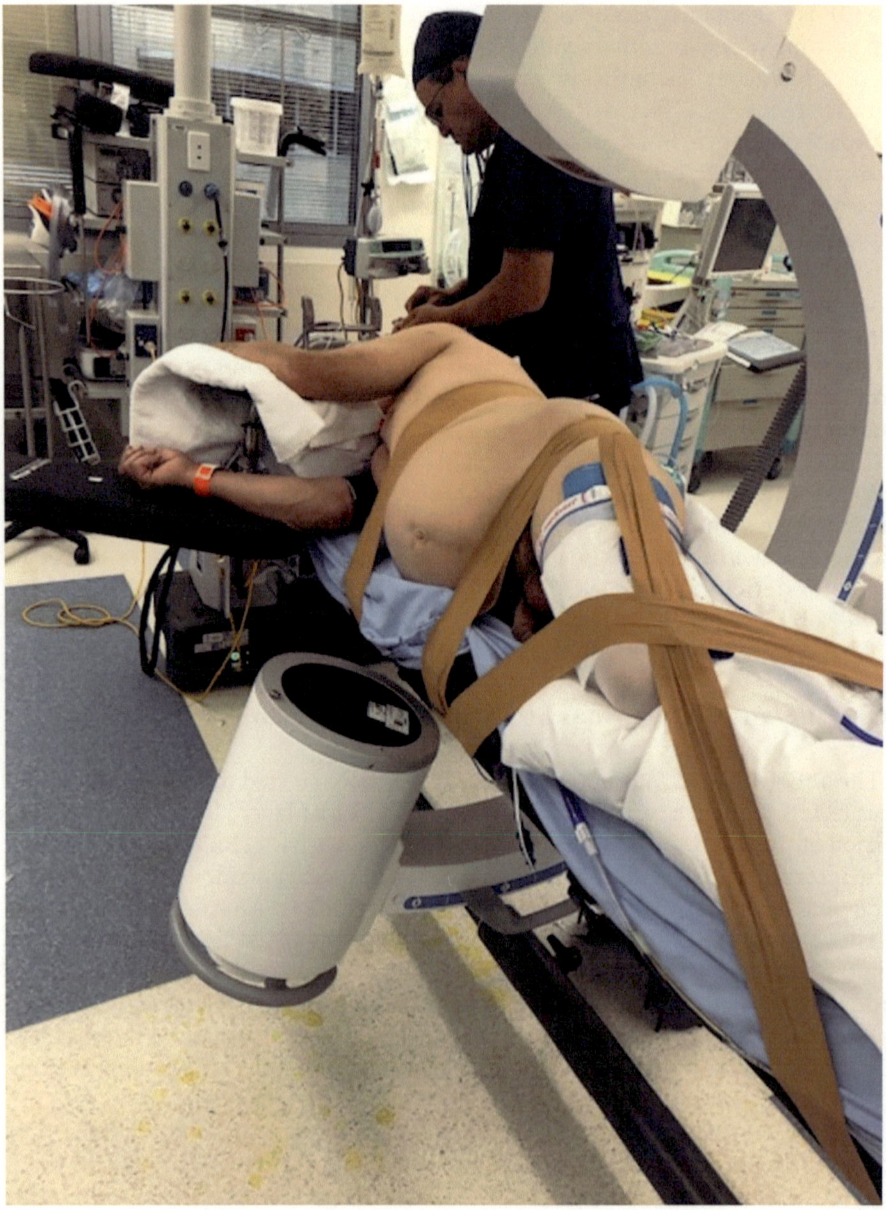

Figure 5.
Patient positioning for an Oblique/ATP interbody fusion.

complications. A large series by Abe [15] reported an overall perioperative complication rate of 48.3%, but only 1.9% of cases resulting in permanent neurological injury among 155 patients. Other significant reported complications included endplate fractures or subsidence (18.7%), and segmental artery injury (2.6%) (**Figure 6**).

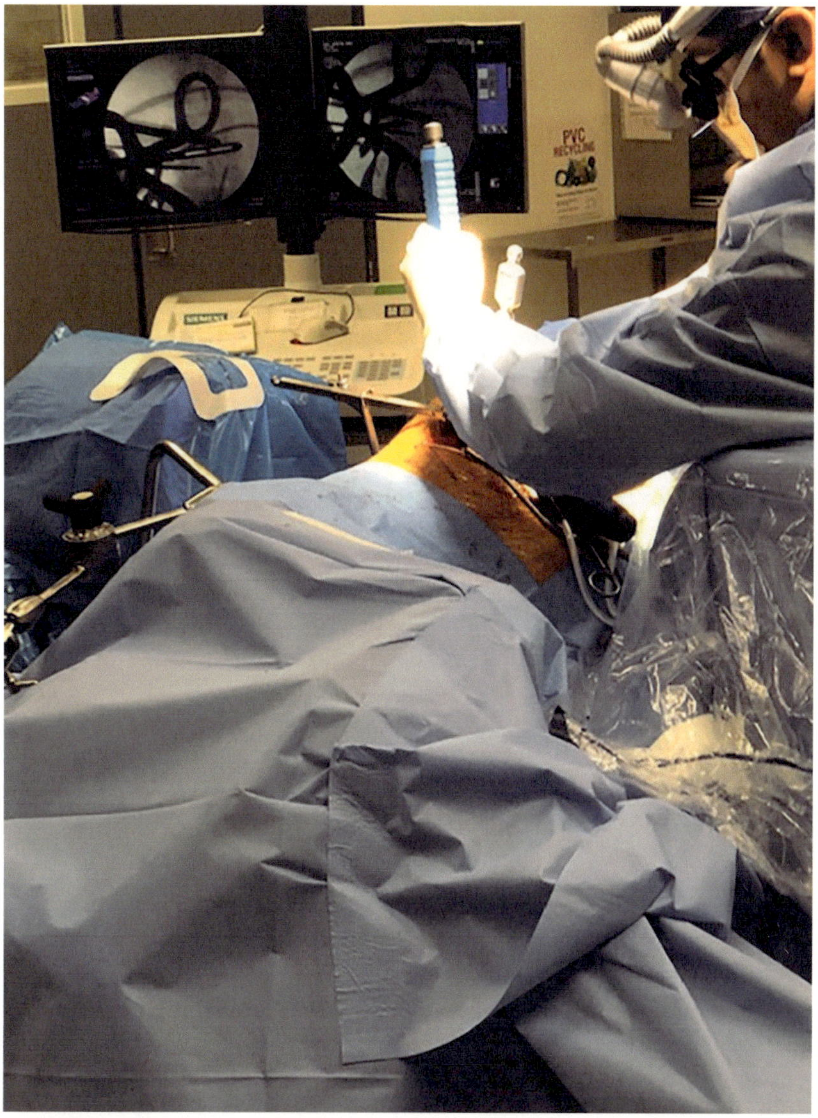

Figure 6.
Oblique approach, surgeon position relative to C-arm and fluoroscopy.

7. Comparison of techniques

7.1 Outcomes: Fusion rates

Evidence in the literature for satisfactory fusion rates is promising for all approaches. In one study [16] focusing on PLIF, researchers reported a spinal fusion success rate of 88.4–96.3%. For ALIF, a fusion rate of 95.3% among 43 patients, with successful fusion at 97% of the assessed levels has been described [17]. OLIF has been shown to achieve fusion rates exceeding 84% [18].

More recently, a systematic review and meta-analysis conducted by John Rathbone and colleagues in 2023 [19] further explored the effectiveness of stand-alone ALIF compared to various posterior fusion techniques for patients with spondylolisthesis and degenerative disc disease. This comprehensive analysis included 21 studies involving 3686 patients who underwent either ALIF, PLIF or TLIF. Fusion rates were not significantly different between ALIF and PLIF at 1 year (5 studies, n = 187, RR 0.92, CI 0.68, 1.24) or 2 years (2 studies, n = 109, RR 1.06, CI 0.97, 1.17). Fusion rates at 1 year (2 studies, n = 111, RR 1.00, CI 0.95, 1.05) and 2 years (n = 17, MD 0.95 CI 0.57 to 1.59) indicated no significant difference between ALIF and TLIF.

7.2 Outcomes: Pain and function

Current evidence largely supports equivalence between techniques for outcomes regarding pain and function. When comparing ALIF with transforaminal lumbar interbody fusion (TLIF), there were no significant differences in Visual Analogue Scale (VAS) scores for back pain at 1 year (four studies, n = 1192, mean difference confidence interval [CI] −0.30 to 0.70) or 2 years (three studies, n = 1507, CI −0.50 to 0.14). Similarly, VAS scores for leg pain did not show significant differences at 1 year (three studies, n = 1060, CI −0.53 to 0.09) or 2 years (three studies, n = 1507, CI −0.59 to 0.06) [19]. In the ALIF versus posterior lumbar interbody fusion (PLIF) comparisons, VAS scores for both back pain (n = 56, CI −0.04 to 1.56) and leg pain (n = 74, CI 0.85 to 1.25) were also not significantly different [19].

Regarding ODI scores, no significant differences were found between ALIF and TLIF at 1 year (four studies, n = 1217, CI −6.76 to 1.50) or 2 years (three studies, n = 1507, CI −1.90 to 1.86). Additionally, ODI scores up to 18 months (n = 58, CI −0.51 to 10.71) and at 2 years (n = 74, CI −6.40 to 11.20) did not show significant differences between ALIF and PLIF. The proportion of patients classified as 'not improved' on the ODI also did not differ significantly between ALIF and PLIF (n = 74, relative risk [RR] 1.03, CI 0.41 to 2.54) [19].

In Yan's retrospective comparison [20] of 176 patients with grade 1-2 degenerative spondylosis at L4/5 or L5/S1, both posterior lumbar interbody fusion (PLIF) and transforaminal lumbar interbody fusion (TLIF) were evaluated. Both techniques resulted in significant reductions in pain, with visual analog scale (VAS) scores showing similar improvements. Additionally, the Japanese Orthopedic Association (JOA) scores indicated a high success rate for both procedures, with no significant difference in outcomes between the two groups. Overall, both PLIF and TLIF were effective in alleviating pain and improving clinical results.

7.3 Additional outcomes: Operative time, blood loss, length of stay

Rathbone's meta-analysis [19] argued that anterior lumbar interbody fusion (ALIF) had notable advantages over both transforaminal lumbar interbody fusion (TLIF) and posterior lumbar interbody fusion (PLIF) regarding operative time and blood loss.

Specifically, surgical times were significantly reduced for ALIF (average 114–159 minutes) compared to PLIF (average 164–180 minutes), with an average difference of approximately 41 minutes [21, 22]. Similarly, ALIF patients experienced a shorter procedure duration than those undergoing TLIF (average 118–236 minutes), with an average reduction of 48 minutes [23, 24].

Blood loss during ALIF surgeries (mean blood loss 212–522 ml) was significantly less than that associated with PLIF, with a mean reduction of 186 ml (mean blood loss

341-725 ml) [21, 25]. ALIF also resulted in lower blood loss compared to TLIF (mean blood loss 210–548 ml, mean reduction 192mls), although this finding was marked by high variability among the studies [19]. In comparison, literature regarding OLIF has operative times ranging from 55 to 145 minutes and blood loss between 67 and 260 milliliters.

When examining hospital stays, the analysis indicated that while lengths of stay were not significantly different between ALIF and PLIF. ALIF patients did have shorter stays compared to those undergoing TLIF with an average difference of 0.71 days, albeit with substantial heterogeneity in the results. Overall, the study highlights ALIF as a more efficient option in terms of surgical time and blood loss, alongside a tendency for reduced hospitalization compared to TLIF.

8. Comparison of complications

Adverse events were infrequent across techniques and showed no significant differences between ALIF and TLIF. Readmission rates were also similar, although TLIF tended to have slightly lower rates. Complications directly related to surgery, postoperative problems, and adjacent segment disease occurring within 2 years did not differ significantly between ALIF and TLIF. Additionally, the incidence of deep vein thrombosis, hematoma, the necessity for revision surgery, and ileus was low and comparable between ALIF and PLIF. There were no significant differences in adjacent segment degeneration, postoperative complications, the need for blood transfusions, or dural tears when comparing ALIF with PLIF.

In Deng-lu Yan's 2008 study [20], despite greater neural retraction associated with PLIF, the complication rates were similar for both PLIF and TLIF. The PLIF group experienced four adverse events, including three cases of radiculitis and one related to a medial pedicle screw. In contrast, the TLIF group reported three complications, also featuring two cases of radiculitis and one medial pedicle screw.

8.1 Vertebral level of pathology

Mobbs [4] made the following useful recommendations for techniques which vary depending on the specific level and condition being treated.

At the L5/S1 level, Anterior Lumbar Interbody Fusion (ALIF) was the suggested approach for managing discogenic low back pain and restoring natural lordosis. Posterior Lumbar Interbody Fusion (PLIF) and Transforaminal Lumbar Interbody Fusion (TLIF) were considered suitable options for addressing issues such as central canal stenosis or recurrent disc herniation. PLIF was recommended for cases of isthmic spondylolisthesis due to the heightened risk of injury to the L5 nerve. In addition, preliminary data indicates that Oblique Lateral Interbody Fusion (OLIF) may be beneficial, whereas Lateral Lumbar Interbody Fusion (LLIF) was not recommended due to anatomic restrictions.

For the L4/5 level, both PLIF and TLIF were thought to be effective choices for treating degenerative spondylolisthesis. ALIF, OLIF, and LLIF could also be utilized for correcting lordosis and spinal deformities, although LLIF presents a risk of injuring the lumbar plexus and psoas muscle.

In the case of L2/3 and L3/4 levels, most surgical techniques are appropriate except for ALIF, which is discouraged due to the significant risk and need for specialized vascular surgical support for access to this level. For correcting deformities at these levels, antero-lateral techniques such as LLIF and OLIF are preferred.

At the T12/L1 and L1/2 levels, ALIF is not a viable option, while PLIF and TLIF may be complicated if the spinal cord or conus interferes with dural retraction during implant placement. LLIF is recommended, especially for deformity correction.

For multilevel surgeries, which typically involve correcting deformities resulting from degenerative conditions, a combination of anterior/lateral and posterior surgical methods is thought to be effective. Multilevel interventions employing ALIF, LLIF, and OLIF can achieve both sagittal and coronal alignment corrections, although they may require additional posterior stabilization.

9. Conclusion

This article provides a review of the surgical techniques employed in lumbar interbody fusion for the treatment of spondylosis. We compare five prominent methods: transforaminal lumbar interbody fusion (TLIF), posterior lumbar interbody fusion (PLIF), extreme lateral lumbar interbody fusion (XLIF), oblique/anterior to psoas lumbar interbody fusion (OLIF/ATP), and anterior lumbar interbody fusion (ALIF). Each technique is described, outlining its specific surgical approach, indications, advantages, and associated risks. The discussion highlights the crucial role of meticulous surgical planning and the importance of selecting the optimal technique based on individual patient anatomy, the specific pathology presented, and the surgeon's expertise.

We analyze the available evidence regarding fusion rates, pain reduction, and functional outcomes following each surgical approach. The data presented suggest that while fusion rates are generally high across all techniques, there is no statistically significant difference in pain relief or functional improvement at one or two-year follow-up assessments among the different techniques. The review highlights the advantages of ALIF in terms of reduced operative time and blood loss, yet acknowledges the associated risks, such as potential vascular injury and visceral complications. Conversely, techniques like TLIF and PLIF, while effective, may involve more extensive dissection and retraction, potentially leading to increased postoperative pain and recovery time. The OLIF/ATP approach, a minimally invasive option, is presented as a viable alternative that may minimize tissue trauma and hasten recovery. XLIF's unique lateral access is detailed, showing its effectiveness in addressing certain sagittal and coronal deformities but emphasizing the potential risks related to the proximity of the psoas major muscle and neural structures.

This article emphasizes the absence of a universally superior technique. The optimal choice is contingent upon a careful consideration of the patient's specific circumstances, including the involved vertebral level(s), the extent of the pathology, and the surgeon's expertise with each method. This personalized approach, thorough preoperative planning and an understanding of both the benefits and limitations of each technique, is crucial for achieving the best possible clinical outcomes in lumbar interbody fusion for spondylosis.

Acknowledgements

The authors would like to thank Mr. Panagiotis Liantis from Guy`s Hospital (London) for his support in the production of this chapter.

Conflict of interest

The authors declare no conflict of interest.

Author details

Bhoresh Dhamija[1*] and Steven Tominey[2]

1 National Hospital for Neurology and Neurosurgery, London, United Kingdom

2 Royal London Hospital, London, United Kingdom

*Address all correspondence to: bhoresh.dhamija1@nhs.net

References

[1] Middleton K, Fish DE. Lumbar spondylosis: Clinical presentation and treatment approaches. Current Reviews in Musculoskeletal Medicine. 2009;**2**(2):94-104

[2] Prabhu MC, Jacob KC, Patel MR, Pawlowski H, Vanjani NN, Singh K. History and evolution of the minimally invasive transforaminal lumbar interbody fusion. Neurospine [Internet]. 2022;**19**(3):479-491. Available from: https://pubmed.ncbi.nlm.nih.gov/36203277/

[3] Jin Y, Chen Q, Chen C, Lyu J, Shi B, Yang C, et al. Clinical research and technique note of TLIF by Wiltse approach for the treatment of degenerative lumbar. Orthopaedic Surgery. 2021;**13**(5):1628-1638

[4] Mobbs RJ, Phan K, Malham G, Seex K, Rao PJ. Lumbar interbody fusion: Techniques, indications and comparison of interbody fusion options including PLIF, TLIF, MI-TLIF, OLIF/ATP, LLIF and ALIF. Journal of Spine Surgery. 2015;**1**(1):2-18

[5] D'Souza M, Macdonald NA, Gendreau JL, Duddleston PJ, Feng AY, Ho AL. Graft materials and biologics for spinal interbody fusion. Biomedicine. 2019;7(4):75

[6] Blume HG, Rojas CH. Unilateral lumbar interbody fusion (posterior approach) utilizing dowel grafts: Experience in over 200 patients. The Journal of Neurological and Orthopaedic Surgery. 1981;**2**:171-175

[7] Harms J, Rolinger H. A one-stager procedure in operative treatment of spondylolistheses: Dorsal traction-reposition and anterior fusion (author's transl). Zeitschrift für Orthopädie und Ihre Grenzgebiete. 1982;**120**(3):343-347

[8] John D, Lane J, Emory S, Moore J. Transperitoneal approach to the intervertebral disc in the lumbar area. Annals of Surgery. 1948;**127**(3):537

[9] Kim YH, Ha KY, Rhyu KW, Park HY, Cho CH, Kim HC, et al. Lumbar interbody fusion: Techniques, pearls and pitfalls. Asian Spine Journal. 2020;**14**(5):730-741

[10] Caiazzo F, Capo L, Bago J. Intraoperative complications of the anterior retroperitoneal approach to the lumbosacral spine in the supine position: A proposal for an algorithm to predict the degree of difficulty of the surgical procedure. Surgical Techniques Development. 2023;**12**(4):188-198

[11] Garg J, Woo K, Hirsch J, Bruffey JD, Dilley RB. Vascular complications of exposure for anterior lumbar interbody fusion. Journal of Vascular Surgery. 2010;**51**(4):946-950

[12] Ozgur BM, Aryan HE, Pimenta L, Taylor WR. Extreme lateral interbody fusion (XLIF): A novel surgical technique for anterior lumbar interbody fusion. The Spine Journal. 2006;**6**(4):435-443

[13] Kono Y, Gen H, Sakuma Y, Koshika Y. Comparison of clinical and radiologic results of mini-open transforaminal lumbar interbody fusion and extreme lateral interbody fusion indirect decompression for degenerative lumbar spondylolisthesis. Asian Spine Journal. 2018;**12**(2):356

[14] Mayer HM. A new microsurgical technique for minimally invasive anterior

lumbar interbody fusion. Spine (Phila Pa 1976). 1997;**22**(6):691-699

[15] Abe K, Orita S, Mannoji C, Motegi H, Aramomi M, Ishikawa T, et al. Perioperative complications in 155 patients who underwent oblique lateral Interbody fusion surgery: Perspectives and indications from a retrospective, multicenter survey. Spine. 2017;**42**(1):55-62

[16] Karki S, Zhang S, Wang X, Sinkemani A, Sah GK. Comparison of clinical outcomes of cortical bone trajectory and traditional pedicle screw fixation in posterior lumbar interbody fusion. Open Journal of Orthopedics. 2019;**9**(3):31-47

[17] Jackson KL, Yeoman C, Chung WM, Chappuis JL, Freedman B. Anterior lumbar interbody fusion: Two-year results with a modular interbody device. Asian The Spine Journal. 2014;**8**(5):591

[18] Li HM, Zhang RJ, Shen CL. Differences in radiographic and clinical outcomes of oblique lateral interbody fusion and lateral lumbar interbody fusion for degenerative lumbar disease: A meta-analysis. BMC Musculoskeletal Disorders. 2019;**20**(1):582

[19] Rathbone J, Rackham M, Nielsen D, Lee SM, Hing W, Riar S, et al. A systematic review of anterior lumbar interbody fusion (ALIF) versus posterior lumbar interbody fusion (PLIF), transforaminal lumbar interbody fusion (TLIF), posterolateral lumbar fusion (PLF). European Spine Journal. 2023;**32**(6):1911-1926

[20] Deng-Lu Y, Fu-xing P, Jian L, Cheng-long S. Comparative study of PILF and TLIF treatment in adult degenerative spondylolisthesis. European Spine Journal. 2008;**17**(10):1311

[21] Freudenberger C, Lindley EM, Beard DW, Reckling WC, Williams A, Burger EL, et al. Posterior versus anterior lumbar interbody fusion with anterior tension band plating: Retrospective analysis. Orthopedics. 2009;**32**(7):492-496

[22] Lee N, Kim KN, Yi S, Ha Y, Shin DA, Yoon DH, et al. Comparison of outcomes of anterior, posterior, and transforaminal lumbar interbody fusion surgery at a single lumbar level with degenerative spinal disease. World Neurosurgery. 2017;**1**(101):216-226

[23] Bozzio AE, Johnson CR, Fattor JA, Kleck CJ, Patel VV, Burger EL, et al. Stand-alone anterior lumbar interbody, transforaminal lumbar interbody, and anterior/posterior fusion: Analysis of fusion outcomes and costs. Orthopedics. 2018;**41**(5):e655-e662

[24] Udby PM, Bech-Azeddine R. Clinical outcome of stand-alone ALIF compared to posterior instrumentation for degenerative disc disease: A pilot study and a literature review. Clinical Neurology and Neurosurgery. 2015;**1**(133):64-69

[25] Klara PM, Freidank SA, Rezaiamiri S. Comparison of lumbar interbody fusion techniques using ray threaded fusion cages and pedicle screw fixation systems. Neurosurgery Quarterly-LWW. 2003;**13**(1):20

Section 3

Emerging Technologies in Neurosurgery

Chapter 10

Advanced Imaging and Augmented Reality in Neurosurgery: Bridging Innovation and Precision

Elad Mashiach, Sauson Soldozy, Ariel Sacknovitz, Ankita Jain, Hayley Donaldson, Sabrina Zeller, Geet Shukla, Cameron Rawanduzy, Fernando De Nigris Vasconcellos, Chirag Gandhi and Justin Santarelli

Abstract

The evolution of advanced imaging technologies has profoundly impacted neurosurgery, enabling greater precision, safety, and improved outcomes in complex procedures. This chapter provides a comprehensive overview of key imaging modalities such as MRI, CT, fMRI, DTI, and iMRI, emphasizing their roles in neurosurgical planning, navigation, and real-time monitoring. Building on these technologies, the advent of augmented reality (AR) has introduced transformative tools that overlay digital information onto the surgical field, allowing neurosurgeons to visualize critical anatomical structures with unprecedented clarity. The integration of AR with imaging systems enhances preoperative planning, intraoperative navigation, and postoperative assessment across various neurosurgical domains, from tumor resections to minimally invasive spinal surgeries. Despite these advancements, the chapter also examines technical and practical challenges, including AR system latency, high implementation costs, and training demands. Ethical and regulatory considerations are also discussed, underscoring the need for stringent data security and alignment with healthcare regulations. The chapter concludes by exploring the potential of integrating AI-driven AR and emerging imaging modalities, highlighting the continuous innovations shaping the future of neurosurgical precision, safety, and patient care.

Keywords: augmented reality, virtual reality, 3D visualization, imaging, neurosurgery, precision, innovation, fluoroscopy, remote surgery

1. Introduction: The role of advanced imaging in modern neurosurgery

Advanced imaging has revolutionized the field of neurosurgery, enabling unprecedented precision, safety, and efficacy in surgical interventions. Over the past few decades, technological advancements in imaging modalities such as magnetic resonance imaging (MRI), computed tomography (CT), and functional imaging techniques have significantly enhanced the capabilities of neurosurgeons. These innovations have allowed for detailed visualization of anatomical structures and critical functional regions, aiding in the development of effective treatment strategies and improving clinical outcomes. With the advent of augmented reality (AR) and its integration with conventional imaging methods, the surgical landscape is transforming even further, allowing neurosurgeons to navigate complex anatomical territories with real-time guidance and visual augmentation. This chapter delves into the role of advanced imaging techniques in modern neurosurgery and explores the impact of AR on surgical procedures, providing a comprehensive review of the latest developments and their clinical implications.

1.1 Evolution of imaging techniques in neurosurgery

The evolution of imaging techniques in neurosurgery has been instrumental in the field's progress. Initially, neurosurgeons relied on basic radiographic techniques that offered limited visualization of the brain and spinal structures. These early methods lacked the resolution necessary for precise localization of lesions, making it difficult to plan surgical interventions effectively. The introduction of CT scanning in the 1970s marked a turning point, as it provided high-resolution images of the brain and allowed for the differentiation between various tissue types. CT quickly became the gold standard for diagnosing intracranial hemorrhages, skull fractures, and other conditions requiring immediate surgical intervention [1].

Following the widespread adoption of CT, MRI emerged in the 1980s as a superior modality for visualizing soft tissue structures. With its ability to produce high-contrast images of the brain, spinal cord, and surrounding tissues without the use of ionizing radiation, MRI rapidly gained favor among neurosurgeons. The subsequent development of functional MRI (fMRI) and diffusion tensor imaging (DTI) expanded the scope of MRI beyond anatomical visualization. These advanced modalities enabled the mapping of brain activity and the visualization of white matter tracts, respectively, providing critical information for surgical planning in cases involving eloquent brain areas [2].

Neuroangiography represents another pioneering imaging modality that has revolutionized not only modern cerebrovascular neurosurgery, but other neurosurgical domains as well. Emerging as an extension of cardiac catheterization, which was pioneered in the early twentieth century by German surgical resident Werner Forssman, the first reports of therapeutic application of endovascular techniques were in the 1980s for basilar artery stenosis [3]. This has since expanded to not only include cerebral revascularization, but also embolization of aneurysms and vascular malformations, selective tumor embolization, intra-arterial drug delivery, and more recently described endovascular shunting and brain machine interface implantation and shunting [4, 5]. In addition to its obvious therapeutic benefits, as a diagnostic tool the value of neuroangiography is unmistakable in providing both effective preoperative planning, as well as real-time intraoperative confirmation of eradication of neurovascular pathologies.

The integration of other intraoperative imaging technologies, such as intraoperative MRI (iMRI) and intraoperative ultrasound (iUS), represented another leap forward in neurosurgical practice. These techniques allowed for real-time imaging during surgery, enhancing the surgeon's ability to detect residual tumor tissue and minimize the risk of damaging healthy brain structures. By incorporating real-time feedback, neurosurgeons could adjust their surgical approach dynamically, improving the precision of resection and reducing postoperative complications [6].

1.2 Overview of augmented reality (AR) in surgical procedures

In recent years, augmented reality (AR) has emerged as a transformative tool in neurosurgery, further advancing the capabilities of traditional imaging techniques. AR overlays digital information—such as 3D anatomical models, preoperative imaging data, and surgical landmarks—onto the surgeon's field of view, providing a comprehensive and intuitive understanding of the surgical site. Unlike virtual reality (VR), which immerses the user in a completely virtual environment, AR enhances the real-world environment by superimposing digital elements in real-time, enabling neurosurgeons to maintain direct visual contact with the patient while accessing critical data [7].

The application of AR in neurosurgery extends across various domains, including resident/fellow education, preoperative planning, intraoperative navigation, and postoperative assessment. In the preoperative phase, AR assists in the visualization of complex anatomical structures, aiding in the identification of safe surgical trajectories and potential risks. Neurosurgeons can use AR-based platforms to interact with 3D models of the patient's anatomy, simulating the surgical procedure and refining their strategy before entering the operating room. During surgery, AR can be integrated with intraoperative imaging modalities, providing continuous visual guidance and reducing the need for repetitive imaging. For example, AR-assisted navigation systems project 3D anatomical models directly onto the surgical field, enabling precise localization of tumors and other critical structures without disrupting the surgical workflow [8].

Moreover, AR has shown promise in enhancing the safety and efficacy of complex neurosurgical procedures, such as skull base surgeries and minimally invasive spinal interventions. By providing detailed visualization of critical neurovascular structures and surgical targets, AR reduces the risk of intraoperative complications and facilitates safer, more accurate surgical maneuvers [9]. Postoperatively, AR can be employed to assess surgical outcomes, monitor recovery, and educate patients about their conditions, fostering a better understanding of the surgical process and improving overall patient care.

1.3 Objectives and scope of the chapter

The primary objective of this chapter is to provide a comprehensive review of advanced imaging techniques and their role in modern neurosurgical practice, with a specific focus on the integration of AR in surgical procedures. The chapter begins by tracing the historical evolution of imaging technologies in neurosurgery, highlighting key milestones and their impact on the field. This retrospective analysis sets the stage for a detailed exploration of current imaging modalities, including MRI, CT, PET, and intraoperative imaging techniques, emphasizing their respective strengths and limitations.

Subsequently, the chapter delves into the emergence of AR as a pivotal technology in neurosurgery, examining its various applications and potential to revolutionize surgical practice. By combining real-world scenarios with advanced imaging data, AR offers neurosurgeons a unique opportunity to enhance their spatial understanding of complex anatomical regions, leading to improved surgical precision and patient outcomes. The integration of AR with traditional imaging modalities is explored in depth, focusing on how these hybrid platforms can overcome the limitations of standalone imaging systems and enable more comprehensive surgical planning and execution.

The chapter also addresses the challenges and limitations associated with implementing AR and advanced imaging in neurosurgery, such as technical constraints, cost considerations, and the learning curve for surgeons. A discussion on ethical and regulatory issues surrounding the use of AR in clinical practice is included to provide a balanced perspective on the future of this technology.

Finally, the chapter concludes by offering insights into the future directions of advanced imaging and AR in neurosurgery, with an emphasis on emerging trends such as AI-driven imaging analysis, remote surgery, and the potential for AR to facilitate collaborative and tele-neurosurgical practices. The chapter aims to equip neurosurgeons with a nuanced understanding of the current state and future potential of these technologies, empowering them to leverage these advancements for the benefit of their patients and the broader field of neurosurgery.

Through this comprehensive overview, readers will gain a deeper appreciation of the transformative impact of advanced imaging and AR on neurosurgical practice, as well as an understanding of the ongoing innovations that are poised to shape the future of the field.

1.4 Methods

A comprehensive review of existing literature on artificial AI and AR was done. Relevant studies, articles, and reports were identified through systematic searches across academic databases, including PubMed, IEEE Xplore, and Scopus, using search terms such as "AI," "augmented reality," "AI in neurosurgery and "advanced imaging in neurosurgery." Inclusion criteria focused on peer-reviewed publications from the past decade, emphasizing technological advancements, integration strategies, and applications in healthcare. Key themes and insights were extracted through thematic analysis to identify trends, challenges, and future directions in the convergence of AI and AR technologies. The findings were synthesized into a narrative structure to provide a comprehensive overview of the field.

2. Current state of imaging technologies in neurosurgery

Advanced imaging techniques create the foundation for neurosurgical practice, offering unmatched levels of precision and insight into the complex structures of the brain and spine. Imaging technologies have significantly enhanced both preoperative planning and intraoperative decision-making, leading to better enhanced understanding of both structural and functional relationships in the brain and spine, reduced complication rates, and more efficient and safer procedures. Below is a comprehensive review of the key imaging modalities currently employed in neurosurgery.

2.1 High-resolution MRI: Functional and structural applications

High-resolution MRI continues to be a fundamental tool in neurosurgical imaging, offering exceptional resolution that enables clinicians to detect pathological changes in normal brain tissue [10]. High-resolution 3D MRI sequences, in particular, allow for detailed visualization of both brain and spinal cord anatomy through various sequences that provide specific insights into different tissue types, offering substantial clinical utility [11]. Ongoing advancements in MRI technology, such as improvements in spatial resolution, contrast techniques, and variable sequences, play a crucial role in diagnosing and planning surgeries for neurosurgical patients [11]. This imaging modality is invaluable for studying the microstructural aspects of neuroanatomy, assessing functional activity, analyzing tissue composition, and monitoring blood flow [11]. These capabilities aid in diagnosing and treating a wide range of neurological conditions, including tumors, strokes, and epilepsy, among others.

Standardized MRI protocols currently include sequences such as 3D T1, axial fluid-attenuated inversion recovery (FLAIR), axial diffusion-weighted imaging (DWI), axial gadolinium-enhanced T2, and 3D gadolinium-enhanced T1. These sequences are typically performed on MRI systems with a minimum magnetic field strength of 1.5 tesla [11, 12]. Most clinical MRI scans utilize field strengths between 1.5 and 3 tesla, though research is exploring the use of ultra-high-field MRI scanners with field strengths as high as 10.5 tesla [11, 13]. These high-field scanners aim to improve signal-to-noise ratios, allowing for superior spatial resolution. While ultra-high-field MRI is not yet widely used in everyday neurosurgical practice, it has proven effective in detecting lesions that standard clinical MRI scanners may miss. Even 7 T MRI systems have demonstrated tremendous value in identifying previously undetectable refractory epilepsy lesions lesions as well as unruptured intracranial aneurysms at resolutions comparable to gold standard diagnostic subtraction angiography (DSA) [13, 14].

MRI functions by manipulating the magnetic fields of hydrogen ions and observing how they return to their normal magnetic orientation. When tissue is placed within a strong magnetic field, the protons within that tissue align with the external field. A radiofrequency (RF) pulse then disrupts this alignment, generating magnetization in a direction distinct from the primary B0 magnetic field. Once the RF pulse ceases, the protons gradually realign [11]. The T1 signal represents the longitudinal relaxation rate, measured along the z-axis, while the T2 signal reflects the transverse relaxation rate, where protons lose phase coherence in the x-y plane. Differences in the relaxation rates of various molecules produce distinct signals, creating unique imaging characteristics for different tissue types [11].

Different MRI sequences provide valuable information to clinicians regarding potential pathologies. For instance, when assessing an intracranial mass, T1-weighted, T2-weighted, and FLAIR imaging offer precise localization and definition of tumor boundaries, helping to distinguish between tumor progression and treatment effects, such as radiation necrosis. These techniques are critical for preoperative planning in gliomas and contribute to improving outcomes in complex procedures like skull base tumor resections by providing surgeons with accurate anatomical details. The ability to differentiate between tissue types enhances the formulation of differential diagnoses and a deeper understanding of the specific pathology a patient may have. For example, tumors often result in vasogenic edema, best visualized with T2-weighted imaging, while specific diffusion-weighted sequences are instrumental in the early detection of ischemic infarcts, revolutionizing ischemic stroke treatment protocols [15]. Gadolinium contrasted studies further enhance the ability to distinguish pathologic tissues from adjacent normal structures, with unique patterns of contrast uptake characteristic of certain disease states aiding in diagnosis, operative planning, and surgical resection strategies.

2.2 Diffusion tensor imaging (DTI) for tractography

DTI tractography enables visualization of white matter tracts and functional networks which is of particular interest for pathologies near critical motor, language, or visual pathways (**Figure 1**). Traditional dogma suggests unique brain functions are localized to distinct anatomical locations; however, DTI mapping has contributed largely to the human connectome project, which seeks to map

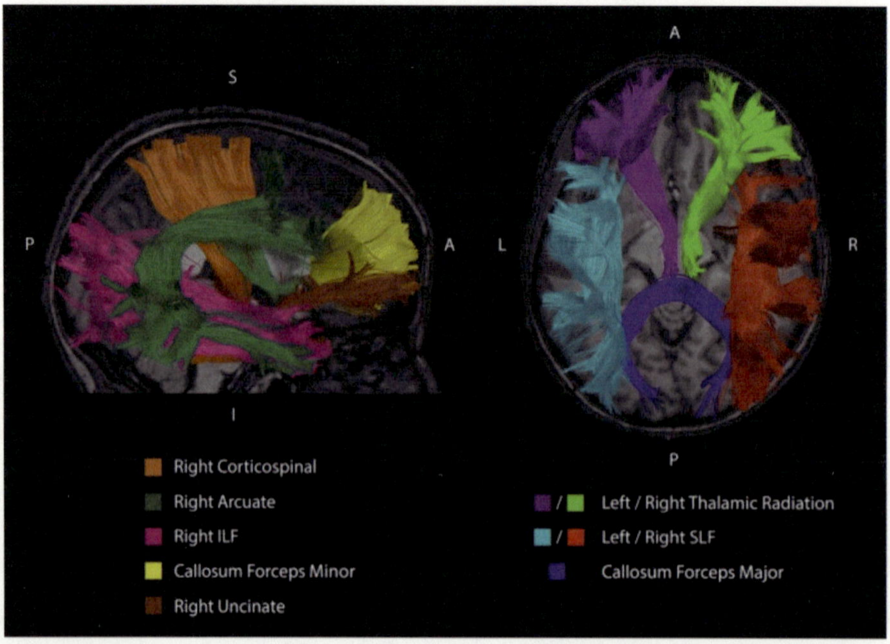

Figure 1.
Axial and sagittal views of MRI tractography showing selection of fiber bundles [16].

the human brain. Connectomics has thus emerged as a burgeoning field that has shed light on the exceedingly complex and integrated structural and functional connectivity of the brain. By detecting the diffusion of water molecules flowing in parallel with axonal fibers, DTI produces fiber maps, the orientation of which allow neurosurgeons to plan resection strategies that aim to preserve structural integrity [17, 18]. This approach has been particularly valuable for intra-axial lesions, where tumor boundaries are often intimately involved with if not invading essential white matter tracts [19]. Several studies have shown that using DTI, in conjunction with other functional imaging modalities, significantly reduces postoperative neurologic deficits [20].

However, DTI tractography is not without its challenges. In isolation, DTI tractography provides information regarding structural relationships and connectivity only. As a result, it is susceptible to shifts or compression of adjacent parenchyma rendering the image acquired tracts inaccurate. Mass lesions or significant peritumoral edema must be accounted for when interpreting these structural data, which ongoing software advancements aim to address. Given that tractography relies on anatomical landmarks to seed regions of interest, it does not account for functional connectivity across anatomically distinct brain regions [19]. In fact, studies have demonstrated functional mapping to reveal subtle changes in functional connectivity in mild traumatic brain injury patients that would otherwise not be delineated with anatomic based tractography [21]. Additionally, functional connectivity may serve to redefine anatomical eloquence in patients with otherwise inoperable or high-risk lesions who have demonstrated cortical reorganization [22]. As a result, the notion of "eloquent noneloquence" further highlights the limitations of DTI and other structural based mapping techniques which fail to account for the presence of highly complex and integrated functional brain networks [23, 24].

While these limitations remain, the continued advancement of imaging technologies is expected to improve the accuracy and reliability of tractography, further enhancing its role in neurosurgical planning and patient outcomes.

2.3 Intraoperative MRI (iMRI) for real-time monitoring

Intraoperative MRI (iMRI) has become a groundbreaking tool in neurosurgery, addressing several critical challenges, such as detecting residual tumor tissue after resection. As technology has advanced and neuronavigation systems have become standard in neurosurgical procedures, iMRI has proven particularly valuable in compensating for brain shift that occurs during intracranial surgeries [25]. By providing real-time imaging, iMRI offers essential intraoperative feedback that can inform further surgical intervention [26]. Since its introduction into operating rooms in the 1990s, the use of iMRI has become more prevalent. However, its widespread adoption remains limited by the substantial costs and infrastructure required for installation [25]. Despite these challenges, iMRI has significantly impacted the field of neuro-oncology, with studies demonstrating that its use enhances the extent of tumor resection, thus reducing the need for repeat operations [26].

2.4 Arterial spin labeling (ASL)

Arterial spin labeling (ASL) is an MRI technique that non-invasively measures cerebral blood flow (CBF), playing a critical role in assessing tumor perfusion, ischemia, and vascular malformations. One of ASL's main advantages is its ability to evaluate brain tumor perfusion without requiring contrast agents, making it particularly beneficial for patients with renal insufficiency who may be considered high risk for cerebral angiography [27]. It allows clinicians to assess microvascular density and perfusion characteristics in brain tumors, offering an alternative to more invasive methods like dynamic susceptibility contrast (DSC) MRI.

In neurosurgical planning, ASL is instrumental in identifying hypoperfused regions and distinguishing between low- and high-grade gliomas. It provides valuable perfusion data, helping surgeons make informed decisions regarding revascularization procedures and the best approach to minimize risk during resection. Studies have demonstrated ASL's strong correlation with histopathological markers like microvascular density, which is critical for assessing tumor aggressiveness and planning treatment strategies [28]. While ASL and DSC-MRI both offer valuable perfusion data, ASL provides an edge in certain clinical settings due to its non-invasive nature and lack of reliance on exogenous tracers [28].

Additionally, ASL has proven valuable in tumor grading, with hyperperfused lesions often correlating with high-grade tumors and hypoperfused regions indicating lower grades [29]. This makes ASL a critical tool in monitoring tumor progression and planning interventions in both primary and metastatic brain tumors [30].

2.5 CT angiography in vascular neurosurgery

CTA (CT angiography) has become an essential tool in vascular neurosurgery, particularly for the diagnosis and treatment of vascular conditions such as aneurysms, arteriovenous malformations (AVMs), and ischemic stroke. It provides high-resolution images of cerebral vasculature, delivering crucial data for both open and endovascular procedures. In cases of aneurysmal subarachnoid hemorrhage, CTA is often the first-line diagnostic imaging tool, offering reliable visualization of the ruptured aneurysm and streamlining pretreatment planning [31]. Studies have shown that CTA-guided aneurysm surgeries can significantly reduce operative time and enhance the clarity of aneurysm morphology, leading to better surgical outcomes. However, when CTA imagery is inadequate or unclear, complementary pretreatment digital subtraction angiography (DSA) may be necessary to ensure the precise evaluation of aneurysm characteristics, further guiding surgical or interventional decision-making [32].

2.6 3D reconstructions for cranial and spinal procedures

3D CT reconstructions are invaluable in cranial and spinal neurosurgery, offering enhanced anatomical visualization and spatial understanding [33]. In skull base surgery, 3D reconstructions enable surgeons to plan precise approaches to tumors located near critical neurovascular structures. A recent study demonstrated that the use of 3D printed reconstructions reduced operative time and improved accuracy in placing spinal instrumentation during complex deformity corrections [34]. This is especially beneficial in deformity cases or traumatic fractures, where detailed preoperative planning is essential [35].

2.7 Positron emission tomography (PET) and SPECT

Positron emission tomography (PET) and single-photon emission computed tomography (SPECT) have become indispensable tools in brain tumor imaging, offering metabolic and functional information that complements structural imaging modalities like MRI and CT. PET, particularly when using tracers such as Fluorodeoxyglucose (FDG) or amino acids, plays a crucial role in differentiating tumor recurrence from radiation necrosis in gliomas, a distinction that can be difficult to make using MRI alone [36]. By mapping metabolic activity, PET enhances surgical precision, improving tumor resection outcomes and contributing to long-term disease control in glioblastoma patients. Studies have demonstrated that PET-guided surgeries result in better tumor delineation and more targeted treatment strategies [36].

Similarly, SPECT, although less frequently employed than PET, is highly valuable in functional imaging, particularly in the context of epilepsy surgery, where it helps localize seizure foci during preoperative evaluations [37]. SPECT can also assess cerebral perfusion, providing critical insights in traumatic brain injury cases, which may in the future be able to help guide surgical and therapeutic interventions [38].

Neuroimaging, including PET and SPECT, is crucial for accurate diagnosis, treatment planning, and monitoring of brain tumors. PET and SPECT improve the ability to localize tumors, evaluate tumor perfusion, and distinguish between tumor types and grades, thus enhancing biopsy precision and optimizing radiotherapy planning. With dual-modality hybrid systems such as PET-CT, PET-MRI, and SPECT-MRI, anatomical and functional data are seamlessly integrated, further refining surgical and treatment approaches [39]. These systems provide superior tumor margin delineation and facilitate stereotactic biopsies, improving accuracy of histologic diagnosis [39].

2.8 Intraoperative ultrasound

Applications in Tumor Resection and Hemorrhage Evacuation.

Intraoperative ultrasound (iUS) has become a valuable tool in neurosurgery due to its portability, cost-effectiveness, and ability to provide real-time imaging without requiring patient repositioning. This is particularly advantageous in brain tumor resections and hemorrhage evacuations, where iUS delivers dynamic feedback during surgery, enhancing precision [40]. Compared to more traditional intraoperative imaging methods like MRI, iUS offers similar efficacy in guiding the extent of resection but is faster and less expensive.

Studies have shown that iUS-guided resections of gliomas can achieve outcomes comparable to intraoperative MRI (iMRI)-guided procedures in terms of tumor removal, while significantly reducing both the time and cost involved [41]. Additionally, iUS is increasingly applied in spinal surgeries, where it assists in localizing tumors and aiding decompression procedures [42]. More advanced techniques, such as multiparametric ultrasound, offer the added advantage of providing both structural and functional information during surgeries, further enhancing its utility in identifying residual tumor tissue and vascularization patterns in a variety of neurosurgical contexts [41].

2.9 Functional imaging and neurophysiological mapping

Mapping Brain Functions and Planning Safe Surgical Trajectories.

Functional MRI, along with intraoperative neurophysiological monitoring (IONM), are critical in neurosurgical procedures involving eloquent brain regions. IONM allows real-time monitoring of motor and sensory pathways, reducing postoperative deficits in surgeries like those for brain tumors, AVMs, and epilepsy. The integration of imaging and mapping techniques is the gold standard for navigating complex brain areas.

fMRI, which measures brain activity through blood flow changes, has been instrumental in preoperative planning, especially near eloquent cortices. fMRI is essential for surgical planning, especially for mapping cortical regions like motor and language areas. While fMRI is non-invasive, the combination of various techniques, such as direct cortical stimulation (DCS) and DTI, offers an enhanced understanding of white matter tracts and eloquent cortex functionality [41]. This multimodal approach optimizes surgical precision while minimizing neurological risks.

However, limitations do exist, for example, brain shift during surgery affecting accuracy and the inability of fMRI to map white matter tracts effectively on its own [41]. Techniques like DTI provide detailed mapping of these tracts, improving the understanding of how functional regions are interconnected. Combining structural and functional imaging—despite being resource-intensive—can significantly improve outcomes by offsetting the limitations of each individual method.

3. Augmented reality (AR) in neurosurgery: Bridging digital and physical worlds

Augmented reality (AR) technology has recently been adopted in neurosurgery to enhance the surgeon's ability to visualize and navigate complex anatomy in real time. By overlaying digital information onto the physical operative field, AR enables surgeons to maintain focus on the patient while receiving critical visual feedback, improving both precision and safety.

3.1 What is AR?

Augmented Reality (AR) in neurosurgery allows surgeons to superimpose digital 3D models of anatomical structures, including vasculature, tumors, or white matter tracts, onto the real-time surgical view. This overlay enhances spatial awareness and enables safer navigation around critical regions. AR-assisted surgeries not only improve accuracy during tumor resections but also reduce operative times, particularly in challenging cases such as subcortically located tumors [43]. AR technology can reduce surgical risks by refining neuronavigation and improving overall precision during intricate procedures.

3.2 Differences between AR, virtual reality (VR), and mixed reality (MR)

Virtual reality (VR) creates an entirely digital environment, immersing the user away from the real world, whereas AR allows surgeons to interact with both digital and physical environments simultaneously. Mixed Reality (MR) further merges these experiences, allowing interaction with both real and virtual objects. Unlike VR, which is primarily used for simulations and training, AR and MR have found growing clinical utility, as they offer real-time surgical guidance without interrupting workflow [43].

3.3 The rise of AR in neurosurgical procedures

AR technology in neurosurgery has evolved from simple 2D image overlays to sophisticated 3D visualizations, combining MRI, CT, and DTI data to produce real-time models of critical structures during surgery [44]. This capability has become especially transformative in skull-base and spinal surgeries, where navigating tight anatomical spaces while preserving function is paramount. AR platforms enhance surgical planning by projecting key structures in real-time, aiding precise decision-making and increasing safety [44].

3.4 Development of AR-based surgical assistance systems

AR systems now seamlessly integrate preoperative imaging with neuronavigation tools, significantly improving the accuracy of tasks such as spinal screw placement in complex deformity surgeries. Recent studies show AR's potential to reduce complications like nerve damage, offering a practical solution to enhance precision. Ongoing research aims to further optimize these systems for widespread intraoperative use through refining their effectiveness and adaptability to diverse neurosurgical scenarios.

4. Application of AR in neurosurgical procedures

4.1 Preoperative planning

Preoperative planning for neuro-oncological cases requires precise visualization of the target tumor via medical imaging as well as preparation of the computer-assisted surgical navigation system to guide entry and approach for brain tumor resection. Neuronavigation is used to create a three-dimensional, virtual coordinate system that allows surgeons to align imaging data and identify patient-specific neuroanatomical landmarks on an electronic display separate from the patient. However, inherent limitations of neuronavigation systems—including spatial disconnection between the physician and patient as well as three-dimensional representation of a two-dimensional image—lead to possible underestimation or overestimation of tumor margins [45]. Preoperative use of AR can address these limitations by allowing for three-dimensional neuroimaging to be superimposed onto the patient. This prevents the attention shift of the surgeon to and from the neuronavigation display and avoids additional cognitive load on the surgeon [46, 47].

AR models with built-in navigation systems have been created for tumor delineation that yield accurate tumor visualization as well as decreased preoperative planning time. One team of researchers proposed the first reported pilot study of the use of OpenSight software through an AR head-mounted display to project preoperative MR images as holographic objects in anatomically-precise locations on the patient [48]. In this study, eleven patients underwent craniotomy for brain tumor resection. In each case, the surgeon used the AR head-mount to perform circumferential tumor border tracing with a red marker on the patient's scalp. As an advancement of this same technology, another group developed an AR-based navigation system with infrared tracking capabilities that allow for improved accuracy without the requirement of external tracking cameras [45]. These AR models equip surgeons with the capacity to develop preoperative tumor resection strategies characterized by an optimal degree of precision with tumor localization.

4.2 Intraoperative navigation and real-time visualization

Since the early utilization of AR in neurosurgical cases, combined AR navigation systems have evolved and risen to the forefront of intraoperative AR employment (**Figure 2**). Several medical device companies have created technologies that merge AR with neuronavigation to enhance real-time brain tumor visualization during surgery. These technologies use preoperative neuroimaging of the patient to generate 360-degree holographic renderings that are overlaid onto the live image of the patient through AR glasses or head-mount devices. The entire system operates out of the headset, with no external devices or screens required [49]. With both imaging and navigation contained in a singular device, the surgeon is able to visualize otherwise concealed neuroanatomical structures, all the while focusing on their surgical field of view.

An intraoperative AR overlay on a neurosurgical patient is a three-dimensional reconstruction of two-dimensional preoperative MR imaging [50]. This superimposition of a patient's neuroimaging through an AR system allows for a level of neuroanatomical accuracy and surgical efficiency that is required in neurosurgical cases. Augmentation of the neurosurgeon's visual intake with features of virtual reality must occur in a smooth way that upholds surgical workflow with minimal to no disruption of the operation. When optimized, the use of AR overlay in neurosurgical cases has the potential to minimize surgical errors, prevent invasive maneuvers, increase operative success, and ultimately improve postoperative clinical outcomes [49, 51].

4.3 Integration of AR for tumor resection

In the field of neuro-oncology, AR has primarily been utilized in the surgical resection of gliomas and meningiomas. With both physical and virtual objects in the same plane, AR is able to optimize the neurosurgeon's perception of the margins of the brain tumor as well as any relevant soft tissue or vascular structures in the surgical path.

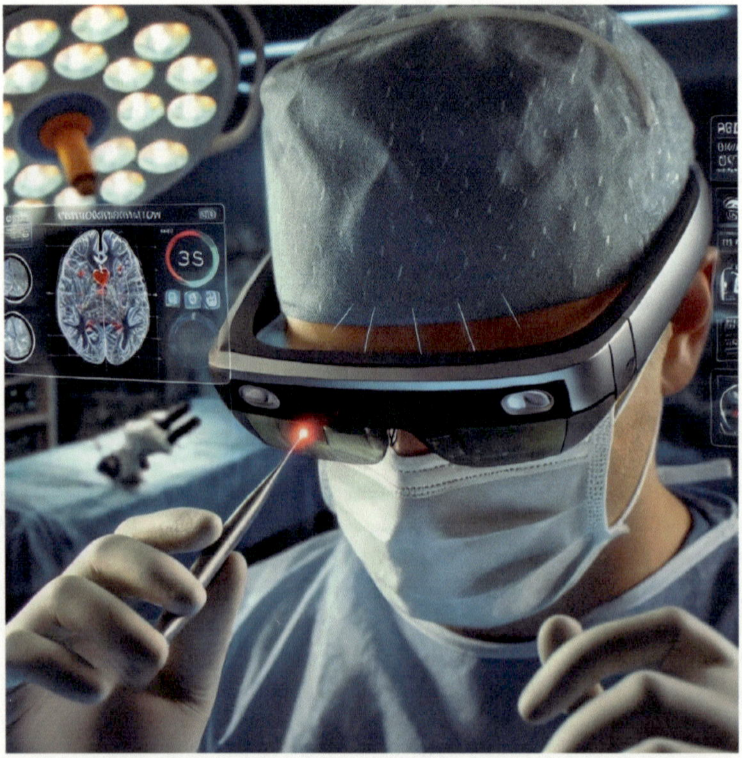

Figure 2.
AI-generated image depicting the use of augmented reality in neurosurgery.

The use of AR in resection of gliomas and meningiomas has demonstrated surgical benefits in safe and precise facilitation of the skin incision and craniotomy, including visualization of the cerebral venous sinuses after dural opening [52]. Furthermore, although studies have shown that AR technology is most beneficial in the surgical resection of gliomas and meningiomas that are located closer to the surface of the brain, the issue of depth perception with brain tumors located in deeper regions of the brain that is posed by traditional two-dimensional navigation systems is overcome with the three-dimensional features offered by AR devices [53].

In the surgical resection of brain tumors, maximizing gross total resection of the tumor while minimizing damage to nearby structures is key to the preservation of function in patients post-operatively. Surgical resection of brain tumors with the assistance of AR technologies has enabled direct view of white matter tracts, which helps guide real-time surgical strategy and decision-making in the operating room [54]. With treatment of brain tumors situated in eloquent areas of the brain, AR devices facilitate the level of exactitude required to ensure reduction of location-dependent functional deficits—including language, memory, and attention—in neurosurgical patients.

4.4 Vascular neurosurgery: AR-assisted visualization for aneurysm clipping and AVM resection

In cerebrovascular neurosurgery, AR may be utilized to treat cerebral aneurysms and brain arteriovenous malformations (AVM) through both open and endoscopic approaches. Preoperative neuroimaging is used to create virtual renderings of the patient's head, skull, vessels, and aneurysms [55]. In open surgery, AR helps with planning of the incision, harvesting the donor vessels, conducting the craniotomy, determining the recipient vessel, and establishing the anastomosis of the vessels [56]. The images are then projected through the surgeon's microscope eyepiece to create a field of view that incorporates the physical and virtual elements in one plane. With brain AVM resection, AR is able to assist with the same visualization. Additionally, it helps to localize the major draining vein [57]. However, AR systems are not yet able to provide detailed information regarding surrounding vessels or feeder vessels in surgical treatment of AVMs [8]. With the endovascular application of AR in aneurysm treatment, different methodologies—including X-ray fluoroscopy and screen mesh deformation—are used to display the virtual models onto the surgical field [58]. The three-dimensional visual capabilities of AR serve as valuable tools for cerebrovascular surgery.

AR imaging optimizes microsurgery in neurosurgical cases, through projection of a virtual anatomical hologram into the microscope that allows the surgeon to easily identify complex neuroanatomical architecture. By providing information on location, size, structure, and flow directionality of cerebral vasculature, AR imaging improves spatial orientation for the surgeon, which minimizes intraoperative complications, such as bleeding. The three-dimensional element of AR technology used in microsurgeries creates a color discrepancy that allows for depth perception in a manner that two-dimensional images are unable to achieve. Furthermore, contrast of colors can be adjusted to account for user differences in color vision. The combination of physical and virtual features in AR imaging through the microscope allows the surgeon to maintain focus on the surgery with minimal interruptions, thereby increasing accuracy and safety in the operating room [59].

4.5 AR in minimally-invasive spine surgery: Pedicle screw placement and spinal fusion

For the purpose of spinal fusion and stabilization in minimally-invasive spine surgery, safe and accurate pedicle screw placement is critically important. Neurosurgeons utilize various methods for the insertion of pedicle screws during spinal fusion surgery, including free-hand technique, intraoperative fluoroscopic guidance, and two-dimensional spinal navigation [60]. In order to address the challenges and complications of traditional pedicle screw placement—including malpositioning of screws and the potential for subsequent neurological injury and compromised spinal stability—AR has emerged as a viable methodology [61]. In the process of insertion of pedicle screws for spinal fusion, AR helps visualize the anatomical landmarks for skin incision as well as the starting point and entry of the screw path [62]. For spine surgery, the advantages of AR technology lie in its ability to integrate preoperative imaging into the field of view to enhance operative precision with spinal instrumentation.

AR-assistance in spine surgery helps prevent complications in spinal fusion procedures. The most commonly reported complication in spinal fusion surgery is the misplacement of pedicle screws [63]. This can result in injury of neural elements, nearby vasculature, or compromise of spinal column integrity leading to increased instability [64]. Although clinically-apparent complications of pedicle screw misplacement are rare, AR-supported visualization of the entry and pathway of the pedicle screw as part of preoperative planning and intraoperative technique helps minimize the complications overall. Currently AR guided technology is capable of mediating pedicle screw placement with greater than 90% accuracy [65]. Furthermore, AR technology utilization in spine surgery addresses the limitations presented by traditional neuronavigation devices, including intraoperative blocked field of view, accidental shifting of reference frames, and unstable connection between the reference base and surgical site [64]. The use of AR in spine surgery serves to optimize real-time visualization of critical neuroanatomical structures and improve clinical decision-making in the operating room.

4.6 Using AR to improve precision in complex Skull Base tumor resection

The standard approach in complex skull base tumor resection cases utilizes neuronavigation to support the surgeon's anatomical orientation through the skull base [66]. However, the use of a bayonet probe in neuronavigation through skull base surgeries presents inherent challenges, including the surgeon's shift of focus from the surgical field to the neuronavigation display as well as mental matching of the physical and virtual elements. AR-assisted neuronavigation in skull base tumor resection directly addresses the shortcomings of traditional neuronavigation. Its projection of the virtual, three-dimensional image directly onto the surgical field allows the surgeon's full attention to remain on the patient. Additionally, it provides the important advantages of enhanced spatial perception and orderly workflow for the operating surgeon. Studies have shown that the use of AR in complex skull base tumor resection is especially beneficial in patients who have had previous operations [66]. With the facilitation of precise preoperative planning and approach to complex skull base tumor resection, AR technology allows for a heightened degree of accuracy, safety, and efficiency in the operating room [67].

The use of AR in endoscopic skull base surgeries has primarily been concentrated in the settings of endoscopic endonasal transsphenoidal surgery for resection of pituitary tumors [68, 69]. One study found that AR-assisted endoscopic endonasal skull base approaches improved neuroanatomical landmark identification via neuronavigation [68]. AR has been shown to increase intraoperative patient safety, even in patient-specific circumstances where the skull base structures are challenging to traverse [70]. It does so by providing enhanced recognition of neuroanatomical structures and vasculature. Through this, it decreases postoperative complication rates [71]. With the complexity of skull base surgeries, surgeon confidence and performance is of utmost importance. Previous studies have shown that the employment of AR in endoscopic skull base procedures—specifically with intraoperative navigation—bolsters surgeons' self-assurance and focus, which subsequently improves operative accuracy [72].

5. Integrating AR and advanced imaging for improved outcomes

5.1 Hybrid imaging-AR platforms

Through combining AR with advanced imaging modalities, including MRI, CT, and DTI, neurosurgeons are able to achieve a level of surgical strategy and precision that traditional multimodal fusion imaging alone has been unable to accomplish. In conjunction with MRI, CTA, and DTI, AR has been used as a tool for preoperative planning and visualization, particularly with surgical resection of extracerebral tumors [73]. For deep-seated meningioma removal, AR has assisted multimodal fusion imaging to identify critical structures, including feeding arteries, perforators, and veins [74]. Furthermore, the merging of different imaging modalities into a single fused view allows for decreased manual editing of imaging [75]. Although still emerging in its combined utilization with MRI, CT, and DTI, AR has strong potential to revolutionize the manner in which various neurosurgical subspecialties navigate preoperative, intraoperative, and postoperative management of patients.

Three-dimensional anatomical modeling has been used to identify critical structures in the brain and assist in minimally-invasive neurosurgical operations [76]. Interactive intraoperative adjustment of three-dimensional visualization allows for direct, microscopic observation of brain tumors, cerebrovasculature, and functional areas of the brain. The utilization of three-dimensional renderings in surgical resection of brain tumors has optimized flexibility, safety, and postoperative outcomes [75]. In addition, studies have found that three-dimensional exoscopes provide neurosurgeons with the benefits of tactile dexterity, surgical comfort, and enhanced performance in a way that two-dimensional exoscopes do not. These advantages of three-dimensional devices allow for better intraoperative visualization of the neuroanatomical features, ultimately increasing surgical precision [77].

5.2 Integrating neurophysiological monitoring with AR to protect critical brain functions

In order to ensure patient safety and preservation of neurological function, best practice of AR in neurosurgical procedures is accompanied by neurophysiological monitoring. The standard of care in any neurosurgical procedure that could potentially cause inadvertent damage to critical neuroanatomical structures is to assess and protect neurological functions intraoperatively through the use of neurophysiological monitoring. An application of AR with neurophysiological monitoring is combined AR and electroencephalogram (EEG) through Neuromonitoring Goggles [78]. This captures intraoperative neuroelectrical changes that represent rational cognitive functions, such as decision-making and reward anticipation [79]. Alterations of EEG signals could indicate disruption in these cognitive functions. Although the current literature on the integration of neurophysiological monitoring with AR is still in development, the simultaneous intraoperative use of the two technologies will serve as a critical consideration in neurosurgical practice in the future.

Intraoperative decision support systems, including neuronavigation, are powerful tools that neurosurgeons use to strategically and safely traverse complex neuroanatomy during a case. AR-assisted neuronavigation is one of the primary uses of AR in neurosurgical procedures. As intraoperative decision support systems advance into anticipatory surgical guidance based on neuroanatomical structures and vasculature, the three-dimensional capability of AR-based devices will further elevate these systems. In the future, AR-based intraoperative decision support systems may have the ability to map out the surgical approach from beginning to end, which would generate a patient-specific, three-dimensional guide of the entire operation that would maximize surgical success and enhance clinical outcomes.

5.3 Reducing surgical risks with image-guided AR systems

AR devices have successfully supported surgeries in a variety of neurosurgical subspecialties, including neuro-oncology, endovascular, and spine surgery. In one patient case, the use of AR neuronavigation assisted with the resection of a patient's left temporal meningioma. AR allowed easy identification of the nearby MCA branches and bifurcation, preventing arterial damage during tumor removal [80]. Within the realm of cerebrovascular surgery, AR technology was employed in the microsurgical resection of a ruptured brain AVM in a patient's right parietal region. At six-month follow-up, the patient remained in stable condition and without any recurring symptoms. Furthermore, neuroimaging revealed complete obliteration of the AVM [59]. In a posterior spinal fixation case at the C1-C2 level, microscope-based AR technology helped to properly position C1 lateral mass and C2 pedicle screws with real-time active visualization of the vertebral artery course via virtual onlay, thereby greatly minimizing vertebral artery injury risk [81]. With the steady increase in utilization of AR devices in neurosurgery, our understanding of the impact of AR on operative success and patient outcomes will continue to evolve over time.

6. Challenges and limitations of AR and imaging in neurosurgery

Advanced imaging and augmented reality (AR) are transforming neurosurgery, but their integration into routine practice necessitates careful consideration of inherent limitations and challenges. Overcoming these obstacles is crucial to fully leverage the precision and capabilities of these technologies.

6.1 Technical limitations

AR devices, such as headsets and displays, need to provide high-resolution, real-time overlays without introducing latency, which could lead to inaccuracies during delicate surgeries [51]. Currently, there is substantial computational power required to support these real-time updates, posing a limitation for both device size and heat generation [51, 82].

Moreover, the integration of AR software with existing neurosurgical platforms remains underdeveloped. Surgical platforms, such as Medtronic StealthStation and Brainlab, offer advanced intraoperative navigation systems but are not optimized to mesh with AR overlays. The lag between AR visualizations and intraoperative actions could lead to impaired surgical performance. Future research is needed to refine the technology to minimize any latency or error and create a more seamless integration with existing neurosurgical tools [50].

AR systems rely heavily on precise imaging data to superimpose digital information onto the physical environment. However, imprecise image registration while aligning preoperative images with real-time anatomical landmarks can reduce the reliability of AR guidance. Even small discrepancies in image alignment can have drastic consequences during procedures that require millimeter-level precision, such as aneurysm clipping or tumor resection [83, 84].

Another current limitation is the inability to adapt to anatomical changes during surgery. As tissue is removed or manipulated, the brain may shift, changing the reality from the preoperative scans. The technology for compensating for intraoperative brain shift is still in its infancy, making it challenging to maintain reliable AR guidance throughout the entire procedure [84].

However, a study analyzing the effect of AR on EVD placement found a significant improvement in target error in the AR cohort (11.9) vs. the freehand cohort (19.9). In addition, the quality of EVD placement was also better in the AR cohort (59.4% mKS grade 1) vs. the freehand cohort (25.0% mKS grade 1) [85]. Similarly, a study was conducted looking at the effect of AR on the accuracy of pedicle screw placement, finding AR-assisted screw placement to be 98% accurate [86].

6.2 Training and learning curve for neurosurgeons

The integration of AR in neurosurgery presents significant challenges for practicing neurosurgeons. Neurosurgeons must navigate complex 3D digital interfaces while performing intricate procedures, necessitating a substantial learning curve [87, 88]. Mastery of these systems–and understanding their limitations–is crucial for effective utilization in the operating room (OR). Surgeons must develop the ability to interpret augmented data superimposed on live anatomical structures, demanding both technical expertise and situational awareness in high-pressure environments [88]. Additionally, there is a risk of over-reliance on AR, potentially compromising independent critical assessment of a patient [87].

These challenges underscore the importance of comprehensive training programs and ongoing education to ensure that neurosurgeons can effectively leverage AR technologies while maintaining fundamental surgical skills and judgment [87, 88].

To promote AR adoption, neurosurgical training programs need to incorporate comprehensive AR education. Simulation-based platforms are essential for providing hands-on, practical experience with AR systems in controlled settings [7]. These platforms enable trainees to practice surgeries using realistic 3D models and AR overlays, developing essential skills for AR-assisted surgeries without real-life consequences [89]. The implementation of AR in neurosurgical education has shown promise in enhancing student training, particularly in neuro-oncology, spinal neurosurgery, and neurovascular procedures [7, 90]. Implementing AR early in training can develop the skills needed for the later operative years in training. For example, students and residents incorporated an AR system to assist and monitor bedside EVD placement. On average, the system improved EVD placement for "year 1 students by 39.4%, the year 2 -4 students by 45.7%, and of the neurosurgeons by 16.7%" [91]. However, the emphasis on cross-referencing the technological overlay with existing anatomical knowledge must be stressed to prevent over-reliance on technology and to help develop the critical thinking and judgment needed as a neurosurgeon [7]. Especially when implemented in early training, surgeons should use AR to augment the existing training without using the technology as a crutch [89]. Additionally, similar to previous new technological advances in neurosurgery, such as stealth navigation and robotics, there is an expected learning curve with slow integration before surgeons become comfortable enough to include them in standard practice. As AR technology continues to evolve, its integration into training programs will be essential for preparing the next generation of neurosurgeons.

6.3 Costs and accessibility

There are high costs associated with purchasing and maintaining AR hardware, advanced imaging systems, and necessary software licenses, creating substantial barriers to widespread adoption [51]. The financial burden extends beyond initial investments, including ongoing costs for training surgeons and OR staff [88]. These expenses can be particularly prohibitive for resource-constrained healthcare institutions such as rural or safety-net hospitals [92]. This challenge is also especially pronounced in developing countries, where limited resources may impede access to cutting-edge neurosurgical care [92].

A crucial consideration when implementing AR is the potential to enhance surgical precision and training in the future. In practice, however, that benefit may not be seen on a financial statement, requiring a more long-term outlook on the return on investment. The immediate result may be a financial loss, adding that barrier to systems unable to absorb that loss [50].

6.4 Global disparities in access to cutting-edge technologies

75% of the world's population lives in low- and middle-income countries, where access to essential neurosurgical care is often limited [88]. There is a scarcity of neurosurgeons, with only one surgeon per 10 million people in some African countries compared to 1 per 80,000 in developed nations, which further compounds this issue [93]. While AR and advanced imaging technologies are increasingly more prevalent in leading neurosurgical centers in high-income countries, access remains limited in developing nations [94]. This disparity exacerbates global inequality in neurosurgical care, particularly for complex cases such as tumors or vascular malformations [95].

Addressing global disparities requires international collaboration to reduce costs and develop affordable, portable versions of AR technology [94]. Telemedicine and remote training programs can be useful in the dissemination of the knowledge and skills to incorporate AR into neurosurgery worldwide [96].

6.5 Ethical and regulatory issues

Similar to the transition to electronic medical records, the integration of AR systems into neurosurgical workflows will require significant data security to prevent breaches in patient privacy and maintain compliance with HIPAA and other privacy statutes. AR relies extensively on confidential patient data, including high-resolution imaging and private medical records, and ensuring the safety and security of the data will be essential as more data is transitioned to cloud management [97, 98]. The constantly developing field of cybersecurity will continue to incorporate new encryption systems to maintain the highest levels of data security as new technologies continue to be introduced.

Government agencies such as the FDA and EMA determine regulatory guidelines and classifications for devices. AR technologies must have medical device approval to be utilized in healthcare settings [99]. These guidelines ensure that AR systems meet rigorous safety and efficacy standards before widespread clinical adoption [100, 101].

7. Artificial intelligence and machine learning in AR

Artificial Intelligence (AI) and Machine Learning (ML) are increasingly integrated with Augmented Reality (AR) systems in neurosurgery, adding automated processes and enhancing real-time decision-making. This ultimately enables more personalized surgical interventions, incorporating vast amounts of information into AR [102].

7.1 AI-driven augmented reality for real-time decision-making

AI systems are being developed to provide real-time, adaptive decision support during neurosurgical procedures. These models can analyze vast amounts of data from multiple inputs, including preoperative imaging, intraoperative monitoring and live visual input to offer valuable insights and options to the surgeon. One promising application is using AI together with AR to suggest optimal surgical trajectories, particularly valuable in challenging cases involving deep tumors, eloquent cortex or intricate vascular malformations [33]. Additionally for pituitary lesions, machine learning can be applied to predict tumor aggressiveness or risk of CSF leak based on imaging information alone [102].

A study evaluating an AI-driven AR system in brain tumors demonstrated significant improvements in accuracy, efficiency, and reduced cognitive load and stress levels for neurosurgeons. The system showed an average Dice similarity coefficient of 0.87 in identifying and localizing brain tumors [103].

AI-powered AR can also provide real-time alerts for critical brain regions/structures during tumor resection. These systems analyze intraoperative imaging and neuromonitoring data to identify and highlight functional areas at risk in the surgeon's view, aiding them in avoiding potential complications [104].

7.2 Machine learning for personalized surgical interventions

ML models are trained to identify patterns and predict outcomes based on large neurosurgical databases. These models can analyze diverse data formats, such as imaging studies and clinical records, to generate predictions and suggested courses of action for a specific patient based on their medical history and presentation [104]. By correlating imaging characteristics with surgical outcomes, AI-driven AR could tailor surgical strategies and planning to each patient's unique anatomy and pathology, increasing both the precision and safety of surgery. For example, a model may analyze a patient's data and scans and assign the likelihood of complete tumor resection with clear margins or the risk of a complication [105].

7.3 Challenges and future perspectives

While AI and ML in AR-assisted neurosurgery have great potential, there are also several challenges to integrating into AR technology. For example, using proprietary data to train the algorithms can be complex, as much of this information can be covered under HIPAA privacy laws. Additionally, algorithm transparency is a crucial limiting factor in the overall expansion of this technology as companies do not want to share their proprietary algorithm, limiting the reproducibility and even the reliability of the model [106]. A review of existing AI models found that just 15% are externally validated on independent cohorts of patients [107]. AI and ML as with any new technology in the healthcare field, also require regulatory approval by governmental agencies such as the FDA and EMA. As these challenges are addressed, the combination of AI, ML, and AR can transform neurosurgical precision beyond what a surgeon alone can do, improve patient outcomes, and pave the road for truly personalized surgical interventions.

7.4 Virtual reality (VR) and mixed reality (MR) in neurosurgical training

VR simulations provide a risk-free environment for neurosurgical trainees to practice complex procedures and surgeries. These systems allow for repetitive practice of intricate techniques, such as aneurysm clipping or spinal fusion, without the pressure of real-world consequences. Additionally, they allow trainees to train for surgeries that rarely occur in the real world. This can lead to more well-rounded neurosurgeons, trained in techniques they would otherwise never have been able to learn. A systematic review evaluating the role of VR in surgical training found that VR-based training was both well-received and effective in teaching acute and trauma-surgical scenarios [108].

While there are no controlled studies or trials comparing VR to standard training, many small individual studies and industry-sponsored studies have shown the benefit of early VR training in neurosurgery [109].

7.5 MR for hybrid learning environments

MR combines both virtual and physical worlds, creating interactive holographic models enhancing spatial awareness and decision-making through real-time visualization on physical surfaces. MR platforms allow trainees to interact with these holographic models of brain structures and pathologies while still working with physical instruments, and brain models. This melds the detail available in the virtual world with the tactile feeling of surgery and tissue, potentially improving hand-eye coordination and spatial awareness without losing the "feel" of surgery [110].

7.6 Integration into neurosurgical residency programs

Integrating VR and MR as standard training tools in neurosurgical residency programs is gaining traction in programs across the country and the world. These technologies offer the potential to standardize training experiences and provide objective assessments of resident performance [109]. They also allow opportunities to learn from complex cases found only in large urban specialty centers, expanding training opportunities to more remote programs. Early implementation can have wide-ranging impacts on residents, giving residents access to surgical skill building at earlier stages than previously possible [109]. However, challenges remain regarding implementation costs, curriculum integration, and validation of training efficacy.

As these technologies continue to evolve, they promise to play an increasingly important role in preparing neurosurgery residents for the complexities of modern surgical practice. Future research should focus on long-term outcomes and the actualization of skills learned in virtual environments to real-world surgical scenarios.

7.7 Remote surgery and tele-neurosurgery using AR

Advancements in AR are paving the road for remote neurosurgery and tele-neurosurgery, offering the potential to extend specialized neurosurgical care across the country and the world.

AR-assisted remote neurosurgery facilitates visual guidance and interaction over long distances, allowing trained neurosurgeons to provide real-time guidance to more local surgeons during complex procedures. A systematic review of remote AR and VR in neurosurgery found the primary use was in cranial procedures (77.8%), with tele-surgical assistance accounting for 18.2% of the applications [109]. This concept is being explored for remote endovascular thrombectomy as well [111].

One study demonstrated the use of AR glasses in a remote operating room, enabling neurosurgeons to guide local surgeries through both voice and visual cues superimposed on the local surgeon's field of view. This approach was successfully implemented in a series of lumbar arthrodesis procedures, showcasing its potential in spine surgery [112]. This approach could be utilized to monitor and guide trainees through operations, and represents a future domain of further research.

Remote surgery can significantly increase access to specialized neurosurgical care in underserved regions. Leveraging AR, expert neurosurgeons can provide guidance and support to local surgeons, potentially improving patient outcomes in areas with limited access to specialized care both in more remote parts of the US and in other countries [113]. The integration of AR improves real-time visualization, enabling surgeons to better assess the spatial relationship between different anatomical structures during remote procedures [109].

7.8 Challenges and future perspectives

However, the implementation of tele-neurosurgery faces several challenges: The first is reliable internet connections. A prerequisite to remote operations is high-speed, stable internet for communication, data transmission and general connectivity [109]. New advancements such as the adoption of satellite internet access in rural geographies is an advancement which may help remedy this issue. A second challenge is the inherent latency in the software. Minimizing delay in video and data transmission is essential for precise surgical guidance, particularly in the neurosurgical field [51]. However, the most considerable challenge will be building the technology infrastructure in these locations. AR hardware and software must be available at both the remote and local sites for this to become a reality [113].

Despite these challenges, the potential benefits of AR-assisted remote neurosurgery can change access to proper neurosurgical care worldwide. As technology continues to advance, tele-neurosurgery may become an increasingly viable option for expanding access globally, offering the potential for more equitable access to advanced neurosurgical care [114].

7.9 Next-generation imaging techniques

7.9.1 Quantum imaging for unprecedented precision

Quantum imaging technology is an experimental technology offering the potential to achieve molecular-level resolution, identifying neural pathways with extraordinary detail. This emerging field leverages quantum mechanical effects to overcome the classical limitations of imaging resolution and sensitivity. For example, quantum dots (Qdots) have shown promise in neurosurgical applications due to their unique optical properties and biocompatibility, potentially enabling the visualization of individual neurons and their connections without the undesired radiation effects of other imaging modalities. These Qdots can be created to emit specific wavelengths of light on excitation, giving minute, granular detail to structures such as brain tumors [115].

7.9.2 7-tesla MRI for ultra-high-resolution imaging

7-Tesla MRI scanners offer significant advantages over conventional 3-Tesla scanners, particularly in preoperative planning for complex cases such as brainstem tumors. The higher field strength provides improved signal-to-noise ratio, allowing for superior spatial resolution and improved contrast. It also creates a greater chemical shift dispersion, leading to increased sensitivity to heterogenous substrates of neurological diseases [116]. A study evaluating the role of 7-Tesla MRI in neurosurgery found that it offers better visualization of microvasculature and subtle lesions, crucial for precise surgical planning [117].

The integration of these highly detailed imaging techniques with AR can create highly detailed anatomical maps. Neurosurgeons can combine the ultra-high-resolution data from 7-Tesla MRI with the real-time visualization of AR, to navigate complex anatomical structures with unprecedented accuracy during surgery in addition to preoperative planning [116].

However, while 7-Tesla imaging can be found in large academic research centers, they are not in widespread use or available for standard clinical care. These imaging modalities will be used in the future for the development and integration with AR, creating a more precise, accurate, and complex system that will change and augment the reality of neurosurgery.

8. Conclusion

The integration of AR and advanced imaging technologies has profoundly reshaped modern neurosurgery, enhancing the precision, safety, and efficacy of surgical interventions. As discussed, AR's ability to superimpose real-time digital information onto the surgeon's field of view has revolutionized neurosurgical practice, improving intraoperative navigation and facilitating complex procedures, such as tumor resections and vascular surgeries. This transformation, combined with advancements in imaging modalities like MRI, CT, and DTI, has equipped neurosurgeons with tools that allow for greater visualization and spatial understanding of critical anatomical structures, ultimately leading to improved patient outcomes.

However, while these technologies offer immense promise, the path forward presents a number of challenges. Technical limitations, such as latency in real-time overlays and difficulties in adapting to intraoperative anatomical changes, remain significant hurdles that must be addressed to fully capitalize on AR's potential. Additionally, the high costs of implementing AR systems, combined with the need for comprehensive training, limit their accessibility in many healthcare settings. Despite these challenges, AR's proven impact on reducing surgical errors and enhancing precision underscores its importance in the future of neurosurgical practice.

In conclusion, the fusion of AR and advanced imaging technologies is not a distant prospect but an emerging reality that is already revolutionizing neurosurgery. As AR continues to evolve, with future developments in artificial intelligence and machine learning, its ability to provide real-time decision-making and personalized surgical interventions will further enhance its role in neurosurgical innovation. The continued refinement and integration of these technologies hold immense potential to shape the future of neurosurgery, offering unprecedented precision, safety, and patient care.

Conflict of interest disclosure and funding information

The authors report no conflict of interest, this was the authors' own work and no funding was received to carry out this project. The manuscript was not created or edited using any AI tools or software.

DOI: http://dx.doi.org/10.5772/intechopen.1008969

Author details

Elad Mashiach[1*], Sauson Soldozy[1], Ariel Sacknovitz[1,2], Ankita Jain[1,2], Hayley Donaldson[3], Sabrina Zeller[1], Geet Shukla[1], Cameron Rawanduzy[1], Fernando De Nigris Vasconcellos[4], Chirag Gandhi[1] and Justin Santarelli[1]

1 Department of Neurosurgery, Westchester Medical Center, Valhalla, NY, USA

2 New York Medical College, Valhalla, NY, USA

3 Rutgers Robert Wood Johnson Medical School, New Brunswick, NJ, USA

4 Boston Medical Center, Boston, MA, USA

*Address all correspondence to: elad.mashiach@wmchealth.org

References

[1] Kim JJ, Gean AD. Imaging for the diagnosis and management of traumatic brain injury. Neurotherapeutics. 2011;**8**:39-53. DOI: 10.1007/s13311-010-0003-3

[2] Rizea RE, Ciurea AV, Onose G, Gorgan RM, Tascu A, Brehar F. New application of diffusion tensor imaging in neurosurgery. Journal of Medicine and Life. 2011;**4**:372-376

[3] Costello JS, Soldozy S, Norat P, Sokolowski JD, Yağmurlu K, Sharifi K, et al. Endovascular approach to cerebral revascularization: Historical vignette. World Neurosurgery. 2020;**136**:258-262. DOI: 10.1016/j.wneu.2020.01.072

[4] Soldozy S, Young S, Kumar JS, Capek S, Felbaum DR, Jean WC, et al. A systematic review of endovascular stent-electrode arrays, a minimally invasive approach to brain-machine interfaces. Neurosurgical Focus. 2020;**49**:E3. DOI: 10.3171/2020.4.Focus20186

[5] Lylyk P, Lylyk I, Bleise C, Scrivano E, Lylyk PN, Beneduce B, et al. First-in-human endovascular treatment of hydrocephalus with a miniature biomimetic transdural shunt. Journal of NeuroInterventional Surgery. 2022;**14**:495-499. DOI: 10.1136/neurintsurg-2021-018136

[6] Dixon L, Lim A, Grech-Sollars M, Nandi D, Camp S. Intraoperative ultrasound in brain tumor surgery: A review and implementation guide. Neurosurgical Review. 2022;**45**:2503-2515. DOI: 10.1007/s10143-022-01778-4

[7] Hey G, Guyot M, Carter A, Lucke-Wold B. Augmented reality in neurosurgery: A new paradigm for training. Medicina (Kaunas, Lithuania). 2023;**59**:1-16. DOI: 10.3390/medicina59101721

[8] Meola A, Cutolo F, Carbone M, Cagnazzo F, Ferrari M, Ferrari V. Augmented reality in neurosurgery: A systematic review. Neurosurgical Review. 2017;**40**:537-548. DOI: 10.1007/s10143-016-0732-9

[9] Tagaytayan R, Kelemen A, Sik-Lanyi C. Augmented reality in neurosurgery. Archives of Medical Science. 2018;**14**:572-578. DOI: 10.5114/aoms.2016.58690

[10] Leung D, Han X, Mikkelsen T, Nabors LB. Role of MRI in primary brain tumor evaluation. Journal of the National Comprehensive Cancer Network. 2014;**12**:1561-1568. DOI: 10.6004/jnccn.2014.0156

[11] Segar DJ, Thum JA, Bastos D, Golby AJ. Magnetic resonance imaging in neurosurgery. In: Akter F, Emptage N, Engert F, Berger MS, editors. Neuroscience for Neurosurgeons. Cambridge: Cambridge University Press; 2024. pp. 398-409

[12] Villanueva-Meyer JE, Mabray MC, Cha S. Current clinical brain tumor imaging. Neurosurgery. 2017;**81**:397-415. DOI: 10.1093/neuros/nyx103

[13] Duyn JH. The future of ultra-high field MRI and fMRI for study of the human brain. NeuroImage. 2012;**62**:1241-1248. DOI: 10.1016/j.neuroimage.2011.10.065

[14] Wrede KH, Matsushige T, Goericke SL, Chen B, Umutlu L, Quick HH, et al. Non-enhanced magnetic resonance imaging of unruptured intracranial aneurysms at 7 tesla: Comparison with digital subtraction

angiography. European Radiology. 2017;**27**:354-364. DOI: 10.1007/s00330-016-4323-5

[15] Aoyama T, Miyaoka Y, Ogiwara T, Ito K, Seguchi T, Hongo K. Long segment spinal Dural cyst: A case report. World Neurosurgery. 2016;**88**:686.e613-686.e617. DOI: 10.1016/j.wneu.2015.11.008

[16] Sommer S, Kozerke S, Seifritz E, Staempfli P. Fiber up-sampling and quality assessment of tractograms – Towards quantitative brain connectivity. Brain and Behavior. 2017;**7**:e00588. DOI: 10.1002/brb3.588

[17] Donaldson H, Golub D, Placantonakis DG. Staged intervention to enable the resection of a large left temporoinsular cystic glioblastoma with language preservation: Illustrative case. Journal of Neurosurgery: Case Lessons. 2024;**8**:CASE24362. DOI: 10.3171/CASE24362

[18] Henderson F, Abdullah KG, Verma R, Brem S. Tractography and the connectome in neurosurgical treatment of gliomas: The premise, the progress, and the potential. Neurosurgical Focus. 2020;**48**:E6. DOI: 10.3171/2019.11.Focus19785

[19] Costabile JD, Alaswad E, D'Souza S, Thompson JA, Ormond DR. Current applications of diffusion tensor imaging and tractography in intracranial tumor resection. Frontiers in Oncology. 2019;**9**:426. DOI: 10.3389/fonc.2019.00426

[20] Kokkinos V, Chatzisotiriou A, Seimenis I. Functional magnetic resonance imaging and diffusion tensor imaging-tractography in resective brain surgery: Lesion coverage strategies and patient outcomes. Brain Sciences. 2023;**13**:1574

[21] Reynolds BB, Stanton AN, Soldozy S, Goodkin HP, Wintermark M, Druzgal TJ. Investigating the effects of subconcussion on functional connectivity using mass-univariate and multivariate approaches. Brain Imaging and Behavior. 2018;**12**:1332-1345. DOI: 10.1007/s11682-017-9790-z

[22] Soldozy S, Akyeampong DK, Barquin DL, Norat P, Yağmurlu K, Sokolowski JD, et al. Systematic review of functional mapping and cortical reorganization in the setting of arteriovenous malformations. Redefining Anatomical Eloquence. Front Surg. 2020;**7**:514247. DOI: 10.3389/fsurg.2020.514247

[23] Hendricks BK, Scherschinski L, Jubran JH, Dadario NB, Karahalios K, Benner D, et al. Eloquent noneloquence: Redefinition of cortical eloquence based on outcomes of superficial cerebral cavernous malformation resection. Journal of Neurosurgery. 2024;**141**:291-305. DOI: 10.3171/2023.12.Jns232588

[24] Chohan MO, Flores RA, Wertz C, Jung RE. "Non-eloquent" brain regions predict neuropsychological outcome in tumor patients undergoing awake craniotomy. PLoS One. 2024;**19**:e0284261. DOI: 10.1371/journal.pone.0284261

[25] Begley SL, McBriar JD, Pelcher I, Schulder M. Intraoperative MRI: A review of applications across neurosurgical specialties. Neurosurgery. 2024;**95**:527-536. DOI: 10.1227/neu.0000000000002933

[26] Bunyaratavej K, Siwanuwatn R, Tuchinda L, Wangsawatwong P. Impact of intraoperative magnetic resonance imaging (i-MRI) on surgeon decision making and clinical outcomes in cranial tumor surgery. Asian Journal

of Neurosurgery. 2022;**17**:218-226. DOI: 10.1055/s-0042-1751008

[27] Petcharunpaisan S, Ramalho J, Castillo M. Arterial spin labeling in neuroimaging. World Journal of Radiology. 2010;**2**:384-398. DOI: 10.4329/wjr.v2.i10.384

[28] Noguchi T, Yoshiura T, Hiwatashi A, Togao O, Yamashita K, Nagao E, et al. Perfusion imaging of brain tumors using arterial spin-labeling: Correlation with histopathologic vascular density. American Journal of Neuroradiology. 2008;**29**:688-693. DOI: 10.3174/ajnr.A0903

[29] Kikuchi K, Hiwatashi A, Togao O, Yamashita K, Yoshimoto K, Mizoguchi M, et al. Correlation between arterial spin-labeling perfusion and histopathological vascular density of pediatric intracranial tumors. Journal of Neuro-Oncology. 2017;**135**:561-569. DOI: 10.1007/s11060-017-2604-8

[30] ElBeheiry AA, Emara DM, Abdel-Latif AA-B, Abbas M, Ismail AS. Arterial spin labeling in the grading of brain gliomas: Could it help? Egyptian Journal of Radiology and Nuclear Medicine. 2020;**51**:235. DOI: 10.1186/s43055-020-00352-6

[31] Anderson GB, Steinke DE, Petruk KC, Ashforth R, Findlay JM. Computed tomographic angiography versus digital subtraction angiography for the diagnosis and early treatment of ruptured intracranial aneurysms. Neurosurgery. 1999;**45**:1315-1320; discussion 1320-1312. DOI: 10.1097/00006123-199912000-00008

[32] Dehdashti AR, Rufenacht DA, Delavelle J, Reverdin A, de Tribolet N. Therapeutic decision and management of aneurysmal subarachnoid haemorrhage based on computed tomographic angiography. British Journal of Neurosurgery. 2003;**17**:46-53

[33] Isikay I, Cekic E, Baylarov B, Tunc O, Hanalioglu S. Narrative review of patient-specific 3D visualization and reality technologies in skull base neurosurgery: Enhancements in surgical training, planning, and navigation. Frontiers in Surgery. 2024;**11**:1427844. DOI: 10.3389/fsurg.2024.1427844

[34] Kabra A, Mehta N, Garg B. 3D printing in spine care: A review of current applications. Journal of Clinical Orthopaedics and Trauma. 2022;**35**:102044. DOI: 10.1016/j.jcot.2022.102044

[35] Bamba Y, Nonaka M, Nakajima S, Yamasaki M. Three-dimensional reconstructed computed tomography-magnetic resonance fusion image-based preoperative planning for surgical procedures for spinal lipoma or tethered spinal cord after myelomeningocele repair. Neurologia Medico-Chirurgica (Tokyo). 2011;**51**:397-402. DOI: 10.2176/nmc.51.397

[36] Frosina G. Positron emission tomography of high-grade gliomas. Journal of Neuro-Oncology. 2016;**127**:415-425. DOI: 10.1007/s11060-016-2077-1

[37] Pittau F, Grouiller F, Spinelli L, Seeck M, Michel CM, Vulliemoz S. The role of functional neuroimaging in pre-surgical epilepsy evaluation. Frontiers in Neurology. 2014;**5**:31. DOI: 10.3389/fneur.2014.00031

[38] Raji CA, Tarzwell R, Pavel D, Schneider H, Uszler M, Thornton J, et al. Clinical utility of SPECT neuroimaging in the diagnosis and treatment of traumatic brain injury: A systematic review. PLoS One. 2014;**9**:e91088. DOI: 10.1371/journal.pone.0091088

[39] Zhang J, Traylor KS, Mountz JM. PET and SPECT imaging of brain tumors. Seminars in Ultrasound, CT and MRI. 2020;**41**:530-540. DOI: 10.1053/j.sult.2020.08.007

[40] Gong M, Zhang H, Shi Z, Yuan Q, Su X. Application of intraoperative ultrasound in neurosurgery for hypertensive intracerebral hemorrhage. Journal of Clinical Neuroscience. 2021;**90**:251-255. DOI: 10.1016/j.jocn.2021.06.008

[41] Prada F, Ciocca R, Corradino N, Gionso M, Raspagliesi L, Vetrano IG, et al. Multiparametric intraoperative ultrasound in oncological neurosurgery: A pictorial essay. Frontiers in Neuroscience. 2022;**16**:1-11. DOI: 10.3389/fnins.2022.881661

[42] Patel MR, Jacob KC, Parsons AW, Chavez FA, Ribot MA, Munim MA, et al. Systematic review: Applications of intraoperative ultrasonography in spinal surgery. World Neurosurgery. 2022;**164**:e45-e58. DOI: 10.1016/j.wneu.2022.02.130

[43] Ragnhildstveit A, Li C, Zimmerman MH, Mamalakis M, Curry VN, Holle W, et al. Intra-operative applications of augmented reality in glioma surgery: A systematic review. Frontiers in Surgery. 2023;**10**:1245851. DOI: 10.3389/fsurg.2023.1245851

[44] Hey G, Guyot M, Carter A, Lucke-Wold B. Augmented reality in neurosurgery: A new paradigm for training. Medicina. 2023;**59**:1721

[45] Van Gestel F, Frantz T, Buyck F, Geens W, Neuville Q, Bruneau M, et al. Neuro-oncological augmented reality planning for intracranial tumor resection. Frontiers in Neurology. 2023;**14**:1104571. DOI: 10.3389/fneur.2023.1104571

[46] Léger É, Drouin S, Collins DL, Popa T, Kersten-Oertel M. Quantifying attention shifts in augmented reality image-guided neurosurgery. Healthcare Technology Letters. 2017;**4**:188-192. DOI: 10.1049/htl.2017.0062

[47] Cutolo F, Meola A, Carbone M, Sinceri S, Cagnazzo F, Denaro E, et al. A new head-mounted display-based augmented reality system in neurosurgical oncology: A study on phantom. Computer Assisted Surgery (Abingdon). 2017;**22**:39-53. DOI: 10.1080/24699322.2017.1358400

[48] Ivan ME, Eichberg DG, Di L, Shah AH, Luther EM, Lu VM, et al. Augmented reality head-mounted display-based incision planning in cranial neurosurgery: A prospective pilot study. Neurosurgical Focus. 2021;**51**:E3. DOI: 10.3171/2021.5.Focus20735

[49] Janssen A, Wang A, Dumont AS, Delashaw J. Augmented reality-guided external ventricular drain placement: A case report. Cureus. 2024;**16**:e64403. DOI: 10.7759/cureus.64403

[50] Olexa J, Cohen J, Alexander T, Brown C, Schwartzbauer G, Woodworth GF. Expanding educational Frontiers in neurosurgery: Current and future uses of augmented reality. Neurosurgery. 2023;**92**:241-250. DOI: 10.1227/neu.0000000000002199

[51] Sharma N, Mallela A, Khan T, Canton S, Kass N, Steuer F, et al. Evolution of the meta-neurosurgeon: A systematic review of the current technical capabilities, limitations, and applications of augmented reality in neurosurgery. Surgical Neurology International. 2024;**15**:146. DOI: 10.25259/SNI_167_2024

[52] Kockro RA, Tsai YT, Ng I, Hwang P, Zhu C, Agusanto K, et al. Dex-

ray: Augmented reality neurosurgical navigation with a handheld video probe. Neurosurgery. 2009;**65**:795-807; discussion 807-798. DOI: 10.1227/01.Neu.0000349918.36700.1c

[53] Inoue D, Cho B, Mori M, Kikkawa Y, Amano T, Nakamizo A, et al. Preliminary study on the clinical application of augmented reality neuronavigation. Journal of Neurological Surgery Part A: Central European Neurosurgery. 2013;**74**:71-76. DOI: 10.1055/s-0032-1333415

[54] Mofatteh M, Mashayekhi MS, Arfaie S, Chen Y, Mirza AB, Fares J, et al. Augmented and virtual reality usage in awake craniotomy: A systematic review. Neurosurgical Review. 2022;**46**:19. DOI: 10.1007/s10143-022-01929-7

[55] Cabrilo I, Bijlenga P, Schaller K. Augmented reality in the surgery of cerebral aneurysms: A technical report. Neurosurgery. 2014;**10**(Suppl. 2):252-260; discussion 260-251. DOI: 10.1227/neu.0000000000000328

[56] Cabrilo I, Schaller K, Bijlenga P. Augmented reality-assisted bypass surgery: Embracing minimal invasiveness. World Neurosurgery. 2015;**83**:596-602. DOI: 10.1016/j.wneu.2014.12.020

[57] Cabrilo I, Bijlenga P, Schaller K. Augmented reality in the surgery of cerebral arteriovenous malformations: Technique assessment and considerations. Acta Neurochirurgica. 2014;**156**:1769-1774. DOI: 10.1007/s00701-014-2183-9

[58] Masutani Y, Dohi T, Yamane F, Iseki H, Takakura K. Augmented reality visualization system for intravascular neurosurgery. Computer Aided Surgery. 1998;**3**:239-247. DOI: 10.1002/(sici)1097-0150(1998)3:5<239::Aid-igs3>3.0.Co;2-b

[59] Li CR, Shen CC, Yang MY, Tsuei YS, Lee CH. Intraoperative augmented reality in microsurgery for intracranial arteriovenous malformation: A case report and literature review. Brain Sciences. 2023;**13**. DOI: 10.3390/brainsci13040653

[60] Butler AJ, Colman MW, Lynch J, Phillips FM. Augmented reality in minimally invasive spine surgery: Early efficiency and complications of percutaneous pedicle screw instrumentation. The Spine Journal. 2023;**23**:27-33. DOI: 10.1016/j.spinee.2022.09.008

[61] Costa F, Villa T, Anasetti F, Tomei M, Ortolina A, Cardia A, et al. Primary stability of pedicle screws depends on the screw positioning and alignment. The Spine Journal. 2013;**13**:1934-1939. DOI: 10.1016/j.spinee.2013.03.046

[62] Wiltse LL, Bateman JG, Hutchinson RH, Nelson WE. The paraspinal sacrospinalis-splitting approach to the lumbar spine. The Journal of Bone and Joint Surgery. American Volume. 1968;**50**:919-926

[63] Hicks JM, Singla A, Shen FH, Arlet V. Complications of pedicle screw fixation in scoliosis surgery: A systematic review. Spine (Phila Pa 1976). 2010;**35**:E465-E470. DOI: 10.1097/BRS.0b013e3181d1021a

[64] Gautschi OP, Schatlo B, Schaller K, Tessitore E. Clinically relevant complications related to pedicle screw placement in thoracolumbar surgery and their management: A literature review of 35,630 pedicle screws. Neurosurgical Focus. 2011;**31**:E8. DOI: 10.3171/2011.7.Focus11168

[65] Youssef S, McDonnell JM, Wilson KV, Turley L, Cunniffe G, Morris S, et al. Accuracy of augmented

reality-assisted pedicle screw placement: A systematic review. European Spine Journal. 2024;**33**:974-984. DOI: 10.1007/s00586-023-08094-5

[66] Cabrilo I, Sarrafzadeh A, Bijlenga P, Landis BN, Schaller K. Augmented reality-assisted skull base surgery. Neurochirurgie. 2014;**60**:304-306. DOI: 10.1016/j.neuchi.2014.07.001

[67] Schwam ZG, Kaul VF, Bu DD, Iloreta AC, Bederson JB, Perez E, et al. The utility of augmented reality in lateral skull base surgery: A preliminary report. American Journal of Otolaryngology. 2021;**42**:102942. DOI: 10.1016/j.amjoto.2021.102942

[68] Thavarajasingam SG, Vardanyan R, Arjomandi Rad A, Thavarajasingam A, Khachikyan A, Mendoza N, et al. The use of augmented reality in transsphenoidal surgery: A systematic review. British Journal of Neurosurgery. 2022;**36**:457-471. DOI: 10.1080/02688697.2022.2057435

[69] Soldozy S, Young S, Yağmurlu K, Norat P, Sokolowski J, Park MS, et al. Transsphenoidal surgery using robotics to approach the Sella turcica: Integrative use of artificial intelligence, realistic motion tracking and telesurgery. Clinical Neurology and Neurosurgery. 2020;**197**:106152. DOI: 10.1016/j.clineuro.2020.106152

[70] Caversaccio M, Langlotz F, Nolte LP, Häusler R. Impact of a self-developed planning and self-constructed navigation system on skull base surgery: 10 years experience. Acta Oto-Laryngologica. 2007;**127**:403-407. DOI: 10.1080/00016480601002104

[71] Black PM, Zervas NT, Candia GL. Incidence and management of complications of transsphenoidal operation for pituitary adenomas. Neurosurgery. 1987;**20**:920-924. DOI: 10.1227/00006123-198706000-00017

[72] Vávra P, Roman J, Zonča P, Ihnát P, Němec M, Kumar J, et al. Recent development of augmented reality in surgery: A review. Journal of Healthcare Engineering. 2017;**2017**:4574172. DOI: 10.1155/2017/4574172

[73] Hou X, Xu R, Chen L, Yang D, Li D. 3D color multimodality fusion imaging as an augmented reality educational and surgical planning tool for extracerebral tumors. Neurosurgical Review. 2023;**46**:280. DOI: 10.1007/s10143-023-02184-0

[74] Sato M, Tateishi K, Murata H, Kin T, Suenaga J, Takase H, et al. Three-dimensional multimodality fusion imaging as an educational and planning tool for deep-seated meningiomas. British Journal of Neurosurgery. 2018;**32**:509-515. DOI: 10.1080/02688697.2018.1485877

[75] Tanrikulu L, Hastreiter P, Troescher-Weber R, Buchfelder M, Naraghi R. Intraoperative three-dimensional visualization in microvascular decompression. Journal of Neurosurgery. 2007;**107**:1137-1143. DOI: 10.3171/jns-07/12/1137

[76] Singh S, Singh R, Kumar S, Suri A. A narrative review on 3-dimensional visualization techniques in neurosurgical education, simulation, and planning. World Neurosurgery. 2024;**187**:46-64. DOI: 10.1016/j.wneu.2024.03.134

[77] Raheja A, Mishra S, Garg K, Katiyar V, Sharma R, Tandon V, et al. Impact of different visualization devices on accuracy, efficiency, and dexterity in neurosurgery: A laboratory investigation. Neurosurgical Focus. 2021;**50**:E18. DOI: 10.3171/2020.10.Focus20786

[78] Zao J, Jung T-P, Chang H-M, Gan T-T, Wang Y-T, Lin Y-P, et al. Augmenting VR/AR Applications with EEG/EOG Monitoring and Oculo-Vestibular Recoupling. Springer; 2016

[79] Decety J, Jackson PL. The functional architecture of human empathy. Behavioral and Cognitive Neuroscience Reviews. 2004;**3**:71-100. DOI: 10.1177/1534582304267187

[80] Lavé A, Meling TR, Schaller K, Corniola MV. Augmented reality in intracranial meningioma surgery: Report of a case and systematic review. Journal of Neurosurgical Sciences. 2020;**64**:369-376. DOI: 10.23736/s0390-5616.20.04945-0

[81] Li CR, Chang YJ, Lin MS, Tsou HK. Augmented reality in spine surgery: A case study of atlantoaxial instrumentation in Os Odontoideum. Medicina (Kaunas, Lithuania). 2024;**60**. DOI: 10.3390/medicina60060874

[82] Khan T, Zhu TS, Downes T, Cheng L, Kass NM, Andrews EG, et al. Understanding effects of visual feedback delay in AR on fine motor surgical tasks. IEEE Transactions on Visualization & Computer Graphics. 2023;**29**:4697-4707. DOI: 10.1109/tvcg.2023.3320214

[83] Bopp MHA, Grote A, Gjorgjevski M, Pojskic M, Saß B, Nimsky C. Enabling navigation and augmented reality in the sitting position in posterior fossa surgery using intraoperative ultrasound. Cancers (Basel). 2024;**16**. DOI: 10.3390/cancers16111985

[84] Huang C-H, Hsieh C-H, Lee J-D, Huang W, Lee S, Wu C, et al. A CT-ultrasound-coregistered augmented reality enhanced image-guided surgery system and its preliminary study on brain-shift estimation. Journal of Instrumentation - J INSTRUM. 2012;**7**:1-12. DOI: 10.1088/1748-0221/7/08/P08016

[85] Van Gestel F, Frantz T, Vannerom C, Verhellen A, Gallagher AG, Elprama SA, et al. The effect of augmented reality on the accuracy and learning curve of external ventricular drain placement. Neurosurgical Focus. 2021;**51**:1-9. DOI: 10.3171/2021.5.FOCUS21215

[86] Liu A, Jin Y, Cottrill E, Khan M, Westbroek E, Ehresman J, et al. Clinical accuracy and initial experience with augmented reality-assisted pedicle screw placement: The first 205 screws. Journal of Neurosurgery. Spine. 2022;**36**:351-357. DOI: 10.3171/2021.2.Spine202097

[87] Guha D, Alotaibi NM, Nguyen N, Gupta S, McFaul C, Yang VXD. Augmented reality in neurosurgery: A review of current concepts and emerging applications. The Canadian Journal of Neurological Sciences. 2017;**44**:235-245. DOI: 10.1017/cjn.2016.443

[88] Jean WC, Piper K, Felbaum DR, Saez-Alegre M. The inaugural "century" of mixed reality in cranial surgery: Virtual reality rehearsal/augmented reality guidance and its learning curve in the first 100-case, single-surgeon series. Operative neurosurgery (Hagerstown). 2024;**26**:28-37. DOI: 10.1227/ons.0000000000000908

[89] Truckenmueller P, Krantchev K, Rubarth K, Früh A, Mertens R, Bruening D, et al. Augmented 360° three-dimensional virtual reality for enhanced student training and education in neurosurgery. World Neurosurgery. 2024;**186**:e35-e47. DOI: 10.1016/j.wneu.2024.01.092

[90] Cannizzaro D, Zaed I, Safa A, Jelmoni AJM, Composto A, Bisoglio A, et al. Augmented reality in neurosurgery, state of art and future projections. A Systematic Review. Front Surg. 2022;**9**:864792. DOI: 10.3389/fsurg.2022.864792

[91] Eom S, Kim S, Jackson J, Sykes D, Rahimpour S, Gorlatova M. Augmented reality-based contextual guidance through surgical tool tracking in neurosurgery. IEEE Transactions on Visualization and Computer Graphics Publishes Papers; 2024. pp. 1-16. DOI: 10.1109/tvcg.2024.3390680

[92] Kazemzadeh K, Akhlaghdoust M, Zali A. Advances in artificial intelligence, robotics, augmented and virtual reality in neurosurgery. Frontiers in Surgery. 2023;**10**:1241923. DOI: 10.3389/fsurg.2023.1241923

[93] Dewan MC, Rattani A, Fieggen G, Arraez MA, Servadei F, Boop FA, et al. Global neurosurgery: The current capacity and deficit in the provision of essential neurosurgical care. Executive summary of the global neurosurgery initiative at the program in global surgery and social change. Journal of Neurosurgery. 2019;**130**:1055-1064. DOI: 10.3171/2017.11.Jns171500

[94] Punchak M, Mukhopadhyay S, Sachdev S, Hung YC, Peeters S, Rattani A, et al. Neurosurgical care: Availability and access in low-income and middle-income countries. World Neurosurgery. 2018;**112**:e240-e254. DOI: 10.1016/j.wneu.2018.01.029

[95] Zhalmukhamedov E. Application of modern neurosurgical technologies in low and middle-income countries. Journal on Surgery. 2022;**2**:1063. DOI: 10.52768/2691-7785/1063

[96] Paro MR, Hersh DS, Bulsara KR. History of virtual reality and augmented reality in neurosurgical training. World Neurosurgery. 2022;**167**:37-43. DOI: 10.1016/j.wneu.2022.08.042

[97] Sri Vigna Hema V, Kesavan R. Augmented security for healthcare data using obfuscation and elliptic curve cryptography algorithm in health cloud environment. Concurrency and Computation: Practice and Experience. 2022;**34**. DOI: 10.1002/cpe.7275

[98] Kiania K, Jameii SM, Rahmani AM. Blockchain-based privacy and security preserving in electronic health: A systematic review. Multimedia Tools and Applications. 2023;**82**:28493-28519. DOI: 10.1007/s11042-023-14488-w

[99] FDA. Augmented Reality and Virtual Reality in Medical Devices. 2024. Available from: https://www.fda.gov/medical-devices/digital-health-center-excellence/ augmented-reality-and-virtual-reality-medical-devices

[100] Yau S, Pandya K, Choudhary S. Regulatory Compliance in Software Services Using Emerging Technologies. IEEE; 2024

[101] Farouk G, Alsamara T. Legal view on blockchain technologies in healthcare: A European states case study. International Journal of Sociotechnology and Knowledge Development. 2023;**15**:1-13. DOI: 10.4018/IJSKD.333154

[102] Soldozy S, Farzad F, Young S, Yağmurlu K, Norat P, Sokolowski J, et al. Pituitary tumors in the computational era, exploring novel approaches to diagnosis, and outcome prediction with machine learning. World Neurosurgery. 2021;**146**:315-321.e311. DOI: 10.1016/j.wneu.2020.07.104

[103] Zeineldin RA, Junger D, Mathis-Ullrich F, Burgert O. Development of an AI-driven system for neurosurgery with a usability study: A step towards minimal invasive robotics. Automatisierungstechnik. 2023;**71**:537-546. DOI: 10.1515/auto-2023-0061

[104] Ramirez M DJE, Chmutin G, Nurmukhametov R, Soto GR,

Kannan S, Piavchenko G, et al. Integrating augmented reality in spine surgery: Redefining precision with new technologies. Brain Sciences. 2024;**14**:645

[105] Baker CR, Pease M, Sexton DP, Abumoussa A, Chambless LB. Artificial intelligence innovations in neurosurgical oncology: A narrative review. Journal of Neuro-Oncology. 2024;**169**:489-496. DOI: 10.1007/s11060-024-04757-5

[106] Khalid N, Qayyum A, Bilal M, Al-Fuqaha A, Qadir J. Privacy-preserving artificial intelligence in healthcare: Techniques and applications. Computers in Biology and Medicine. 2023;**158**:106848. DOI: 10.1016/j.compbiomed.2023.106848

[107] Warman A, Kalluri AL, Azad TD. Machine learning predictive models in neurosurgery: An appraisal based on the TRIPOD guidelines. Systematic Review. Neurosurgical FOCUS. 2023;**54**:E8. DOI: 10.3171/2023.3.FOCUS2386

[108] Kavallieros K, Tran M-T, Ahmad M, Ahmad B, Shalhoub J, Davies A. O262: Evaluating the role and efficacy of virtual reality and simulation in teaching acute and trauma scenarios – A systematic review. British Journal of Surgery. 2024;**111**. DOI: 10.1093/bjs/znae046.060

[109] Mishra R, Narayanan MDK, Umana GE, Montemurro N, Chaurasia B, Deora H. Virtual reality in neurosurgery: Beyond neurosurgical planning. International Journal of Environmental Research and Public Health. 2022;**19**:1-14

[110] Pettinelli NJ, Lee AY, Lee MS, Mahatme RJ, Gillinov SM, Jimenez AE. Virtual reality is an effective tool for learning techniques in arthroplasty: A systematic review and meta-analysis. JAAOS Global Research & Reviews. 2023;7(e23):00078. DOI: 10.5435/JAAOSGlobal-D-23-00078

[111] Singer J, VanOosterhout S, Madder R. Remote robotic endovascular thrombectomy for acute ischaemic stroke. BMJ Neurology Open. 2021;**3**:e000141. DOI: 10.1136/bmjno-2021-000141

[112] Lai M, Skyrman S, Kor F, Homan R, El-Hajj VG, Babic D, et al. Development of a CT-compatible, anthropomorphic skull and brain phantom for neurosurgical planning, training, and simulation. Bioengineering. 2022;**9**:537

[113] Marunganathan V, Guru A. Tele-neurosurgery: Expanding access and expertise through remote consultation and virtual surgery. Brain and Spine. 2024;**4**:102920. DOI: 10.1016/j.bas.2024.102920

[114] Patel SA, Covell MM, Patel S, Kandregula S, Palepu SK, Gajjar AA, et al. Advancing endovascular neurosurgery training with extended reality: Opportunities and obstacles for the next decade. Frontiers in Surgery. 2024;**11**:1440228. DOI: 10.3389/fsurg.2024.1440228

[115] Karthik A, Shiek Aalam S, Sivakumar M, Rama Sundari MV, Dafni Rose J, Elangovan M, et al. Improving brain tumor treatment with better imaging and real-time therapy using quantum dots. Biomedical Signal Processing and Control. 2024;**95**:106286. DOI: 10.1016/j.bspc.2024.106286

[116] Filippi M, Evangelou N, Kangarlu A, Inglese M, Mainero C, Horsfield MA, et al. Ultra-high-field MR imaging in

multiple sclerosis. Journal of Neurology, Neurosurgery & Psychiatry. 2014;**85**:60-66. DOI: 10.1136/jnnp-2013-305246

[117] Perera Molligoda Arachchige AS, Meuli S, Centini FR, Stomeo N, Catapano F, Politi LS. Evaluating the role of 7-tesla magnetic resonance imaging in neurosurgery: Trends in literature since clinical approval. World Journal of Radiology. 2024;**16**:274-293. DOI: 10.4329/wjr.v16.i7.274

Chapter 11

Foundations of Robotic Spine Surgery: Emerging Technologies and Future Directions

Fernando Terry, Alejandro Enriquez-Marulanda, Punit Pandya, Forough Yazdanian, Efstathios Papavassiliou and Ziev B. Moses

Abstract

Robotic technology is increasingly employed in minimally invasive spine surgery (MISS) to mitigate morbidity, operative duration, radiation exposure, and complications. The first FDA-approved (2004) robotic platform was the SpineAssist by Mazor Robotics, followed by the Mazor Renaissance (2011), and the Mazor X Stealth System (2016). These sequential Mazor generations featured enhancements in human interface, hardware, software, range of motion and system capacity. Additional robotic spine surgery systems are the ROSA robot by Zimmer Biomet, the ExcelsiusGPS by Globus Medical and REMI by Alphatec Spine. Some modern stations like the TiRobot have been approved by their country's governmental regulatory agencies. As spine surgery increasingly transitions to outpatient settings, there is a growing preference for smaller robotic platforms. Lastly, robot-guided endoscopic spine surgery (ESS) represents a significant advancement in ultra-minimally invasive techniques, combining robotic precision with endoscopic methods to enhance surgical outcomes. While it offers benefits like reduced recovery time and improved visualization, challenges such as the steep learning curve and high costs exist, necessitating further long-term studies to evaluate its efficacy and viability. Based on this foundation, this chapter will delineate the historical progression of robotic spine surgery techniques, as well as explore the continuous emergence of novel modalities through rigorous methodological assessment.

Keywords: spine, minimally invasive surgical procedures, robotic surgical procedures, endoscopy, artificial intelligence

1. Introduction

The integration of robotics in surgical practice, driven by advancements in surgical instrumentation and current technology, has significantly increased over the past decade [1]. Initially introduced in 1985, surgical robots have become utilized across various specialties, including general surgery, urology, gynecology, orthopedics, and spine surgery [2]. The original robotic surgery concept–automatic machines able to perform human tasks–stems from more than 60 years ago in the military field, relying on the difficult-to-access hostile war environments and need for surgical assistance during polytrauma and hypovolemic hemorrhagic shock after gunshot wounds. Nevertheless, the first robotic platform appeared in early 1980s and was called the "Programmable Universal Machine for Assembly 200 (PUMA)" [3] whose primary objective was to increase the efficiency of neurosurgical biopsies [4].

Approximately five million spinal surgeries are annually performed worldwide, with nearly one million occurring in the United States alone [2]. Lumbar spinal surgeries, particularly robotic guided instrumented fusions, have experienced an increased rate of nearly 62% between 2004 and 2015 [5]. Furthermore, recent projections estimate that the demand for thoracolumbar spine fusion surgeries are experiencing a steep increase in the following years. For instance, anterior lumbar interbody fusion (ALIF) surgeries are expected to increase from 49,205 to 55,528 between 2020 and 2040; while posterior lumbar interbody fusion (PLIF) surgeries will present an increase from 255,319 to 297,994 cases just in the United States throughout the same time period [6]. Within this context, spinal pathologies encompass a diverse range of conditions that require a broad range of therapeutic approaches such as stabilization via interbody fusion utilizing pedicle screws and rods, which is a commonly employed technique [1]. However, precise placement is essential for optimal postoperative outcomes, as misalignment can jeopardize adjacent neurovascular structures, lead to iatrogenic injuries, and potentially compromise fusion rates [7]. Published literature states that serious screw-related complications, such as neurological, visceral or vascular are seldom reported; however, this underreporting may be limited by authors' medicolegal considerations [8–11].

Surgical robots can be classified into three main types: Supervisory controlled systems, which allow for surgeon's surgical pre-planning while the robot executes the intraoperative steps; tele surgical systems, which enable the surgeon to manipulate the surgical instrumentation remotely; and shared control systems, which alternate both the surgeon's and robot participation [12, 13]. The recent integration of computer and robotic navigation, stemming from the need to improve precision and mitigate complications, has substantially increased the accuracy of the pedicle screw trajectory [5]. Robot-assisted pedicle screw placement offers significant advantages over traditional methods such as free-hand placement, CT navigation, and 2D fluoroscopy [14]. These advantages account for enhanced accuracy of screw placement and a reduced incidence of surgical complications. Likewise, it enhances the safety of surgical procedures while reducing intraoperative radiation exposure for patients and healthcare providers. Indeed, robotic spine surgery enables minimally invasive techniques, resulting in smaller incisions, reduced blood loss, less postoperative pain, faster recovery, and shorter hospital stays [15].

Given that, this chapter aims to provide an overview of the available surgical robotic navigation systems in the healthcare market, outlining their advantages and limitations, as well as our institutional clinical experience with the Mazor X Stealth Edition and the Excelsius GPS Robotic Navigation platform, two of the latest robotic systems used in the spine surgery field.

2. Current applications of robotic spine surgery

2.1 Mazor X (Medtronic)

In 2001, Medtronic Robotics developed a small-spine mounted robot whose main purpose was to increase pedicle screw instrumentation accuracy [16]. The first FDA-approved spine robot, SpineAssist (Mazor Robotics Ltd., Caesarea, Israel), was introduced to the market in 2004. It consisted of a small, spine-mounted robot-assisted platform that had an attached arm with six degrees of freedom. This shared-control robot offers enhanced navigation capabilities compared to traditional computer-assisted systems and remains one of the most widely used spine robots, especially in small medical centers. During the preoperative phase, SpineAssist's software acquires CT images of the targeted spinal levels to generate a virtual map following registration. A plan for the desired screw entry point, size, and screw trajectory can be conducted either preoperatively or intraoperatively. The final registration point is established using anteroposterior (AP) and oblique fluoroscopic images for calibration. Once the mounting system is affixed to the patient's spinous process or the surgical table, the robotic arm can be guided along its predetermined trajectory to facilitate drilling [13, 17, 18].

Introduced in 2011, the Renaissance Robotic System represents the second generation of Mazor's SpineAssist technology. Although it is smaller, lighter, and features upgraded software, both the Renaissance and SpineAssist systems have faced criticism regarding potential skiving, which could lead to incorrect screw trajectories. Finally, in 2016 the Mazor X Stealth Edition (MXSE) was launched, incorporating a workstation and a mechanical surgical arm equipped with a linear optical camera that enables volumetric assessment of the surgical field and facilitates intraoperative collision avoidance. Additionally, the MXSE allows for the registration of individual vertebral bodies, significantly enhancing accuracy in screw placement [17, 18].

Mazor robotic systems are the most widely used spinal robots in the United States and in the whole world, being present in at least 250 medical centers across the globe during 2018. Recent reports are focusing on evaluating cortical bone trajectory (CBT) screws using robotic assistance, rather than traditional pedicle screw trajectory [19–21], showcasing several advantages for the MXSE, such as having an inferomedial entry point with a more superolateral trajectory, thus, requiring a smaller incision for the instrumentation. Some of the purported benefits of CBT screws include a higher insertional torque and pullout strength [22–24], improved accuracy and safety during the screw placement; higher precision during the screw size selection and surgical planning, reduction of operating room time, intraoperative radiation and enhanced operator's ergonomics.

2.2 Excelsius GPS (Globus medical)

The Globus Medical Excelsius GPS (Globus Medical, Inc., Audubon, PA), which received FDA clearance in 2017, represents a notable advancement in spinal surgery technology by addressing several limitations of earlier robotic systems, such as inaccuracies in registration and navigation, loss of tactile feedback and extended operative times. This innovative robotic navigation system employs a floor-mounted robotic arm and utilizes surveillance markers positioned at the posterior superior iliac spine. It integrates real-time preoperative or intraoperative CT imaging, thereby obviating the need for extensive preoperative scans and reducing patient radiation exposure. Additionally, it allows for automatic adjustments during surgery, enabling direct screw insertion without K-wires and providing immediate feedback on potential skiving or movement of the reference array, which enhances surgical safety and offers real-time visualization of instrument positioning and screw placement in relation to the patient's anatomy [13, 17, 18, 25].

The Excelsius GPS system is further distinguished by its sophisticated software, which delivers real-time visualizations of instrument positioning and screw placement aligned with the patient's anatomical structures. Equipped with advanced sensors, the system can detect drill skiving and the sliding of the reference frame while automatically compensating for any patient movements. A cadaveric study validated the system's efficacy, demonstrating 100% accuracy in screw placement, with no breaches exceeding 2 mm, along with reduced insertion times and decreased radiation exposure compared to traditional methods. Subsequent studies evaluating the performance of Excelsius GPS have reported a screw placement success rate graded A by the Gertzbein and Robbins classification in over 96% of patients treated, underscoring the system's effectiveness in enhancing surgical outcomes [26–31].

2.3 REMI system (AlphaTec spine)

The REMI system, developed by Accelus, is another competitor in spinal robotics. This innovative platform integrates intra-operative deep navigation with both 3D imaging and 2D fluoroscopic scans, employing a compact, table-mounted navigation system that directs surgical instrumentation and implants with precision. The REMI system not only enhances the efficiency and cost-effectiveness of surgical procedures but also prioritizes a surgeon-centric approach. Its advanced software, in conjunction with the hardware, facilitates streamlined image acquisition, trajectory planning, and navigation workflows, thereby enabling the surgeon to maintain active engagement throughout the surgical process [32–34].

A notable technical feature of the REMI system is its capacity for real-time trajectory adjustments, utilizing optical marker arrays affixed to both the targeting platform and surgical instruments. This capability permits surgeons to position the REMI targeting platform in proximity to the planned surgical site, where it can autonomously micro-adjust its trajectory in accordance with pre-established surgical plans. The system's proprietary effector further allows for surgeon-controlled micro-adjustments, providing a visual representation of instrumentation on a navigation screen. The integration of a near-field monocular camera enhances spatial awareness by continuously monitoring the markers, thus reporting their positions to the workstation. This configuration not only mitigates line-of-sight challenges prevalent in competing systems but also demonstrates an accuracy of less than 2 mm in a pedicle screw placement, ultimately resulting in improved workflow efficiency [35].

The REMI received FDA clearance in February 2021 and is indicated for assisting surgeons in the precise placement of pedicle screws in the posterior lumbar region (L1-S1) during open or percutaneous procedures. Its compatibility with the Accelus LineSider Spinal System, including the unique screw tip geometry and mandible tip designed for optimal bone engagement, underscores its operational efficacy. A landmark surgical event in March 2022 showcased the integration of the REI system with the LineSider Spinal System and the FlareHawk Expandable Interbody Fusion Device, exemplifying a seamless, minimally invasive approach that reduces incision sizes and minimizes the risk of nerve injury. As the system evolves to incorporate 2D fluoroscopic imaging capabilities, its potential impact on spinal surgery is poised to expand further. Being a highly attractive robotic platform, it has recently been acquired by AlphaTec Spine [35, 36].

2.4 VELYS spine surgery robot (Johnson and Johnson)

The VELYS Robotic-Assisted Solution, developed through a collaboration between Johnson and Johnson MedTech, DePuy Synthes (USA), and eCential Robotics (France), represents a novel dual-use robotic and navigation platform for spine surgery. This proprietary system allows spine surgeons the flexibility to utilize either standalone navigation or an active robotic-assisted approach. Previously cleared for unicompartmental knee arthroplasty, the VELYS system recently received FDA 510(k) clearance for planning and executing spinal fusion procedures across the cervical, thoracolumbar, and sacroiliac regions. Early clinical studies suggest that the integration of patient-specific techniques with the VELYS system enhances patient outcomes, minimizes healthcare resource utilization, and facilitates a rapid learning curve for surgeons [37–39].

The VELYS Spine system is distinguished by its active robotic assistance, which accommodates unintentional patient movement, including intraoperative spinal position shifts, while adapting to individual surgeon preferences. This system supports customizable workflows tailored to specific pathologies through features such as adaptive tracking technology and trajectory assistance. Furthermore, it can function either as a standalone navigation aid or as an active robotic platform, enhancing flexibility in surgical planning and execution. The VELYS Spine is compatible with DePuy Synthes' comprehensive product catalog, including the TriALTIS portfolio and FDA-cleared navigation-enabled instruments, which encompass a posterior thoracolumbar pedicle screw system, drills, taps, and screwdrivers, all operable with or without robotic assistance.

2.5 Mako spine system (Stryker)

The Mako Robotic Spine System, developed by Stryker, comprises several subtypes: Mako Total Knee, Mako Total Hip, Mako Partial Knee, Mako Shoulder, and Mako Spine, the latter of which is anticipated to be showcased at this robotic platform has gained significant traction in orthopedic surgery, contributing to an 8% growth in sales of the company's knee replacements in the third quarter. In early 2024, it received FDA clearance for spine surgery. The Mako system's versatility enhances its appeal to Ambulatory Surgical Centers and allows for integration with existing Mako Robots [40].

Stryker's forthcoming comprehensive spine robotic ecosystem, which includes Mako Spine, Q Guidance, and CoPilot, highlights the company's commitment to innovation and improved surgical outcomes. CoPilot, compatible with the Q Guidance camera, provides haptic feedback during procedures, thereby enhancing safety and precision. This technology delivers sensory alerts to surgeons to avoid vital structures during spine surgeries, significantly improving patient safety. Notably, CoPilot automatically halts upon reaching a predetermined depth during surgery, facilitating accurate screw placement [41].

2.6 ROSA (Zimmer Biomet)

The original ROSA robot (Medtech, Montpellier, France), approved by the FDA in 2012, was initially designed for cranial applications. In 2014, it obtained the CE Mark for minimally invasive spine procedures. Later in 2016, the ROSA Spine system (Zimmer Biomet Robotics, formerly Medtech SA, Montpellier, France) received FDA approval, introducing a robotic arm and navigation camera. The device has been approved for minimally invasive lumbar fusion (considering general and percutaneous transpedicular screw insertion); having as main indication the minimally invasive circumferential arthrodesis. Nowadays, it is currently being used in at least 29 US facilities [42].

The device comprises a robotic arm with tracking abilities, combined with a navigation system (optical navigation camera). The main platform includes a robotic arm (with six degrees of freedom), a haptic sensor and a surgical workshop with a touch screen. Its software allows for user registration, surgical planification, and intraoperative imaging. This system necessitates a preoperative CT scan and employs a percutaneous reference pin, typically placed in the iliac bone, to facilitate auto-positioning during surgery. The ROSA robotic arm operates within a three-dimensional plane, synchronized with the patient, and is guided by a tracking camera that monitors real-time data from the percutaneous pin, which moves in conjunction with the robotic arm [17, 18]. The surgical technique for circumferential lumbar arthrodesis with a minimally invasive transforaminal approach remains the main indication for the ROSA robot [43], being a therapeutic option for degenerative lumbar disease such as spondylolisthesis or recurrent herniated disk.

The robotic platform's main advantage is the possibility to track the patient's movements and respiratory motion. The spine is a dynamic entity that can present intraoperative motion because of the respiratory pattern or surgical instrumentation. For that matter, the O-arm CT performs a 30-second 3D beath-hold acquisition, to monitor the patient's movements. Nevertheless, it may present several limitations: The information provided can be biased if the patient moves abnormally, which may result in inaccurate instrumentation; the operator (surgeon) must have a perfect understanding of the device, requiring an in-depth learning curve; and it has not been implemented for cervical spine surgery [42, 43]. Finally, the ROSA robot system's feasibility has been assessed mostly in cadaveric studies [43–45], decreasing its applicability to clinical practice and its comparability with other robotic technologies.

2.7 Da Vinci surgical system (Intuitive surgical)

The Da Vinci surgical robot, approved by the FDA in 2000 for general surgery laparoscopic applications, is the third most used robotic system. Unlike other robotic platforms, it employs a tele surgical model, allowing surgeons to control the robot from a remote booth equipped with joysticks and 3D visualization. In spine surgery, the da Vinci has demonstrated promising clinical outcomes, particularly in laparoscopic anterior lumbar interbody fusion (ALIF). The first reported case utilizing a minimally invasive surgical (MIS) approach with the da Vinci robot occurred in 1991, aiming to reduce vascular complications, retrograde ejaculation, postoperative pain, and to improve incision size and hospital stay. Several case series have documented successful cage exposure and placement using the da Vinci robot; however, its application in other spinal approaches, including posterior techniques, remains unclear [13, 17].

2.8 TiRobot (TINAVI medical)

The TiRobot surgical robotic navigation and positioning system, developed by Beijing TINAVI Medical Technologies (Beijing, China), exemplifies a significant advancement in orthopedic surgery as a third-generation surgical robot. Renowned for its precision and safety, the TiRobot is particularly effective in high-accuracy procedures, including complex spinal surgeries and sacroiliac joint screw fixation. Its modular and miniaturized design enhances surgical planning and spatial mapping, thereby facilitating accurate intraoperative execution and improving overall patient outcomes. The system's minimally invasive approach notably reduces perioperative complications and expedites recovery, positioning it as a critical asset in modern orthopedic practices [46–48].

Empirical studies illustrate that the TiRobot markedly improves screw placement accuracy in various orthopedic applications, surpassing traditional fluoroscopy-guided techniques. For instance, TiRobot-assisted pelvic screw fixation not only enhances precision but also decreases intraoperative radiation exposure and blood loss. Its real-time feedback capabilities allow for immediate corrections during needle insertion, ensuring accurate trajectory planning through computer-reconstructed imaging. The system's optical tracking technology continuously monitors patient movements, allowing for real-time adjustment to surgical approaches, thereby mitigating the variability commonly associated with conventional manual navigation systems [48–50].

Despite its numerous advantages, the TiRobot presents some limitations. Its operational complexity necessitates human assistance, which can hinder ease of use. Although a second-generation TiRobot has been developed to enhance user-friendliness, extensive surgeon training remains essential for effective operation, presenting a barrier to widespread adoption. Thus, while the TiRobot signifies a leap forward in orthopedic surgical technology, the challenges of training and operational complexity must be addressed to fully realize its potential in clinical setting. **Table 1** showcases the main features of the spine robotic navigation systems [46, 47, 50].

Robotic navigation system	Advantages	Disadvantages
Mazor X Stealth Edition (Medtronic) [51]	• Ease of registration. • Integrates sophisticated navigation tools, facilitating precision in complex spinal surgeries. • Streamlines surgical workflow with enhanced planning tools.	• Requires extensive training to maximize system capabilities. • Bed-mounted limits intraoperative mobility. • Cannot re-register once hardware has been placed.
Excelsius GPS (Globus Medical) [51]	• Combines robotics with advanced navigation technologies for real-time feedback for optimal intraoperative decision-making. • Compatible with various imaging modalities (e.g. fluoroscopy, CT), enhancing surgical precision. • Easy to mobilize as not bed mounted. • Can re-register at any time during surgery.	• Require significant time for integration with existing surgical protocols and imaging systems. • Uses two PSIS pins (surveillance and tracking) which can be cumbersome.
REMI (AlphaTec Spine) [32]	• Enhanced dexterity and precision by the employment of an articulated robotic arm with multiple-jointed instruments. • Improved visualization via high-definition 3D stereoscopic optics with real-time advanced haptic feedback.	• Longer setup times, affecting surgical efficiency. • Not all patients are ideal candidates for REMI approaches, based on anatomical constraints.
VELYS Spine Surgery Robot (Johnson & Johnson) [37]	• Focused on usability, features an intuitive interface that simplifies the planning and execution process.	• Effectiveness relies heavily on a robust technological infrastructure.

Robotic navigation system	Advantages	Disadvantages
Mako Spine System (Stryker) [41]	• The Auto-Pilot system is novel and allows for safer, pre-defined drilling corridors • Incorporates haptic feedback • Real-time feedback on surgical progress and implant positioning, allowing for immediate corrections if necessary.	• High capital and operational costs, limiting its adoption in smaller healthcare facilities. • Learning curve is initially slow down surgical throughput. • Effectiveness is contingent upon the quality of preoperative imaging and planning.
ROSA Spine System (Zimmer Biomet) [52]	• Integrates seamlessly with intraoperative imaging technologies. • Adaptability to different surgical approaches and techniques.	• High initial and ongoing costs associated with maintenance. • Fewer number of surgeons are trained in this system (compared to other more popular platforms).
Da Vinci Surgical Robot (Intuitive Surgical) [51]	• Initially designed for general surgery, it has a high versatility for complex spinal procedures requiring soft tissue manipulation. • Superior visualization and instrument control, offering enhanced depth perception and magnification during procedures.	• Lacks dedicated features for spine surgery. • Extremely high cost and ongoing maintenance requirements.
TiRobot Surgical Robotic System (TINAVI Medical) [52]	• Use of artificial intelligence and machine learning for improved surgical outcomes. • Tailor procedures to individual patient anatomy using preoperative data, optimizing surgical approaches and instrument selection.	• Less established presence in the global market. • Fewer available resources for training and ongoing support.

Table 1.
Advantages and Disadvantages of Spine Robotic Navigation Systems.

3. Limitations of robotic navigation

3.1 Cost–benefit analysis of robotic spine surgery

Cost–benefit analysis is a crucial aspect of spine surgery and healthcare management. Between 2001 and 2010, approximately 3.6 million spinal fusions were performed in the United States, with a total cost exceeding $287 billion [2]. The incorporation of robotic systems can positively influence these costs, as robotics are known to reduce operative time, hospital length of stay, rates of misplaced screws, and exposure to fluoroscopy [2]. A retrospective cost-effectiveness analysis demonstrated that robotic spine technology resulted in decreased lengths of stay, fewer revision surgeries, lower infection rates, and shorter operative times, contributing to its cost-effectiveness [53]. Additionally, a retrospective study found that robotic technology significantly improved screw accuracy, reduced radiation exposure, and enhanced perioperative patient outcomes, including decreased postoperative opioid use and shorter hospital stays [54]. The prospective multicenter study MISReFRESH [7] is a robust observational study, partially randomized measuring endpoints at 1-year follow-up like the rates of complications, revision surgery, radiation comparison between Mazor robotic-guidance and fluoro-guidance. The preliminary results have determined a 75% reduction in fluoroscopy need for pedicle screw insertion, significantly less complications and revisions within the robotic group. When accounting for these covariates, the worldwide robotic spine surgery market is expected to reach an annual income of $2.77 billion by 2022 [55].

3.2 Technical limitations

Limitations of robotic spine technology include the learning curve, potential for longer operative times, and associated costs [13]. While reported cases indicate that robotic procedures may take longer than free-hand cases, this difference can often be attributed to the additional time required for operating room setup [13]. The upfront cost of a single spine robot typically ranges from $500,000 to over $1,000,000, not accounting for maintenance, navigation platforms, and other disposable items needed for each procedure. Nevertheless, as demonstrated by Menger et al., the reduction in rates of misplaced screws, infections, and lengths of stay can ultimately result in cost savings over time. The future of robotic spine surgery is promising; however, further rigorous clinical evaluation is necessary to fully realize the potential of this innovative technology [53].

4. The BIDMC/HMS experience

4.1 Illustrative cases

4.1.1 Case 1: Mazor X stealth edition (MXSE) - L2: 5 posterior robotic laminectomy and fusion

A 79-year-old female with history of L4-L5 grade I spondylolisthesis and L2-L5 moderate to severe stenosis, suffers from persistent severe low back pain, bilateral leg pain accompanied by paresthesia, symptoms indicative of lumbar neurogenic claudication. A comprehensive neurological examination showed full motor strength and intact light touch sensation. There were no indications of bowel or bladder dysfunction.

Magnetic resonance imaging (MRI) images were obtained from a prior clinical appointment at an external healthcare facility (**Figure 1**). Nonetheless, the preoperative planning required the obtention on a "Mazor protocol" CT to better assess recent anatomical changes on the lumbar spine (**Figure 2**).

Based on clinical symptomatology and imaging findings, an elective procedure involving posterior L2–5 laminectomy and robotic fusion was performed using the MXSE. No intraoperative complications were reported. A postoperative anteroposterior (AP) and lateral lumbar radiography were obtained on postoperative day 1 (POD1) to verify the adequate placement of the lumbosacral instrumentation (screws, pins and plates) (**Figure 3**). The postoperative course was uneventful, and the patient was subsequently discharged to an extended care facility for physical rehabilitation.

4.1.2 Case 2: Globus medical Excelsius GPS - L4-L5 right robotic TLIF

A 50-year-old female presented with worsening axial low back pain and MRI findings of significant facet fluid at L4-L5, a right synovial cyst, and grade

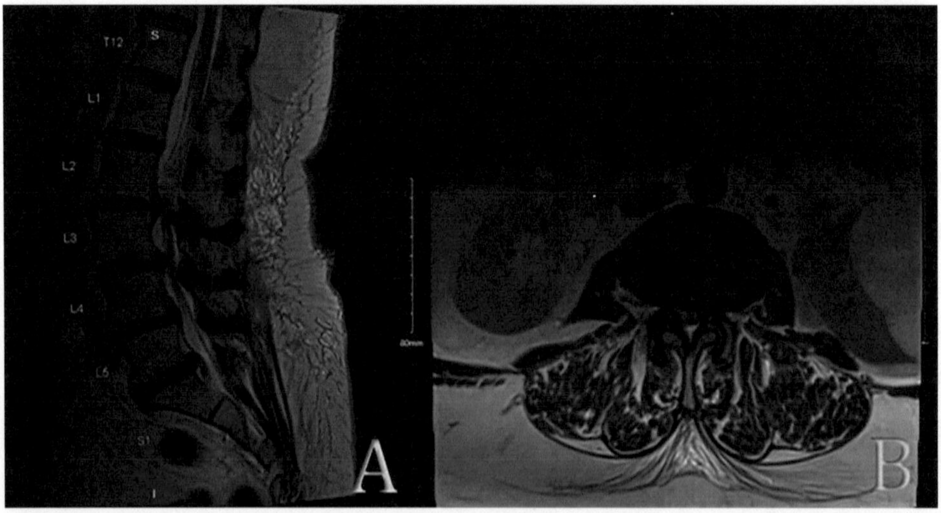

Figure 1.
Lumbar (A) sagittal and (B) L2–3 axial slice T2 MRI reveal multilevel degenerative changes throughout the lumbar spine with L2–5 moderate to severe spinal canal stenosis.

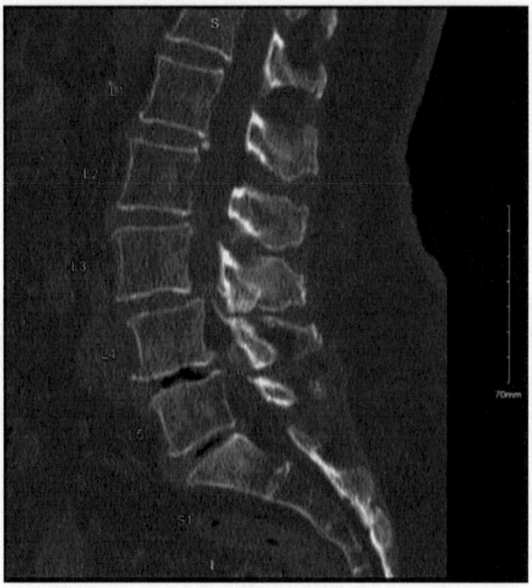

Figure 2.
CT lumbar with 1 mm slices with representative sagittal slice.

I spondylolisthesis, with motion observed on flexion-extension radiographs (**Figure 4**). Previous interventions, including lumbar epidural steroid injections at the L4-L5 level, medial branch blocks, and physical therapy, yielded minimal symptom relief. The initial physical examination revealed full motor strength and intact sensation to light touch in all extremities. Given the progressive clinical course and imaging findings, surgical intervention was deemed the optimal treatment.

The patient underwent an elective L4-L5 right robotic transforaminal lumbar interbody fusion (TLIF) using the Globus Excelsius. No intraoperative complications were reported. A postoperative anteroposterior (AP) and lateral lumbar radiography

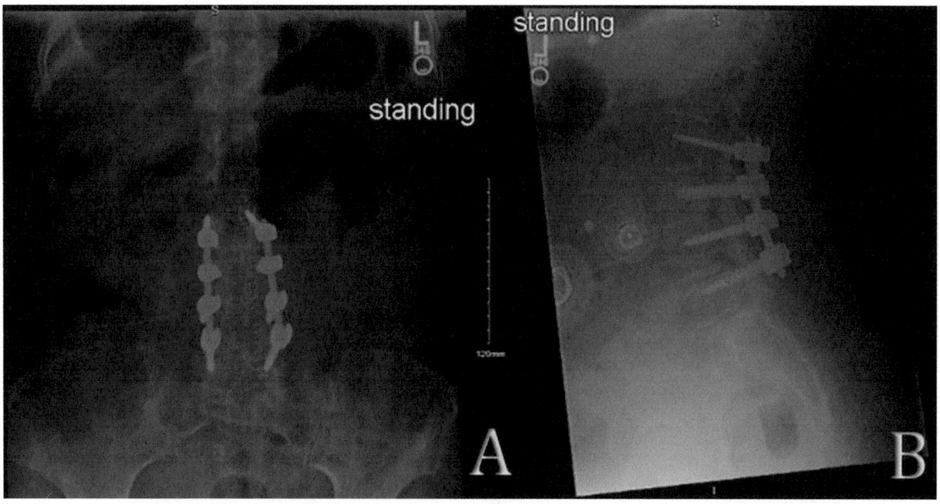

Figure 3.
(A) AP and (B) Post-operative lateral standing x-rays revealing satisfactory hardware placement.

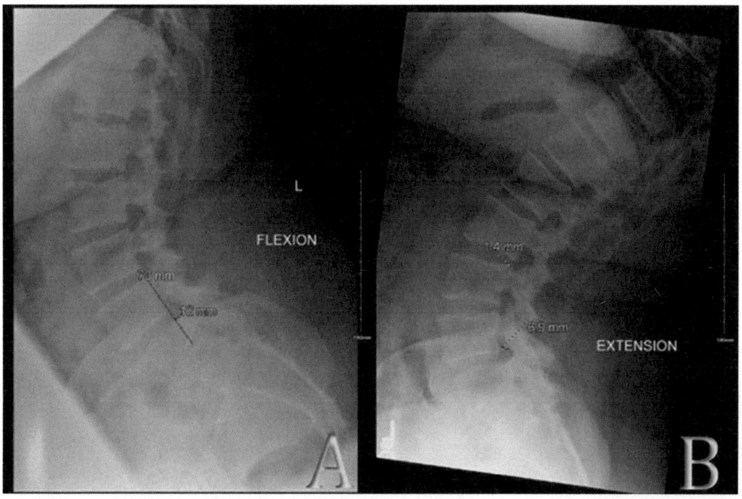

Figure 4.
Preoperative lateral (A) flexion and (B) extension x-rays revealing dynamic instability.

were obtained on POD1 to verify the adequate placement of the lumbosacral instrumentation (screws, pins and plates) (**Figure 5**). The postoperative course was uneventful, and the patient was discharged home.

4.1.3 Case 3: Mazor X stealth edition (MXSE) - minimally invasive Lumbopelvic fixation for unstable sacral fracture

A 69-year-old female presented after a fall while walking backwards with a trash-can. In the subsequent days, she developed significant sacral pain associated symptoms including urinary retention and pain while sitting. During her initial physical examination, she exhibited stable vital signs, was cooperative, alert, and oriented,

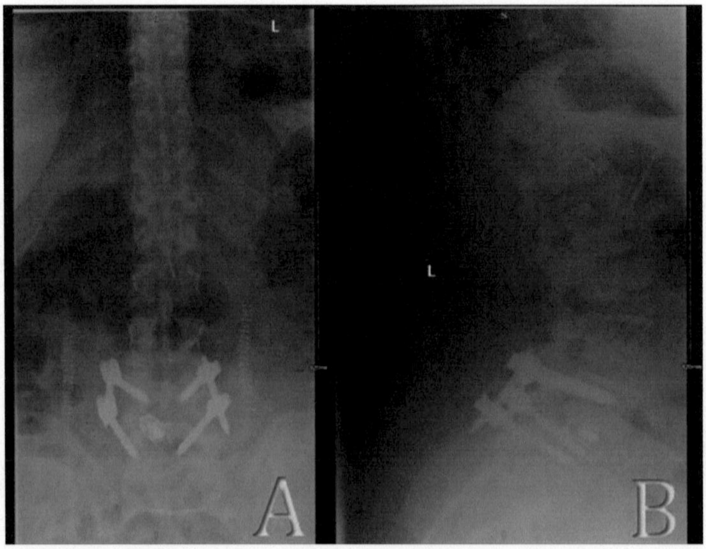

Figure 5.
Postoperative (A) AP and (B) lateral x-rays revealing satisfactory hardware placement.

with no signs of acute distress. Neurological examination revealed intact sensation to light touch and normal rectal tone. Preoperative AP and lateral sacrum CT scans identified combined vertical and transverse sacral fractures, resulting in lumbopelvic dissociation (**Figures 6** and 7).

Traditional open surgical access for iliac screws necessitates large incisions and extensive muscle dissection via a lateral approach to the sacral ala, which can increase postoperative morbidity. Additionally, significant subfascial dissection to expose the posterior superior iliac spine (PSIS) during implant insertion often contributes to intraoperative complications. In this context, preoperative

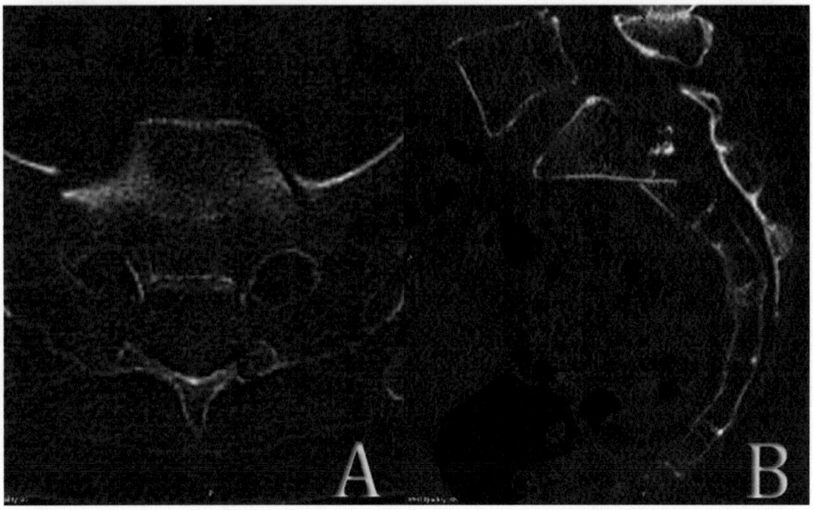

Figure 6.
CT lumbar spine with (A) axial and (B) sagittal slices revealing bilateral vertical fractures through the sacrum alae and a transverse fracture through the sacral body consistent with U-type fracture.

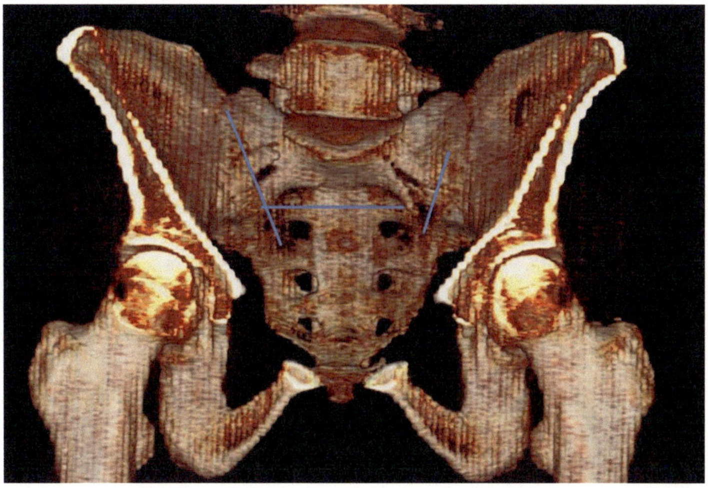

Figure 7.
3D CT reconstruction with U-type fracture (blue lines denote fracture lines).

surgical planning required a thorough analysis of the imaging and the patient's unique anatomy, resulting in the creation of a digital flight plan. In our case, the MXSE robotic navigation system facilitated precise planning for each screw and its associated trajectory (**Figures 8** and **9**).

A thorough literature review revealed two case series with a similar MIS approach reported by Tianjin Hospital (Tianjin, China) [56] and Duke University Medical Center (North Carolina, US) [57]. The first case series examined MIS spinopelvic fixation utilizing the TiRobot System (TINAVI Medical) for patients with high-energy traumatic sacral fractures. Pre-surgical planning involved the placement of bilateral reference arrays on the PSIS and the careful planning of screw trajectories, angles, and depths for both pedicle and S2AI screws. Conversely, the case series from Duke focused on patients with high-energy traumatic spinopelvic dissociation, employing the ExcelsiusGPS (Globus Medical) system. In this study, pre-surgical planning included percutaneous fixation of a navigation tracker on the L3 spinous process, as well as the design of pedicle screws based on the anatomical features of the L5 vertebra, including length, angulation, and direction. Additionally, a sacral laminectomy was performed to address any sacral nerve compression. A Schantz pin was inserted from the PSIS into the iliac wing and rotated to correct rotational displacement of the pelvic ring. Ultimately, bilateral S1 sacroiliac screws were placed under robotic guidance.

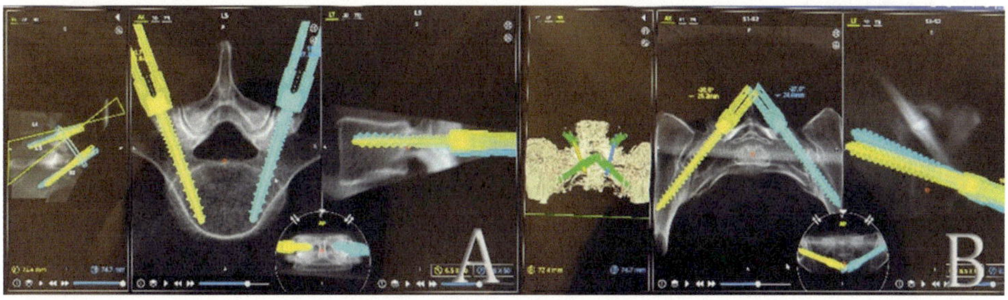

Figure 8.
Digital interface of MXSE robot. (A) Preoperative planning of L5 and (B) S2AI screws.

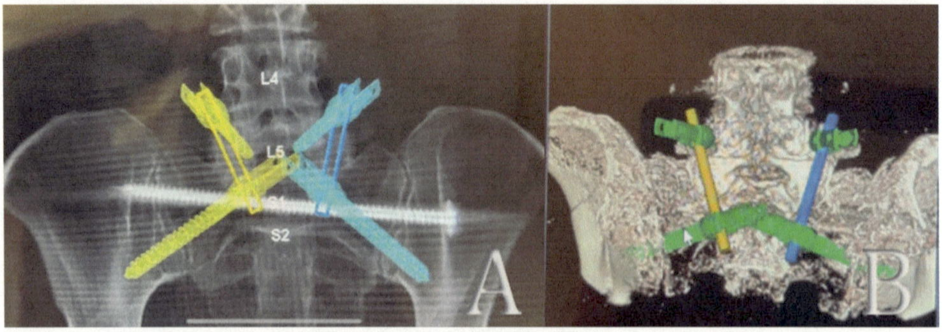

Figure 9.
Digital interface of MXSE robot. (A) 2D and (B) 3D digital screw overlay.

For our patient, based on the preoperative planning and the anatomical features of the L5-sacrum region, the length, angulation, and direction of the bilateral pedicle and iliac screws were simulated to enhance accuracy during placement. No intraoperative complications were reported. AP and lateral x-rays were obtained on POD1 to verify the placement of the instrumentation (**Figure 10**). The postoperative course was uneventful, and the patient was discharged home with minimal functional impact and no esthetic sequel (**Figure 11**).

4.2 Critical analysis

4.2.1 Postoperative clinical outcomes

Spinal fusion is indicated for a variety of conditions, including deformities such as scoliosis and kyphosis, spondylolisthesis, and spinal instability. Several studies have assessed the efficacy of the MXSE and ExcelsiusGPS robotic systems in the postoperative context, demonstrating reductions in operative time, surgeon radiation

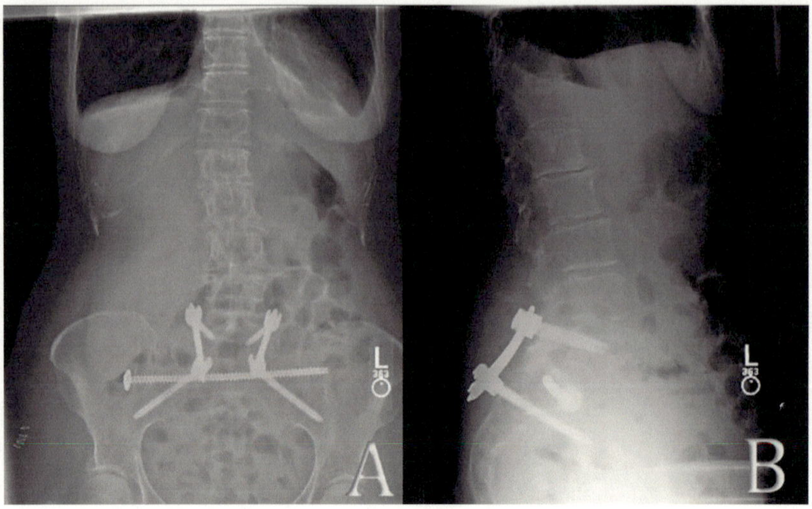

Figure 10.
Postoperative (A) AP and (B) lateral lumbar x-rays reveal satisfactory hardware placement.

DOI: http://dx.doi.org/10.5772/intechopen.1008268

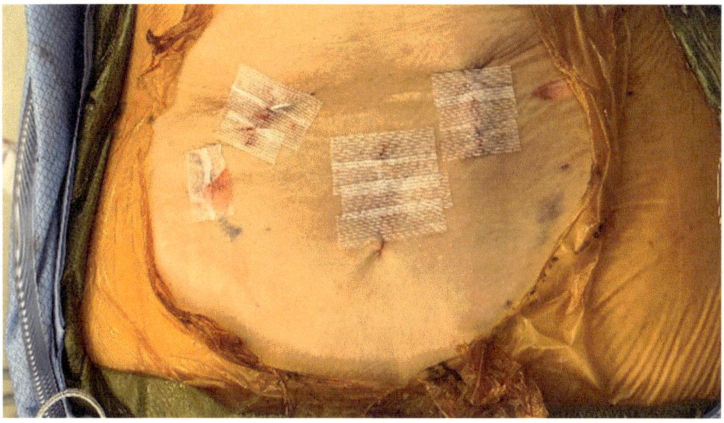

Figure 11.
Esthetic result revealing small MIS incisions for hardware placement.

exposure, and fluoroscopy frequency, along with enhanced accuracy in screw placement [58, 59]. The notable reduction in operative time can be attributed to the minimization of turning, repositioning, and intraoperative fluoroscopy, leading to shorter anesthesia duration and decreased intraoperative patient movement. For instance, a recent metanalysis reported a significant decline in revision surgeries due to screw malposition following thoracolumbar arthrodesis performed with robotic platforms [60]. However, total intraoperative blood loss and blood loss per spinal level may be influenced by the specific spinal pathology, particularly in cases involving oncologic conditions or extensive deformities that require open procedures and substantial osteotomy [28, 58, 59, 61–64].

Robotic systems utilize various imaging modalities, including preoperative CT, intraoperative CT, or fluoroscopy, combined with patient reference and positioning cameras to guide real-time pedicle screw placement. Notably, the two most popular systems, MXSE and ExcelsiusGPS use preoperative (CT or MRI) and intraoperative imaging for trajectory planning, incorporating real-time tracking with dynamic reference markers and camera feedback. Notably, MXSE is table-mounted while the ExcelsiusGPS is mobile, which is a distinct advantage. In addition, MXSE uses a small PSIS pin to attach the patient to the robot which if inadvertently nudged will result in a failure of the robotic system and potentially lead to abortive surgery. Both robotic platforms enhance patient safety by reducing postoperative complications and minimizing surgeon exposure. While pedicle screw placement accuracy can vary, computer-navigated screws generally pose a lower risk of cortical damage compared to freehand techniques. Some inaccuracies may arise from the learning curve associated with adapting to 3D navigation workflows.

The use of Mazor X navigation platform contributes to a significant reduction in operative time by eliminating the need for turning, repositioning, fluoroscopic positioning, and disinfection, which shortens anesthesia duration and decreases intraoperative patient movement, ultimately reducing surgical risks. However, operative time can vary widely based on the complexity of the procedures performed, including posterior column osteotomies, corpectomies, and curve corrections, in addition to pedicle screw fixation. Furthermore, variability in operative time among surgeons is influenced by their prior experience with specific robotic navigation systems.

Patient-reported outcomes are an essential aspect of holistic patient care, yet literature on this subject remains limited. A recent retrospective cohort study indicated that patients undergoing robot-assisted short segment spine fusion experienced significant improvements in health-related quality of life (HRQoL), as evidenced by a greater reduction in the Oswestry Disability Index (ODI) compared to freehand surgery. Additionally, there was a noted decrease in unplanned readmissions within the first year postoperatively [65].

4.2.2 Learning curve

Misplaced pedicle screws can lead to neurovascular injuries, visceral damage, and dural tears [66, 67]. The adoption of robotic platforms in spinal surgery has markedly diminished perioperative complications while also reducing the time required for pedicle screw placement, intraoperative blood loss, and the surgeon's exposure to radiation. However, the benefits of these technologies are largely contingent upon the surgeon's learning curve. Research indicates minimal differences in procedural efficiency between novice and experienced surgeons utilizing robotic guidance for pedicle screw placement. Nonetheless, a trend toward enhanced efficiency emerges after a surgeon performs a specific number of cases; both studies suggest that at least 30 screws must be placed before a significant improvement in efficiency is observed [68, 69].

The use of MXSE and ExcelsiusGPS systems in spine surgery entails a steep learning curve. It is essential for new users to set realistic expectations to mitigate the risk of early abandonment of these technologies. The MXSE platform exhibits a manageable learning curve, achieving consistent successful outcomes after 25 to 30 cases. Conversely, optimal proficiency with the ExcelsiusGPS is generally attained within 15 to 30 cases, with success rates for screw placement markedly improving after 30 procedures. Robotic navigation achieves a 99% success rate in pedicle screw placement, yet the highest rates of abandonment occur within the initial 5 to 25 cases [70–73].

The learning curve for attending surgeons and neurosurgical residents mastering advanced robotic platforms is substantial and is influenced by several factors: years of experience in robotic navigation surgery, duration of general neurosurgical training, time invested per screw placement, and abandonment rates [63, 74]. Interestingly, clinical fellows and residents learning from attending neurosurgeons who have recently acquired robotic skills demonstrate immediate and sustained superior performance compared to their mentors, suggesting that the learning curve can be effectively transferred through observation. This may be facilitated by the real-time visual feedback provided by robotic navigation systems [75].

Recent studies reveal that the average neurosurgery resident graduates with approximately 100 lead or senior-level procedures and 3100 hours of operative time, with a notable increase in operative hours per year, particularly in spinal cases [76]. While operative hours and the volume of spine cases are important metrics, individualized teaching and mentoring are critical to expediting the learning curve. Furthermore, attending neurosurgeons often acquire robotic techniques post-training, while residents and clinical fellows learn these methods at various stages of their education, presenting a unique challenge for neurosurgical educators who must "teach while learning" [77].

The integration of robotic navigation systems in spinal surgery has enhanced the safety and accuracy of various neurosurgical procedures, particularly in pedicle screw placement. While the learning curves for experienced neurosurgeons employing open free-hand techniques and trainees appear similar, surgical skills remain transferable from mentors to mentees, facilitating increased surgical experience and shorter learning curves.

4.2.3 Financial outcomes

The initial acquisition cost of robotic platforms for spine surgery is notably high, and further research is necessary to assess the long-term financial implications of these technologies (**Table 2**). Nonetheless, the integration of robotic systems into spine surgery has the potential to be cost-effective by reducing the rates of revision surgeries, as well as decreasing both the length of hospital stays and operative times. A pioneering cost-effectiveness study by Menger et al. [53] critically evaluated the economic impact of robotic technology within a busy spine neurosurgical practice. This study highlighted the importance of a thorough assessment of both direct costs (initial acquisition expenses) and indirect costs (patient surgical investments and effects on hospitalization duration). In this study, improved screw accuracy (computer-assisted navigation associated with robotic platforms) reduced the number of revision surgeries and conversion rates, as well as, decreased postoperative infection and length of stay. Overall, the use of robotic spine surgery led to a saving of $608,546 during the 1-year follow-up period, compared to free-hand surgery, even after accounting for the initial acquisition charge of the robotic platform and subsequent maintenance fees.

When considering the purchase of robotic navigation spinal systems, several recommendations emerge. It is advisable to select systems that provide comprehensive access to all necessary software and hardware features, regardless of the implant choice, while ensuring maximum compatibility with imaging technologies. The use of 3D fluoroscopy is particularly recommended, as it enhances operational efficiency, speed, and mobility. Despite the promising advantages of robotic-assisted minimally invasive (MIS) spine surgery—including reduced operative time, shorter hospital stays, lower rates of misplaced screws, and decreased exposure to fluoroscopy—more health economic data is essential for evidence-based clinical decision-making. This data is crucial to justify the increased costs associated with robotic interventions compared to traditional free-hand open surgery [78].

Existing literature lacks robust information on decision analysis in robotic spine surgery through frameworks such as cost-effectiveness, cost–benefit, and cost-utility analyses, as well as the application of advanced mathematical models, such as Markov modeling, Monte Carlo simulations, and decision trees. Thus, further investigation is imperative to fully understand the economic implications of robotic spine surgery [2].

Features	Mazor X Stealth Edition (MXSE)	Excelsius GPS
FDA approval year	2016	2017
Preoperative CT required	No	No
Mount	Table-mounted	Floor mounted
Instrument tracking	Yes	Yes
K-wires required	No	No
Cost per unit	$1500, 000	$ 1,000,000–$ 1500, 000

Table 2.
Features of institutional spine robotic systems.

5. Future directions

5.1 Robot-guided endoscopic spine surgery (ESS)

Robot-guided endoscopic spine surgery (ESS) marks a significant advancement in ultra-minimally invasive techniques, merging the precision of robotics with the advantages of endoscopic methods. This innovative approach enables surgeons to perform complex spinal procedures through small incisions, minimizing soft tissue injury, blood loss, and recovery time. The integration of robotic systems enhances the accuracy of instrument placement and mitigates the learning curve associated with traditional ESS. These systems often employ three-dimensional CT navigation, providing real-time imaging and instrument tracking, which reduces radiation exposure for the surgical team compared to conventional fluoroscopy-based techniques [79].

ESS has experienced significant evolution since Parviz Kambin introduced transforaminal lumbar discectomy in the 1980s. Over the decades, the indications for ESS have expanded considerably, now encompassing surgeries across cervical and lumbar segments, including both decompression and fusion procedures. The rapid adoption and increasing popularity of ESS highlight its effectiveness in addressing a wide range of spinal conditions, covering nearly all segments and pathologies [80].

Despite its advantages, robot-guided ESS faces several limitations. A primary challenge is the steep learning curve for surgeons, which can adversely affect initial procedural outcomes. Additionally, the acquisition, maintenance, and operation of robotic systems are costly, requiring specialized training of the surgical team. The reliance on single working instruments, with minimal assistance from a scope retractor, complicates fine tasks such as intramedullary surgery or dura suturing. In contrast, traditional three-portal laparoscopic surgery—with one camera portal and two working portals—allows surgeons to operate with both hands, offering a more dynamic and ergonomic approach that may reduce fatigue and enhance precision [79, 81]. Concerns also exist regarding the adequacy of decompression in certain cases and the potential for technical malfunctions during surgery. Integrating robotic systems into existing surgical workflows can pose challenges, as issues such as system malfunctions or frequent calibration may disrupt the surgical process [80].

In terms of clinical outcomes, studies indicate that robot-guided ESS can enhance visualization of the surgical field, facilitating safer and more effective procedures. Patients typically report better surgical outcomes, including reduced complication and infection rates, alongside improved overall satisfaction. However, as evidence is still evolving, more long-term studies are needed to comprehensively assess the benefits and risks associated with this technique [79].

Overall, robot-guided ESS represents a promising advancement in spine surgery, offering the potential for greater precision, reduced invasiveness, and improved patient outcomes. As technology advances and more surgeons gain experience with these systems, it is likely that robot-guided ESS will become a standard treatment option for various spinal pathologies [49].

5.2 Use of artificial intelligence and augmented reality in robotic spine surgery

The integration of Artificial Intelligence (AI) and Augmented Reality (AR) in robotic spine surgery represents a transformative advancement in medical technology, offering enhanced precision, improved patient outcomes, and optimized surgical workflows. In this context, AI primarily facilitates preoperative planning, intraoperative guidance, and postoperative care. AI algorithms can analyze extensive patient data to predict surgical outcomes, optimize patient selection, and personalize treatment plans. Machine learning models, particularly those employing supervised learning, have demonstrated potential in improving diagnostic accuracy and predicting complications. Intraoperatively, AI supports real-time decision-making, enhancing the surgeon's ability to navigate complex anatomical structures with increased precision [82–84].

Augmented Reality (AR) provides surgeons with immersive, three-dimensional visualizations of the patient's anatomy, overlaying critical information directly onto the surgical field. This technology facilitates precise spinal instrumentation placement, thereby reducing the risk of damage to surrounding tissues. AR systems can display real-time data, such as the positions of surgical instruments and anatomical landmarks, directly in the surgeon's line of sight, which enhances accuracy and reduces operative times. The integration of AR with robotic systems enables a more intuitive and controlled surgical experience [85, 86].

However, the adoption of AI and AR in spine surgery is not without challenges. The high costs associated with AR technology can hinder widespread implementation. Furthermore, concerns about integrating AR into existing surgical workflows and the necessity for extensive surgeon training remain significant barriers. The accuracy and reliability of AI algorithms are contingent upon the quality and diversity of the training data, which can limit their effectiveness in certain cases [82, 83, 87].

AI and AR technologies offer substantial benefits for complex spinal disorders, such as spinal tumors, where precision and enhanced visualization are critical. These innovations are particularly advantageous in scenarios where traditional surgical methods carry higher risks or where improved visualization is essential for successful outcomes. As technology continues to advance, ongoing research and development are expected to address current limitations and expand the applications of AI and AR in spine surgery. It is also crucial to establish ethical and legal frameworks that define practice standards, validate specialist credentials, shape insurance coverage, outline informed consent protocols, and ensure accountability among developers, users, and owners [82, 83, 87–89]. Nowadays, two of the most popular devices available in the market for spine surgery are the Augmedics (Augmented Reality in Spine Surgery – X-Ray Vision device) [90] and the VisAR (Augmented Reality Surgical Navigation) [91].

In conclusion, AI and AR are revolutionizing robotic spine surgery by enhancing precision, safety, and patient outcomes. While challenges to widespread adoption exist, the potential benefits of these technologies in improving surgical accuracy and enhancing patient care are substantial.

Conflict of interest

The authors declare no conflict of interest.

Notes/thanks/other declarations

Not applicable.

Author details

Fernando Terry, Alejandro Enriquez-Marulanda, Punit Pandya, Forough Yazdanian, Efstathios Papavassiliou and Ziev B. Moses*
Division of Neurosurgery, Beth Israel Deaconess Medical Center, Harvard Medical School, Boston, MA, USA

*Address all correspondence to: zmoses@bidmc.harvard.edu

References

[1] Farber SH, Pacult MA, Godzik J, Walker CT, Turner JD, Porter RW, et al. Robotics in spine surgery: A technical overview and review of key concepts. Frontiers in Surgery. 2021;**8**:578674

[2] D'Souza M, Gendreau J, Feng A, Kim LH, Ho AL, Veeravagu A. Robotic-assisted spine surgery: History, efficacy, cost, and future trends. Robotic Surgery: Research and Reviews. 2019;**6**:9

[3] Kwoh YS, Hou J, Jonckheere EA, Hayati S. A robot with improved absolute positioning accuracy for CT guided stereotactic brain surgery. IEEE Transactions on Biomedical Engineering. 1988;**35**(2):153-160

[4] Morrell ALG, Morrell-Junior AC, Morrell AG, Mendes JMF, Tustumi F, De-Oliveira-E-Silva LG, et al. The history of robotic surgery and its evolution: When illusion becomes reality. Revista do Colegio Brasileiro de Cirurgioes. 2021;**48**:e20202798

[5] Abel F, Avrumova F, Goldman SN, Abjornson C, Lebl DR. Robotic-navigated assistance in spine surgery. The Bone and Joint Journal. 2023;**105-B**(5):543-550

[6] Neifert SN, Martini ML, Hanss K, Rothrock RJ, Gilligan J, Zimering J, et al. Large rises in thoracolumbar fusions by 2040: A cause for concern with an increasingly elderly surgical population. World Neurosurgery. 2020;**144**:e25-e33

[7] Good CR, Orosz L, Schroerlucke SR, Cannestra A, Lim JY, Hsu VW, et al. Complications and revision rates in minimally invasive robotic-guided versus fluoroscopic-guided spinal fusions: The MIS ReFRESH prospective comparative study. Spine. 2021;**46**(23):1661-1668

[8] Gautschi OP, Schatlo B, Schaller K, Tessitore E. Clinically relevant complications related to pedicle screw placement in thoracolumbar surgery and their management: A literature review of 35,630 pedicle screws. Neurosurgical Focus. 2011;**31**(4):E8

[9] Lonstein JE, Denis F, Perra JH, Pinto MR, Smith MD, Winter RB. Complications associated with pedicle screws. The Journal of Bone and Joint Surgery. American Volume. 1999;**81**(11):1519-1528

[10] Nottmeier EW, Seemer W, Young PM. Placement of thoracolumbar pedicle screws using three-dimensional image guidance: Experience in a large patient cohort. Journal of Neurosurgery. Spine. 2009;**10**(1):33-39

[11] Functional Outcome of Computer-Assisted Spinal Pedicle Screw Placement: A Systematic Review and Meta-Analysis of 23 Studies Including 5992 Pedicle Screws - PubMed [Internet]. Available from: https://pubmed.ncbi.nlm.nih.gov/20052504/ [Accessed: October 7, 2024]

[12] Thieme USA [Internet]. Corrective Osteotomies for Rigid Spinal Deformi ties|9783131730817|Thieme Webshop. Available from: https://shop.thieme.com/Corrective-Osteotomies-for-Rigid-Spinal-Deformities/9783131730817 [Accessed: September 18, 2024]

[13] Antonacci CL, Zeng F, Block A, Davey A, Makanji H. Robotic-assisted spine surgery-a narrative review. The Journal of Spine Surgery Hong Kong. 2024;**10**(2):305-312

[14] Naik A, Smith AD, Shaffer A, Krist DT, Moawad CM, MacInnis BR, et al. Evaluating robotic pedicle screw

placement against conventional modalities: A systematic review and network meta-analysis. Neurosurgical Focus. Jan 2022;**52**(1):E10. DOI: 10.3171/2021.10.FOCUS21509. PMID: 34973681

[15] Spine SR for the. Global Surgical Robots for the Spine Industry Trend, Growth, [Internet]. 2017. Available from: https://www.openpr.com/news/442943/global-surgical-robots-for-the-spine-industry-trend-growth-shares-strategy-and-forecasts-2016-to-2022.html [Accessed: September 18, 2024]

[16] Shweikeh F, Amadio JP, Arnell M, Barnard ZR, Kim TT, Johnson JP, et al. Robotics and the spine: A review of current and ongoing applications. Neurosurgical Focus. 2014;**36**(3):E10

[17] Communications E. Navigation and Robotics in Spine Surgery [Internet]. Available from: https://medone-neurosurgery.thieme.com/ebooks/cs_10186097#/ebook_cs_10186097_cs475 [Accessed: September 18, 2024]

[18] Gajjar AA, Le AHD, Lavadi RS, Boddeti U, Barpujari A, Abou-Al-Shaar H, et al. Evolution of robotics in spine surgery: A historical perspective. Interdiscipline Neurosurgery. 2023;**33**:101721

[19] Ver MLP, Gum JL, Crawford CH, Djurasovic M, Owens RK, Brown M, et al. Index episode-of-care propensity-matched comparison of transforaminal lumbar interbody fusion (TLIF) techniques: Open traditional TLIF versus midline lumbar interbody fusion (MIDLIF) versus robot-assisted MIDLIF. Journal of Neurosurgery. Spine. 2020;**32**(5):741-747

[20] Le XF, Shi Z, Wang QL, Xu YF, Zhao JW, Tian W. Rate and risk factors of superior facet joint violation during cortical bone trajectory screw placement: A comparison of robot-assisted approach with a conventional technique. Orthopaedic Surgery. 2020;**12**(1):133-140

[21] Santoni BG, Hynes RA, McGilvray KC, Rodriguez-Canessa G, Lyons AS, Henson M, et al. Cortical bone trajectory for lumbar pedicle screws. Spine Journal of Official North American Spine Society. 2009;**9**(5):366-373

[22] Matsukawa K, Yato Y, Kato T, Imabayashi H, Asazuma T, Nemoto K. In vivo analysis of insertional torque during pedicle screwing using cortical bone trajectory technique. Spine (Phila Pa 1976). 15 Feb 2014;**39**(4):E240-5. DOI: 10.1097/BRS.0000000000000116. PMID: 24253778

[23] Perez-Orribo L, Kalb S, Reyes PM, Chang SW, Crawford NR. Biomechanics of lumbar cortical screw-rod fixation versus pedicle screw-rod fixation with and without interbody support. Spine (Phila Pa 1976). 15 Apr 2013;**38**(8):635-641. DOI: 10.1097/BRS.0b013e318279a95e. PMID: 23104197

[24] Baluch DA, Patel AA, Lullo B, Havey RM, Voronov LI, Nguyen NL, et al. Effect of physiological loads on cortical and traditional pedicle screw fixation. Spine. 2014;**39**(22):E1297-E1302

[25] Jiang B, Karim Ahmed A, Zygourakis CC, Kalb S, Zhu AM, Godzik J, et al. Pedicle screw accuracy assessment in ExcelsiusGPS® robotic spine surgery: Evaluation of deviation from pre-planned trajectory. Chinese Neurosurgical Journal. 2018;**4**(1):23

[26] Zygourakis CC, Ahmed AK, Kalb S, Zhu AM, Bydon A, Crawford NR, et al. Technique: Open lumbar decompression and fusion with the Excelsius

GPS robot. Neurosurgical Focus. 2018;**45**(VideoSuppl1):V6

[27] Vaccaro AR, Harris JA, Hussain MM, Wadhwa R, Chang VW, Schroerlucke SR, et al. Assessment of surgical procedural time, pedicle screw accuracy, and clinician radiation exposure of a novel robotic navigation system compared with conventional open and percutaneous freehand techniques: A cadaveric investigation. Global Spine Journal. 2019;**10**(7):814

[28] Huntsman KT, Ahrendtsen LA, Riggleman JR, Ledonio CG. Robotic-assisted navigated minimally invasive pedicle screw placement in the first 100 cases at a single institution. Journal of Robotic Surgery. 2020;**14**(1):199-203

[29] Godzik J, Walker CT, Hartman C, de Andrada B, Morgan CD, Mastorakos G, et al. A quantitative assessment of the accuracy and reliability of robotically guided percutaneous pedicle screw placement: Technique and application accuracy. Operative neurosurgery (Hagerstown, Md.). 2019;**17**(4):389-395

[30] Benech CA, Perez R, Benech F, Greeley SL, Crawford N, Ledonio C. Navigated robotic assistance results in improved screw accuracy and positive clinical outcomes: An evaluation of the first 54 cases. Journal of Robotic Surgery. 2020;**14**(3):431-437

[31] Vardiman AB, Wallace DJ, Crawford NR, Riggleman JR, Ahrendtsen LA, Ledonio CG. Pedicle screw accuracy in clinical utilization of minimally invasive navigated robot-assisted spine surgery. Journal of Robotic Surgery. 2020;**14**(3):409-413

[32] Accelus Announces First Procedure Integrating Remi Robotic Navigation System, LineSider Spinal System, and FlareHawk Expandable Interbody Fusion Device Technologies–Accelus. Available from: https://accelusinc.com/accelus-announces-first-procedure-integrating-remi-robotic-navigation-system-linesider-spinal-system-and-flarehawk-expandable-interbody-fusion-device-technologies/ [Accessed: October 23, 2024]

[33] Vetalice JA. ATEC Spine Acquires the REMI Robotic Navigation System | [Internet]. ORTHOWORLD; 2023. Available from: https://www.orthoworld.com/atec-spine-acquires-the-remi-robotic-navigation-system/

[34] ATEC Acquires Navigation-Enabled Robotics Platform; Raises. Revenue Guidance on Strength of Preliminary First Quarter Revenue Results. 2023. Available from: https://investors.alphatecspine.com/press-releases/news-details/2023/ATEC-Acquires-Navigation-Enabled-Robotics-Platform-Raises-2023-Revenue-Guidance-on-Strength-of-Preliminary-First-Quarter-Revenue-Results/default.aspx [Accessed: October 23, 2024]

[35] Soliman MA, Khan A, O'Connor TE, Foley K, Pollina J. Accuracy and efficiency of fusion robotics™ versus Mazor-X™ in single-level lumbar pedicle screw placement. Cureus. 26 Jun 2021;**13**(6):e15939. DOI: 10.7759/cureus.15939. PMID: 34211815; PMCID: PMC8236238

[36] Iampreechakul P, Chongchokdee C, Tirakotai W. The accuracy of computer-assisted pedicle screw placement in degenerative lumbrosacral spine using single-time, paired point registration alone technique combined with the surgeon's experience. Journal of the Medical Association of Thailand = Chotmaihet Thangphaet. 2011;**94**(3):337-345

[37] Hale C. J&J's DePuy Synthes nets clearance for Velys spine surgery robot [Internet]. Fierce Biotech. 2024. [cited 2024 Dec 4]. Available from: https://www.fiercebiotech.com/medtech/jjs-depuy-synthes-nets-clearance-velys-spine-surgery-robot

[38] Whooley S. MassDevice. J&J's DePuy Synthes Launches Velys Surgical Robot for Spine. 2024. Available from: https://www.massdevice.com/depuy-synthes-launches-velys-spine-robot/ [Accessed: October 29, 2024]

[39] DePuy Synthes Launches Dual Use Spine Robotics and NAV Platform|Orthopedics This Week [Internet]. 2024. Available from: https://ryortho.com/breaking/depuy-synthes-launches-dual-use-spine-robotics-and-nav-platform/ [Accessed: October 29, 2024]

[40] Post, Share, Post, Print, Email, License. MedTech Dive. Stryker touts Mako robot in DTC ads, as device makers eye broader patient populations. Available from: https://www.medtechdive.com/news/SYK-Stryker-Mako-robot-DTC-advertising-marketing/690307/ [Accessed: October 29, 2024]

[41] Mako SmartRobotics Overview [Internet]. Available from: https://www.stryker.com/us/en/joint-replacement/systems/Mako_SmartRobotics_Overview.html [Accessed: October 29, 2024]

[42] Lefranc M, Peltier J. Evaluation of the ROSA™ spine robot for minimally invasive surgical procedures. Expert Review of Medical Devices. 2016;**13**(10):899-906

[43] Chenin L, Peltier J, Lefranc M. Minimally invasive transforaminal lumbar interbody fusion with the ROSA(TM) spine robot and intraoperative flat-panel CT guidance. Acta Neurochirurgica. 2016;**158**(6):1125-1128

[44] Lefranc M, Peltier J. Accuracy of thoracolumbar transpedicular and vertebral body percutaneous screw placement: Coupling the Rosa® spine robot with intraoperative flat-panel CT guidance--a cadaver study. Journal of Robotic Surgery. 2015;**9**(4):331-338

[45] Chenin L, Capel C, Fichten A, Peltier J, Lefranc M. Evaluation of screw placement accuracy in circumferential lumbar arthrodesis using robotic assistance and intraoperative flat-panel computed tomography. World Neurosurgery. 2017;**105**:86-94

[46] Long T, Li K, Gao J, Liu T, Mu J, Wang X, et al. Comparative study of percutaneous sacroiliac screw with or without TiRobot assistance for treating pelvic postẽrior ring fractures. Orthopedic Surgery. 2019;**11**(3):386-396. Available from: https://www.ncbi.nlm.nih.gov/pmc/articles/PMC6595115/ [Accessed: September 21, 2024]

[47] Li N, Zhu Z, Xiao C, Wei D, Wang F, Zhang W, et al. The efficacy of «TiRobot»orthopaedic robot-assisted VS conventional fluoroscopic percutaneous screw fixation of the sacroiliac joint. International Orthopaedics. 2023;**47**(2):351-358

[48] Zhao C, Zhu G, Wang Y, Wu X. TiRobot-assisted versus conventional fluoroscopy-assisted percutaneous sacroiliac screw fixation for pelvic ring injuries: A meta-analysis. Journal of Orthopaedic Surgery. 2022;**17**:525. Available from: https://www.ncbi.nlm.nih.gov/pmc/articles/PMC9721051/ [Accessed: September 19, 2024]

[49] Liounakos JI, Wang MY. Endoscopic robotic spinal surgery: Current status

and future. In: Kim JS, Härtl R, Wang MY, Elmi-Terander A, editors. Technical Advances in Minimally Invasive Spine Surgery: Navigation, Robotics, Endoscopy, Augmented and Virtual Reality. Singapore: Springer Nature; 2022. pp. 321-325. DOI: 10.1007/978-981-19-0175-1_29

[50] Yan K, Zhang Q, Tian W. Comparison of accuracy and safety between second-generation TiRobot-assisted and free-hand thoracolumbar pedicle screw placement. BMC Surgery. 2022;**22**(1):275. Available from. DOI: 10.1186/s12893-022-01723-8 [Accessed: September 19, 2024]

[51] Alluri RK, Avrumova F, Sivaganesan A, Vaishnav AS, Lebl DR, Qureshi SA. Overview of robotic Technology in Spine Surgery. HSS Journal. 2021;**17**(3):308

[52] Wang J, Miao J, Zhan Y, Duan Y, Wang Y, Hao D, et al. Spine surgical robotics: Current status and recent clinical applications. Neurospine. 2023;**20**(4):1256-1271

[53] Menger RP, Savardekar AR, Farokhi F, Sin A. A cost-effectiveness analysis of the integration of robotic spine technology in spine surgery. Neurospine. 2018;**15**(3):216-224

[54] Kantelhardt SR, Martinez R, Baerwinkel S, Burger R, Giese A, Rohde V. Perioperative course and accuracy of screw positioning in conventional, open robotic-guided and percutaneous robotic-guided, pedicle screw placement. Official Publication of the European Spine Society, the European Spinal Deformity Society, and the European Section of the Cervical Spine Research Society. 2011;**20**(6):860-868

[55] Ng KC, Yuan L. Robotic-assisted laparoscopic radical nephrectomy and lymph nodes dissection using Senhance robotic system and Senhance ultrasonic energy device: A case report. Clinical Case Reports. 2024;**12**(8):e9117

[56] Liu ZJ, Cheng HY, Tian W, Jin X, Tian QH, Xi SY, et al. Robot-aided minimally invasive Lumbopelvic fixation in treatment of traumatic spinopelvic dissociation. Orthopaedic Surgery. 2021;**13**(2):563

[57] Hardigan AA, Tabarestani TQ, Dibble CF, Johnson E, Wang TY, Albanese J, et al. Robotic-assisted minimally invasive spinopelvic fixation for traumatic sacral fractures: Case series investigating early safety and efficacy. World Neurosurgery. 2023;**177**:e186-e196

[58] Zhao W, Wang Y, Zhang H, Guo J, Han J, Lin A, et al. Analysis of the screw accuracy and postoperative efficacy of screw placement in single position and bipedal position in robot-assisted oblique lumbar interbody fusion: Preliminary results of Mazor X stealth usage. Orthopaedic Surgery. 2024;**16**(2):401-411

[59] Wallace DJ, Vardiman AB, Booher GA, Crawford NR, Riggleman JR, Greeley SL, et al. Navigated robotic assistance improves pedicle screw accuracy in minimally invasive surgery of the lumbosacral spine: 600 pedicle screws in a single institution. The International Journal of Medical Robotics + Computer Assisted Surgery : MRCAS. 2020;**16**(1):e2054

[60] Staartjes VE, Klukowska AM, Schröder ML. Pedicle screw revision in robot-guided, navigated, and freehand thoracolumbar instrumentation: A systematic review and meta-analysis. World Neurosurgery. 2018;**116**: 433-443.e8

[61] Mao G, Gigliotti MJ, Myers D, Yu A, Whiting D. Single-surgeon direct

comparison of O-arm Neuronavigation versus Mazor X robotic-guided posterior spinal instrumentation. World Neurosurgery. 2020;**137**:e278-e285

[62] Solomiichuk V, Fleischhammer J, Molliqaj G, Warda J, Alaid A, von Eckardstein K, et al. Robotic versus fluoroscopy-guided pedicle screw insertion for metastatic spinal disease: A matched-cohort comparison. Neurosurgical Focus. 2017;**42**(5):E13

[63] Lieberman IH, Hardenbrook MA, Wang JC, Guyer RD. Assessment of pedicle screw placement accuracy, procedure time, and radiation exposure using a miniature robotic guidance system. Journal of Spinal Disorders & Techniques. 2012;**25**(5):241-248

[64] Shi C, Tong Y, Harris L, Owusu-Sarpong S, Goldstein J. Proficiency Development and Learning Curve in Robot-Assisted Spine Surgery Using the ExcelsiusGPS® System: Experience From a Single Institution. Global Spine Journal. 18 Apr 2024:21925682241242449. DOI: 10.1177/21925682241242449. Epub ahead of print. PMID: 38635306; PMCID: PMC11572081

[65] Clinical and Patient-Reported Outcomes after Robot-Assisted Short-Segment Lumbar Fusion with a Minimum 1-Year Follow-Up - ScienceDirect [Internet]. Available from: https://www-sciencedirect-com.echo.louisville.edu/science/article/pii/S2214751921000803 [Accessed: November 2, 2024]

[66] Fan Y, Du JP, Liu JJ, Zhang JN, Qiao HH, Liu SC, et al. Accuracy of pedicle screw placement comparing robot-assisted technology and the free-hand with fluoroscopy-guided method in spine surgery: An updated meta-analysis. Medicine (Baltimore). 2018;**97**(22):e10970

[67] Tian W, Han X, Liu B, Liu Y, Hu Y, Han X, et al. A robot-assisted surgical system using a force-image control method for pedicle screw insertion. PLoS One. 2014;**9**(1):e86346

[68] Urakov TM, Chang KHK, Burks SS, Wang MY. Initial academic experience and learning curve with robotic spine instrumentation. Neurosurgical Focus. 2017;**42**(5):E4

[69] Kam JKT, Gan C, Dimou S, Awad M, Kavar B, Nair G, et al. Learning curve for robot-assisted percutaneous pedicle screw placement in thoracolumbar surgery. Asian Spine Journal. 2019;**13**(6):920-927

[70] Buza JA, Good CR, Lehman RA, Pollina J, Chua RV, Buchholz AL, et al. Robotic-assisted cortical bone trajectory (CBT) screws using the Mazor X stealth edition (MXSE) system: Workflow and technical tips for safe and efficient use. Journal of Robotic Surgery. 2021;**15**(1):13-23

[71] Hu X, Ohnmeiss DD, Lieberman IH. Robotic-assisted pedicle screw placement: Lessons learned from the first 102 patients. Official Publication of the European Spine Society, the European Spinal Deformity Society, and the European Section of the Cervical Spine Research Society. 2013;**22**(3):661-666

[72] Hyun SJ, Kim KJ, Jahng TA, Kim HJ. Minimally invasive robotic versus open fluoroscopic-guided spinal instrumented fusions: A randomized controlled trial. Spine. 2017;**42**(6):353-358

[73] Schatlo B, Molliqaj G, Cuvinciuc V, Kotowski M, Schaller K, Tessitore E. Safety and accuracy of robot-assisted

versus fluoroscopy-guided pedicle screw insertion for degenerative diseases of the lumbar spine: A matched cohort comparison. Journal of Neurosurgery. Spine. 2014;**20**(6):636-643

[74] Torii Y, Ueno J, Iinuma M, Yoshida A, Niki H, Akazawa T. The learning curve of robotic-assisted pedicle screw placements using the cumulative sum analysis: A study of the first 50 cases at a single Center. Spine Surgery and Related Research. 2022;**6**(6):589-595

[75] Siddiqui MI, Wallace DJ, Salazar LM, Vardiman AB. Robot-assisted pedicle screw placement: Learning curve experience. World Neurosurgery. 2019;**130**:e417-e422

[76] West JL, Fargen KM, Aschenbrenner CA, Wilson JA, Branch CL, Wolfe SQ, et al. Commentary: Resident operative experience: Training an expert neurosurgeon. Neurosurgery. 2019;**84**(5):E279-E286

[77] Green CA, Mahuron KM, Harris HW, O'Sullivan PS. Integrating robotic technology into resident training: Challenges and recommendations from the front lines. Academic Medicine: Journal of the Association of American Medical Colleges. 2019;**94**(10):1532-1538

[78] Malham GM, Wells-Quinn T. What should my hospital buy next?-guidelines for the acquisition and application of imaging, navigation, and robotics for spine surgery. Journal of Spine Surgery Hong Kong. 2019;**5**(1):155-165

[79] Derman PB, Satin AM. Navigation, mixed reality, and robotics in endoscopic spine surgery. Minimally Invasive Surgery. 2022;**6**:8. DOI: 10.20517/2574-1225.2021.111

[80] Future of Endoscopic Spine Surgery: Insights from Cutting-Edge Technology in the Industrial Field-PubMed [Internet]. Available from: https://pubmed.ncbi.nlm.nih.gov/38135953/ [Accessed: September 21, 2024]

[81] Kiran Alluri R, Sivaganesan A, Vaishnav AS, Qureshi SA. Robotic Guided Minimally Invasive Spine Surgery [Internet]. Minimally Invasive Spine Surgery - Advances and Innovations. IntechOpen; 2022. DOI: 10.5772/intechopen.97599

[82] Rasouli JJ, Shao J, Neifert S, Gibbs WN, Habboub G, Steinmetz MP, et al. Artificial intelligence and robotics in spine surgery. Global Spine Journal. 2021;**11**(4):556-564. Available from: https://www.ncbi.nlm.nih.gov/pmc/articles/PMC8119909/ [Accessed: September 22, 2024]

[83] Zhou S, Zhou F, Sun Y, Chen X, Diao Y, Zhao Y, et al. The application of artificial intelligence in spine surgery. Frontiers in Surgery. 2022;**9**:885599. DOI: 10.3389/fsurg.2022.885599

[84] Gutman MJ, Schroeder GD, Murphy H, Flanders AE, Vaccaro AR. Artificial Intelligence in Spine Care. Clinical Spine Surgery. 2021;**34**(4):121. Available from: https://journals.lww.com/jspinaldisorders/Abstract/2021/05000/Artificial_Intelligence_in_Spine_Care.2.aspx [Accessed: September 22, 2024]

[85] Knudsen JE, Ghaffar U, Ma R, Hung AJ. Clinical applications of artificial intelligence in robotic surgery. Journal of Robotic Surgery. 2024;**18**(1):102. DOI: 10.1007/s11701-024-01867-0 [Accessed: September 22, 2024]

[86] Vadalà G, Salvatore SD, Ambrosio L, Russo F, Papalia R, Denaro V. Robotic

spine surgery and augmented reality systems: A state of the art. Neurospine. 2020;**17**(1):88-100. Available from: //www.e-neurospine.org/journal/view.php?doi=10.14245/ns.2040060.030 [Accessed: September 22, 2024]

[87] Xiao SX, Wu WT, Yu TC, Chen IH, Yeh KT. Augmenting reality in spinal surgery: A narrative review of augmented reality applications in pedicle screw instrumentation. Medicina (Mex). 2024;**60**(9):1485. Available from: https://www.mdpi.com/1648-9144/60/9/1485 [Accessed: September 22, 2024]

[88] Kuris EO, Veeramani A, McDonald CL, DiSilvestro KJ, Zhang AS, Cohen EM, et al. Predicting readmission after anterior, posterior, and posterior interbody lumbar spinal fusion: A neural network machine learning approach. World Neurosurgery. 2021;**151**:e19-e27

[89] Alves ÓL, Alves ML, Magalhães S. Robotic surgery and artificial intelligence in spine and brain surgery: Ethical challenges. In: Ammar A, editor. Learning and Career Development in Neurosurgery: Values-Based Medical Education. Cham: Springer International Publishing; 2022. pp. 249-261. DOI: 10.1007/978-3-031-02078-0_24 [Accessed: September 22, 2024]

[90] Augmedics [Internet]. Augmented Reality Spine Surgery-X-Ray Vision. Available from: https://augmedics.com/ [Accessed: October 7, 2024]

[91] VisAR: Augmented Reality Surgical Navigation|Novarad [Internet]. Available from: https://www.novarad.net/visar [Accessed: October 7, 2024]